Chapter	Chapter Title	Video Contributor	Vi...
4	Diagnostic Arthroscopy of the Ankle and Subtalar Joints	James W. Stone, MD	Ankle and Subtalar Joint Arthroscopy: Set Up, Portals, Diagnostic Arthroscopy
6	Soft Tissue Impingement Lesions of the Ankle Joint	Michael Tucker, Jr., MD and Champ L. Baker, Jr., MD	Management of Soft Tissue Impingement Lesions of the Ankle and Subtalar Joints
7	Anatomy, Operating Room Set-Up, and Diagnostic Arthroscopy for Posterior Ankle Arthroscopy	David Sitler, MD	Treatment of Posteromedial Soft Tissue Impingement
9	Instability of the Ankle and Subtalar Joints	Sameh A. Labib, MD	Brostrum Repair
		Sameh A. Labib, MD	Repair of Os Subfibulare
10	Ankle Fractures	Beat Hinterman, MD	Ankle Arthroscopy in Acute Ankle Fracture
12	Osteochondral Lesions of the Talar Dome: Debridement, Abrasion, Drilling, and Microfracture	Thomas O. Clanton, MD	Curettage, Drilling and Microfracture for Osteochondral Lesions of the Talus
14	Osteochondral Lesions of the Talar Dome: Cartilage Replacement Using Autologous Chondrocyte Implantation and Allografts	Gregory C. Berlet, MD, FRSC(C)	Chevron Malleolar Osteotomy and OATS
16	Tendoscopy	Prof. Dr. C.N. van Dijk, P.A.J. de Leeuw, MSc and Drs. M.N. van Sterkenburg	Testing Flexor Hallucis Longus
		Prof. Dr. C.N. van Dijk, P.A.J. de Leeuw, MSc and Drs. M.N. van Sterkenburg	Endoscopic Treatment of FHL Tendinopathy
		Prof. Dr. C.N. van Dijk, P.A.J. de Leeuw, MSc and Drs. M.N. van Sterkenburg	Endoscopic Release of Flexor Hallucis Longus
17	Degenerative Arthritis Ankle: Fusion	Troy Gorman, MD	Anterior Ankle Arthroscopy for Fusion
		Troy Gorman, MD	Posterior Ankle Arthroscopy for Fusion: Setup
20	Great Toe Arthroscopy	Phinit Phisitkul, MD	Great Toe Arthroscopy for Soft Tissue Impingement

AANA Advanced Arthroscopy

The Foot and Ankle

Series Editor

Richard K. N. Ryu, MD

President (2009-2010)
Arthroscopy Association of North America
Private Practice
Santa Barbara, California

Other Volumes in the AANA Advanced Arthroscopy Series

The Elbow and Wrist

The Hip

The Knee

The Shoulder

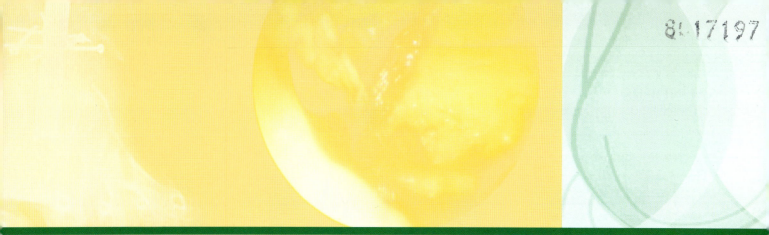

AANA Advanced Arthroscopy

The Foot and Ankle

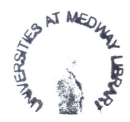

Annunziato Amendola, MD
Professor and Director of University of Iowa Sports Medicine Center
Department of Orthopaedics and Rehabilitation
University of Iowa Hospital and Clinics
Iowa City, Iowa

James W. Stone, MD
Assistant Clinical Professor of Orthopaedic Surgery
Medical College of Wisconsin
Milwaukee, Wisconsin

SAUNDERS

ELSEVIER

SAUNDERS
ELSEVIER

1600 John F. Kennedy Blvd.
Ste 1800
Philadelphia, PA 19103-2899

AANA Advanced Arthroscopy: The Foot and Ankle　　　　　　　ISBN: 978-1-4377-0662-8

Copyright © 2010 Arthroscopy Association of North America. Published by Elsevier Inc.

Notice

Knowledge and best practice in this field are constantly changing. As new research and experience broaden our knowledge, changes in practice, treatment and drug therapy may become necessary or appropriate. Readers are advised to check the most current information provided (i) on procedures featured or (ii) by the manufacturer of each product to be administered to verify the recommended dose or formula, the method and duration of administration, and contraindications. It is the responsibility of the practitioner, relying on their own experience and knowledge of the patient, to make diagnoses, to determine dosages and the best treatment for each individual patient, and to take all appropriate safety precautions. To the fullest extent of the law, neither the Publisher nor the Authors assumes any liability for any injury and/or damage to persons or property arising out of or related to any use of the material contained in this book.

The Publisher

Library of Congress Cataloging-in-Publication Data
AANA advanced arthroscopy. The foot and ankle / [edited by] Annunziato Amendola, James W. Stone. -- 1st ed.
　　p. ; cm.
　Other title: Advanced arthroscopy
　Other title: Foot and ankle
　Includes bibliographical references.
　ISBN 978-1-4377-0662-8
　1. Foot--Endoscopic surgery.　2. Ankle--Endoscopic surgery.　I. Amendola, A. (Annunziato)　II. Stone, James W., 1956-　III. Title: Advanced arthroscopy　IV. Title: Foot and ankle.
　[DNLM: 1. Ankle--surgery.　2. Foot--surgery.　3. Arthroscopy--methods.
　WE 880 A112 2010]　RD563.A16 2010
　617.5'850597--dc22　　　　　　　　　　　2010011087

Publishing Director: Kim Murphy
Developmental Editor: Ann Ruzycka Anderson
Publishing Services Manager: Frank Polizzano
Senior Project Manager: Peter Faber
Design Direction: Ellen Zanolle

Printed in China

Last digit is the print number:　9　8　7　6　5　4　3　2　1

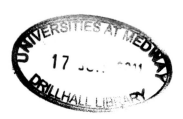

DEDICATION

To all the residents and fellows I have had the privilege of working with

and who have contributed to this work —

We have both taught and learned from each other.

In appreciation.

Ned Amendola, MD

_____

In appreciation to all of the contributors to this volume who have volunteered their time

and effort to produce an excellent text and video series which will be an asset to

orthopedic surgeons who desire to improve their surgical skills in ankle arthroscopy.

Your commitment to improving arthroscopic education is inspiring.

James W. Stone, MD

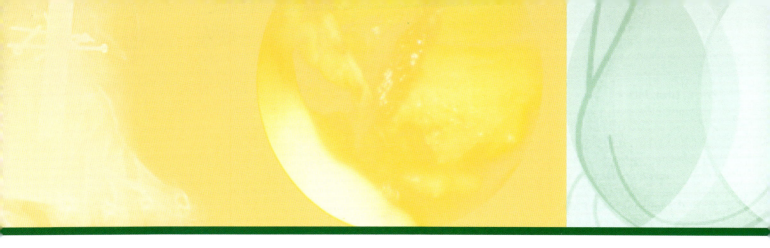

Contributors

Stephen P. Abelow, MD
Professor Honorífico, Department of Orthopaedic Sports
Medicine and Traumatology, Universidad Católica San Antonio
de Murcia; Clinica CEMTRO, Madrid, Spain
*Osteochondral Lesions of the Talar Dome: New Horizons
in Cartilage Replacement*

Jean-Pascal Allard, MD
Assistant Professor, Sherbrooke University; Consultant,
Orthopedic Surgery, CHUS-Hôtel-Dieu, Quebec, Canada
*Osteochondral Lesions of the Talar Dome: Cartilage Replacement
Using Osteochondral Autogenous Transplantation and Mosaicplasty*

Annunziato Amendola, MD
Professor and Director of the University of Iowa Sports
Medicine Center, Department Orthopaedic and Rehabilitation,
University of Iowa Hospital and Clinics, Iowa City, Iowa
Bony Impingement of the Ankle and Subtalar Joints

Champ L. Baker, Jr., MD
Clinical Assistant Professor of Orthopaedics, Medical College
of Georgia, Augusta; Staff Physician, The Hughston Clinic,
Columbus, Georgia
Soft Tissue Impingement of the Ankle Joint

Timothy C. Beals, MD
Associate Professor of Orthopaedics, Co-Director,
Harold K. Dunn Orthopaedic Laboratory, University of Utah
School of Medicine, Salt Lake City, Utah
Fusion for Degenerative Arthritis of the Ankle

Gregory C. Berlet, MD
Chief, Division of Foot and Ankle Surgery, Ohio University
College of Medicine and Public Health, Columbus; Orthopaedic
Surgeon, Orthopedic Foot and Ankle Center, Westerville, Ohio
*Osteochondral Lesions of the Talar Dome: Cartilage Replacement
Using Autologous Chondrocyte Implantation and Allografts*

John H. Brady, MD
Orthopedic Surgeon, Intermountain Medical Group,
Bountiful, Utah
Arthroscopic Fusion for Degenerative Arthritis of the Subtalar Joint

Thomas O. Clanton, MD
Professor of Orthopaedic Surgery, University of Texas Medical
School at Houston, Houston, Texas; Director, Foot and Ankle
Sports Medicine, The Steadman Clinic, Vail, Colorado
*Osteochondral Lesions of the Talar Dome: Débridement, Abrasion,
Drilling, and Microfracture*

Peter A.J. de Leeuw, MD
Resident, Department of Orthopaedic Surgery, Academic
Medical Center, Amsterdam, Netherlands
Tendoscopy

John E. Femino, MD
Associate Clinical Professor, Department of Orthopaedics and
Rehabilitation, University of Iowa Carver College of Medicine;
University of Iowa Hospitals and Clinics, Iowa City, Iowa
*Posterior Ankle Arthroscopy for Conditions Causing Ankle Pain:
Os Trigonum, Posterior Ankle Soft Tissue Impingement, Flexor
Hallucis Longus Stenosis, Haglund's Deformity, and Other
Considerations*

Carol Frey, MD
Assistant Clinical Professor of Orthopaedic Surgery (Volunteer),
UCLA David Geffen School of Medicine, Los Angeles;
Co-Director, Sports Medicine Fellowship and Family Medicine
Sports Medicine Fellowship, West Coast Sports Medicine
Foundation and Harbor General Hospital, Manhattan Beach,
California
Gross Anatomy of the Subtalar Joint

Eric R. Giza, MD
Assistant Professor of Orthopaedic Surgery, University
of California, Davis, School of Medicine; Chief, Foot and Ankle
Service, UC Davis Health System, Sacramento, California
*Osteochondral Lesions of the Talar Dome: Cartilage Replacement
Using Autologous Chondrocyte Implantation and Allografts*

Mark Glazebrook, MD, PhD
Associate Professor of Orthopedic Surgery, Dalhousie
University; Orthopedic Consultant, Queen Elizabeth II Health
Sciences Center, Halifax, Nova Scotia, Canada
*Osteochondral Lesions of the Talar Dome: Anatomy, Etiology,
and Evaluation; Osteochondral Lesions of the Talar Dome: Cartilage
Replacement Using Osteochondral Autogenous Transplantation
and Mosaicplasty*

Jordan L. Goldstein, MD
Orthopedic Sports Medicine Fellow, Emory School of Medicine,
Atlanta, Georgia
Instability of the Ankle and Subtalar Joints

Troy M. Gorman, MD
Department of Orthopaedics, University of Utah School of
Medicine; University Orthopaedic Center, Salt Lake City, Utah
Fusion for Degenerative Arthritis of the Ankle

Isabel Guillén, MD
Staff Physician and Surgeon, Department of Orthopaedic Sports
Medicine and Traumatology, Clinica CEMTRO, Madrid, Spain
*Osteochondral Lesions of the Talar Dome: New Horizons in
Cartilage Replacement*

Marta Guillén, MD
Staff Physician and Surgeon, Department of Orthopaedic Sports
Medicine and Traumatology, Clinica CEMTRO, Madrid, Spain
*Osteochondral Lesions of the Talar Dome: New Horizons in
Cartilage Replacement*

Pedro Guillén, MD
Professor and Chair, Department of Orthopaedic Sports
Medicine and Traumatology, Universidad Católica San Antonio
de Murcia; Medical Director and Chief Traumatologist,
Clinica CEMTRO, Madrid, Spain
*Osteochondral Lesions of the Talar Dome: New Horizons
in Cartilage Replacement*

W. Bryce Henderson, MD
Orthopedic Surgeon, Alberta Health Services, Red Deer,
Alberta, Canada
*Osteochondral Lesions of the Talar Dome: Anatomy, Etiology,
and Evaluation*

Beat Hintermann, MD
Associate Professor, University of Basel; Chair, Clinic of
Orthopaedic Surgery, Kantonsspital, Liestal, Switzerland
Ankle Fractures

Johnny Tak-Choy Lau, MD
Assistant Professor of Orthopedic Surgery, University of Toronto
Faculty of Medicine; Orthopedic Consultant, University Health
Network-Toronto Western Division, Toronto, Ontario, Canada
*Osteochondral Lesions of the Talar Dome: Anatomy, Etiology,
and Evaluation; Osteochondral Lesions of the Talar Dome: Cartilage
Replacement Using Osteochondral Autogenous Transplantation
and Mosaicplasty*

Sameh A. Labib, MD
Assistant Professor of Orthopaedic Surgery, Emory University
School of Medicine; Emory Sports Medicine Center, Emory
Healthcare, Atlanta, Georgia
Instability of the Ankle and Subtalar Joints

Tun Hing Lui, MBBS
Department of Orthopaedics and Traumatology, North District
Hospital, Sheung Shui, Hong Kong SAR, China
Great Toe Arthroscopy

Steven Mussett, MB BCh
Orthopedic Surgeon, Brockville General Hospital, Brockville,
Ontario, Canada
*Osteochondral Lesions of the Talar Dome: Anatomy, Etiology,
and Evaluation*

Florian Nickisch, MD
Assistant Professor of Orthopaedics, University of Utah
School of Medicine; University Orthopaedic Center,
Salt Lake City, Utah
Fusion for Degenerative Arthritis of the Ankle

Fernando Pena, MD
Assistant Professor of Orthopaedic Surgery, University
of Minnesota Medical School, Minneapolis, Minnesota
Gross Anatomy of the Ankle Joint

Phinit Phisitkul, MD
Clinical Professor, Foot and Ankle Surgery, Department of
Orthopaedics and Rehabilitation, University of Iowa Hospitals
and Clinics, Iowa City, Iowa
Great Toe Arthroscopy

Charles L. Saltzman, MD
Professor and Chair, Department of Orthopaedics, University
of Utah School of Medicine, Salt Lake City, Utah
Fusion for Degenerative Arthritis of the Ankle

David Sitler, MD
Orthopedic Surgeon, Foot and Ankle Surgery, Sharp Rees-Stealy
Medical Group, San Diego, California
*Anatomy, Evaluation, and Operative Setup for Posterior Ankle
Arthroscopy*

Bradley E. Slagel, MD
Fellow, Orthopaedic Sports Medicine, Fowler Kennedy Sport Medicine Clinic, The University of Western Ontario, London, Ontario, Canada
Instrumentation and Operative Setup for Ankle and Subtalar Arthroscopy

James W. Stone, MD
Assistant Clinical Professor of Orthopedic Surgery, Medical College of Wisconsin, Milwaukee, Wisconsin
Diagnostic Arthroscopy for the Ankle and Subtalar Joints

James P. Tasto, MD
Clinical Professor, University of California, San Diego, School of Medicine; Founder, San Diego Sports Medicine and Orthopaedic Center, San Diego, California
Arthroscopic Fusion for Degenerative Arthritis of the Subtalar Joint

Michael Tucker, MD
Staff Physician, The Houston Clinic, Columbus, Georgia
Soft Tissue Impingement of the Ankle Joint

John Louis-Ugbo, MD
Orthopedic Resident, Emory School of Medicine, Atlanta, Georgia
Instability of the Ankle and Subtalar Joints

Tanawat Vaseenon, MD
Instructor, Department of Orthopedic Surgery, Faculty of Medicine, Chiang Mai University, Chiang Mai, Thailand
Bony Impingement of the Ankle and Subtalar Joints

C. Niek van Dijk, MD, PhD
Professor, University of Amsterdam; Chief of Service, Department of Orthopaedic Surgery, Academic Medical Center, Amsterdam, Netherlands
Tendoscopy

Maayke N. van Sterkenburg, MD
Fellow, Department of Orthopaedic Surgery, Academic Medical Center, Amsterdam, Netherlands
Tendoscopy

Brian Weatherby, MD
Orthopedic Surgeon, Steadman Hawkins Clinic of the Carolinas, Greenville, South Carolina
Osteochondral Lesions of the Talar Dome: Débridement, Abrasion, Drilling, and Microfracture

Kevin R. Willits, MD
Associate Professor of Orthopedic Surgery, University of Western Ontario, London, Ontario, Canada
Instrumentation and Operative Setup for Ankle and Subtalar Arthroscopy

Alastair S.E. Younger, MB ChB
Associate Professor of Orthopaedics, University of British Columbia; Head, Orthopaedic Research, St. Paul's Hospital, Vancouver, British Columbia, Canada
Complex Ankle, Subtalar, and Triple Fusions

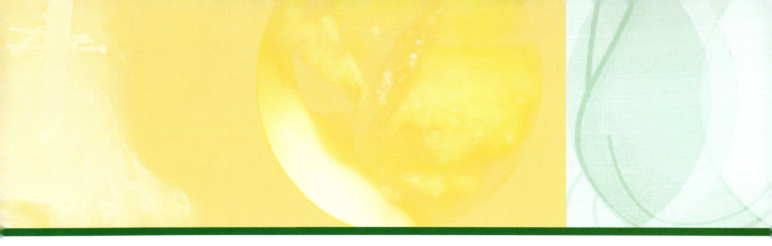

Preface

The Arthroscopy Association of North America (AANA) is a robust and growing organization whose mission, simply stated, is to provide leadership and expertise in arthroscopic and minimally invasive surgery worldwide.

Towards that end, this five-volume series represents the very best that AANA has to offer the clinician in need of a timely, authoritative, and comprehensive arthroscopic textbook. These textbooks covering the shoulder, elbow and wrist, hip, knee, and foot and ankle were conceived and rapidly consummated over a 15-month timeline. The need for an up-to-date and cogent text as well as a step-by-step video supplement was the driving force behind the rapid developmental chronology. The topics and surgical techniques represent the cutting edge in arthroscopic philosophy and technique, and the individual chapters follow a reliable and helpful format in which the pathoanatomy is detailed and the key elements of the physical examination are emphasized in conjunction with preferred diagnostic imaging. Indications and contraindications are followed by a thorough discussion of the treatment algorithm, both nonoperative and surgical, with an emphasis on arthroscopic techniques. Additionally, a Pearls and Pitfalls section provides for a distilled summary of the most important features in each chapter. A brief annotated bibliography is provided in addition to a comprehensive reference list so that those who want to study the most compelling literature can do so with ease. The supporting DVD meticulously demonstrates the surgical techniques, and will undoubtedly serve as a critical resource in preparing for any arthroscopic intervention.

I am most grateful for the outstanding effort provided by the volume editors: Rick Angelo and Jim Esch (shoulder), Buddy Savoie and Larry Field (elbow and wrist), Thomas Byrd and Carlos Guanche (hip), Rob Hunter and Nick Sgaglione (knee), and Ned Amendola and Jim Stone (foot and ankle). Their collective intellect, skill, and dedicaton to AANA made this series possible. Furthermore, I sincerely thank all the chapter contributors whose expertise and wisdom can be found in every page. Elsevier, and in particular Kim Murphy, Ann Ruzycka Anderson, and Kitty Lasinski, was a delight to work with, and deserves our gratitude for a job well done. I would be remiss if I did not acknowledge that the proceeds of this five-volume series will go directly to the AANA Education Foundation, from which ambitious and state-of-the-art arthroscopic educational initiatives will be funded.

RICHARD K.N. RYU, MD
Series Editor

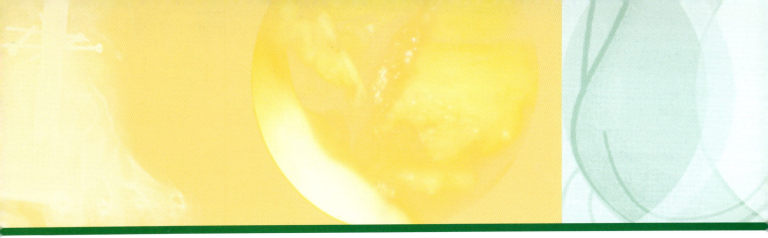

Contents

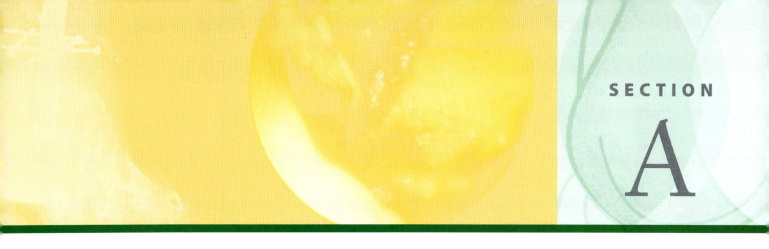

Basics

Gross Anatomy of the Ankle Joint

Fernando Pena

The first attempts of arthroscopic interventions were made in the beginning of the 20th century.[1] Originally, the knee joint was the focus of attention because of its more accessible anatomy than other joints, such as the ankle, shoulder, and smaller joints. Technical difficulties and the lack of appropriate equipment contributed to the late emergence of ankle arthroscopy compared with other joints.

In the late 1970s, Watanabe and subsequently some of his followers reported on the first attempts of ankle arthroscopy.[2] Later, Ferkel, Guhl, and others reported series of ankle arthroscopies, outlining the indications, the type of pathology that could be treated, and long-term outcomes.[3-5] They also reported a methodology to evaluate and address the ankle joint from an arthroscopic approach.

The ankle joint has a well-described and easily identifiable topographic anatomy, which decreases the chances of arthroscopic complications. Most of the vital structures are readily visualized, making ankle arthroscopy a technically reasonable and reliable operation for which the results are easily reproduced. A review of the topographic anatomy and the expected location of vital structures is essential to better understand the ankle joint and guide the operator safely through ankle arthroscopy.

TOPOGRAPHIC ANATOMY

The ankle joint is formed by the distal tibia, fibula, and the talus. Because it is a highly congruent joint with complex, curved articular surfaces tightly bound by ligaments, access to the entirety of the joint from a single portal is not possible. To simplify the description of the ankle joint, it is divided into the anterior and posterior compartments.

Anterior Ankle Topographic Anatomy

The anteromedial aspect of the ankle joint presents the most superficial portion of the distal tibia and the medial malleolus,

whose tip is approximately 1 cm distal to the joint line. Slightly anterior to the medial malleolus are the saphenous nerve and the saphenous vein, both of which are located medial to the anterior tibialis tendon. The saphenous vein is at risk for being punctured during the creation of the anteromedial portal (Fig. 1-1).[3]

The anterior tibialis tendon represents the lateral margin of the so-called soft spot of the ankle joint. The soft spot is delineated by the anterior tibialis tendon laterally, the most distal portion of the tibial plafond superiorly, and the lateral margin of the medial malleolus medially. This soft spot is the site of choice for placement of the anteromedial portal and for performing intra-articular injections of the ankle joint. The distal medial aspect of the tibia demonstrates a superiorly oriented notch of variable height known as the notch of Harty. This notch often affords easier initial placement of the arthroscopic cannula into the joint.

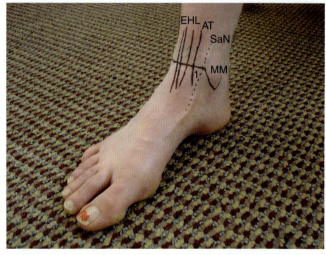

FIGURE 1-1 Anteromedial aspect of the ankle joint. AT, anterior tibialis tendon; EHL, extensor hallucis longus tendon; MM, medial malleolus; SaN, saphenus nerve; 1, soft spot of the ankle joint.

In both applications, penetration of the ankle joint through the soft spot should be as lateral as possible and close to the anterior tibialis tendon to avoid damage to the saphenous vein and possibly to the more medially located saphenous nerve. Portal placement immediately adjacent to the medial border of the tibialis anterior tendon and as far away from the medial malleolus as possible facilitates manipulation of the arthroscope and instruments, avoiding mechanical impingement of the cannula on the medial malleolus.

The extensor hallucis longus (EHL) tendon is located lateral to the anterior tibialis tendon. The EHL tendon is easily palpated and identified by passive range of motion of the great toe. This tendon represents a safe landmark to avoid any damage to the anterior neurovascular bundle, which includes the anterior tibialis artery and veins and the deep peroneal nerve. The anterior neurovascular bundle is located immediately lateral to the EHL tendon. Use of the anterior central portal was advocated in the early arthroscopic ankle literature to allow complete joint access. The combination of noninvasive methods of ankle joint distraction and improved optics that allow excellent picture clarity with 2.7-mm diameter arthroscopes has made this portal, which places the anterior neurovascular bundle at risk for injury, unnecessary.

The extensor digitorum longus (EDL) tendon is located lateral to the anterior neurovascular bundle. Lateral to it, the dorsal cutaneous branch of the superficial peroneal nerve is found, which can be visualized or palpated in most patients by placing the foot in forced maximum plantar flexion and adding maximal plantar flexion of fourth metatarsophalangeal (MTP) joint.[6] At the level of the ankle joint line, the course of the dorsal cutaneous branch of the superficial peroneal nerve ranges from the anterior margin of the lateral malleolus to the lateral aspect of the extensor digitorum longus tendon (Fig. 1-2).[7]

Creation of the anterolateral portal should take the location of the dorsal cutaneous branch of the superficial peroneal nerve into consideration to avoid damage to the nerve. The dorsal cutaneous branch of the superficial peroneal nerve is the neurologic structure at highest risk for complication during ankle arthroscopy.[4] It is important to avoid injury to the superficial peroneal nerve by using proper portal creation technique, known as the *nick and spread technique*. First, only the skin is incised. The knife blade is not allowed to penetrate into the subcutaneous tissues. Second, the subcutaneous tissues are bluntly dissected using a small mosquito forceps. Third, the portal is created using a blunt trocar. The joint capsule is quite thin, and avoiding sharp trocars helps to minimize the likelihood of nerve injury.

The lateral malleolus is the most lateral structure of the ankle joint. It is located slightly posterior to the medial malleolus, which allows a larger exposure of the lateral wall of the talus along the lateral gutter as compared with the medial aspect of the ankle joint. The tip of the lateral malleolus is approximately 2 cm distal to the joint line and 1 cm posterior to the medial malleolus. The peroneal tendons are immediately posterior to the lateral malleolus. The peroneus brevis tendon is the closest one to the posterior margin of the fibula. Posterior to it, the peroneus longus tendon is found.

Posterior Ankle Topographic Anatomy

The sural nerve is located between the peroneal tendons and the Achilles tendon, approximately 1 to 1.5 cm distal to the tip of the fibula and 1.5 to 2 cm posterior to it.[5] The location of the sural nerve has some variability within the posterolateral aspect of the ankle joint. It is always located close to the lesser saphenous vein.[8] These two structures are the only ones at risk in the posterolateral aspect of the ankle joint (Fig. 1-3).

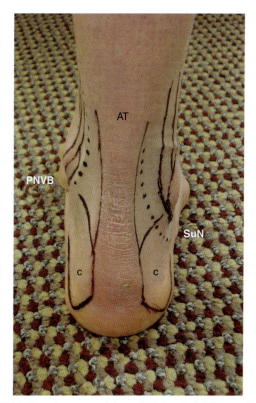

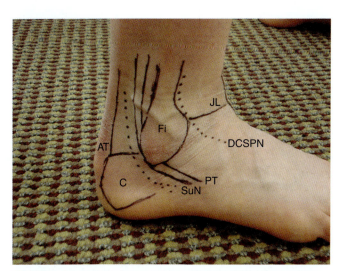

FIGURE 1-2 Anterolateral aspect of the ankle joint. AT, Achilles tendon; C, calcaneus; DCSPN, dorsal cutaneous branch of the superficial peroneal nerve; Fi, fibula; JL, joint line; PT, peroneal tendons; SuN, sural nerve.

FIGURE 1-3 Posterior aspect of the ankle joint. AT, Achilles tendon; C, calcaneus; PNVB, posterior neurovascular bundle; SuN, sural nerve.

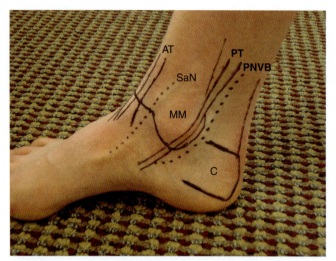

FIGURE 1-4 Posteromedial aspect of the ankle joint. AT, anterior tibialis tendon; C, calcaneus; MM, medial malleolus; PNVB, posterior neurovascular bundle; PT, posterior tibialis tendon; SaN, saphenus nerve.

The Achilles tendon has an average width of 1 to 1.5 cm immediately above the superior margin of the calcaneus tuberosity. The deep flexor tendons are located medial to the Achilles tendon, and the flexor hallucis longus (FHL) tendon is the most lateral of the deep flexor tendons. Identification of this tendon is key to avoiding damage to the posterior neurovascular structures. The posterior neurovascular bundle is located immediately adjacent and medial to the FHL, and it includes the posterior tibial artery, veins, and tibial nerve. The flexor digitorum longus (FDL) tendon is located medial to the posterior neurovascular bundle. The posterior tibialis tendon is anterior and medial to the FDL. The posterior tibialis tendon is located on the medial malleolus at the level of the joint line (Fig. 1-4).

Before performing ankle arthroscopy, the topographic anatomy of the ankle joint should be clearly marked and delineated with a sterile surgical marker to avoid damage to critical structures. This step is of key importance to appreciate the location of the structures at risk during the intervention.

INTRA-ARTICULAR ANATOMY AND ACCESS

Details about the setup, patient position, and instrumentation required for ankle arthroscopy are provided in Chapter ••.

The ankle is a highly constrained joint that may make access to the posterior compartment from the anterior portals technically demanding. Similarly, the operator should not expect to have access to the front of the ankle when performing posterior ankle arthroscopy. The degree of constraint and shallowness of the ankle joint make the location of the portals at an ideal level, neither too proximal nor too distal, a critical feature that enables complete visualization of the joint. If the location of the portals is off by a few millimeters, it will be difficult to evaluate most of the ankle joint, except for its most anterior portion in the case of anterior ankle arthroscopy.

Successful ankle arthroscopy demands placement of the working instrument on the same side where the pathology is located; for example, the medial portal is used to place a working instrument to address medial talar pathology. Any attempt to cross the ankle joint with an instrument may result in iatrogenic damage to the osteochondral structures of the ankle joint.

The ankle joint is inspected first from the anteromedial portal. Ferkel described a 21-point inspection of the intra-articular anatomy.[4] Regardless of the method chosen to inspect the ankle joint, it is crucial to do it in a systematic way to avoid missing any unexpected findings and pathology.

The anterocentral portal has fallen out of favor because of the potential for increased complications associated with it.[8,9] Another feature contributing to its lack of popularity is that most pathology can be visualized through the more standard anteromedial and anterolateral portals and the occasional use of accessory anteromedial and anterolateral portals.

Anterior Access to the Ankle Joint

Anteromedial Portal

The anteromedial portal is created along the soft spot of the ankle joint as close as possible to the anterior tibialis tendon to avoid any damage to the saphenous nerve and vein. On entrance into the ankle joint, the anterior aspect of the tibia and the dorsal and medial aspects of the neck of the talus can be visualized. The most superior aspect of the neck of the talus may reveal some intra-articular dorsal osteophytes. Ankle dorsiflexion helps to visualize the osteophytes by distention of the most anterior and distal portion of the capsule (Fig. 1-5). The distal anterior tibia may also reveal some intra-articular osteophytes. They may require some retraction and elevation of the most superior portion of the capsular attachment for better visualization. Moving laterally, examination of this area of the ankle may be difficult if there is hypertrophic synovitis or lack of sufficient intra-articular fluid pressure while performing the arthroscopy (Fig. 1-6).

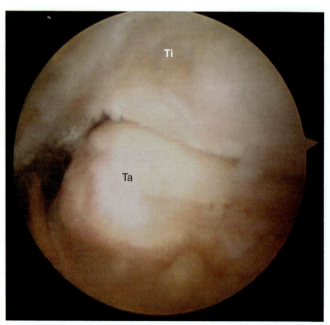

FIGURE 1-5 Intra-articular picture of the ankle joint visualized from the anteromedial portal with the ankle in dorsiflexion. Ta, talus; Ti, tibia.

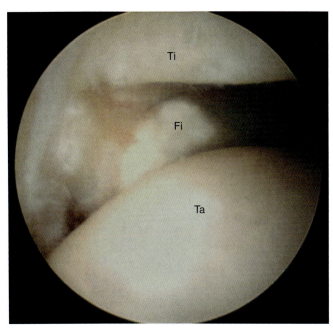

FIGURE 1-6 Intra-articular picture of the ankle joint visualized from the anteromedial portal. Fi, fibula; Ta, talus; Ti, tibia.

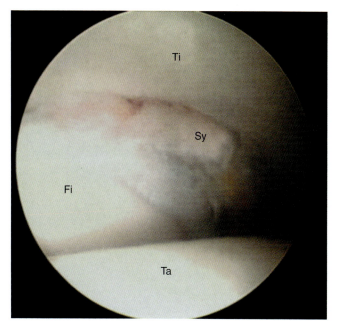

FIGURE 1-8 Lateral aspect of the ankle joint visualized from the anteromedial portal. Fi, fibula; Sy, intra-articular portion of the ankle syndesmosis; Ta, talus; Ti, tibia.

The lateral gutter is difficult to assess from the anteromedial portal, and its inspection is limited to the most anterior portion. The most anterior margin of the distal fibula also is visualized at this level. The anterior-inferior tibiofibular ligament may also be visualized at this point, with its fibers running in an oblique fashion at approximately 45 degrees from proximal and medial to distal and lateral (Fig. 1-7). The lateral malleolus reveals its articular surface against the lateral wall of the talus.

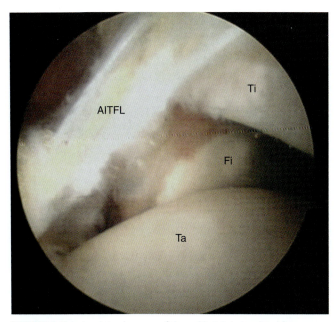

FIGURE 1-7 Anterolateral corner of the ankle joint visualized from the anteromedial portal. AITFL, anterior-inferior tibiofibular ligament; Fi, fibula; Ta, talus; Ti, tibia.

The most distal portion of the ankle syndesmosis can be visualized, and some hypertrophic soft tissue may be seen along the recess located between the fibula and the tibia as a result of previous ankle syndesmosis injuries (Fig. 1-8).

Some degree of traction may be required to better visualize the most posterior aspect of the ankle joint. In some patients, the ankle joint may be so stiff that inspection of the posterior aspect of the ankle joint may be extremely difficult. In this case, options include the application of traction, the use of a 2.7-mm scope, and ensuring that the portals are well placed.

More posteriorly, the posterior-inferior tibiofibular ligament is visualized. The posterior fibers have an oblique arrangement similar to that of their anterior counterpart (Fig. 1-9). The tibial attachment of the posterior-inferior tibiofibular ligament may extend medially all the way to the most medial portion of the tibia (Fig. 1-10). More medially, an invagination of the posterior capsule is visualized, which correlates with the FHL tendon (Fig. 1-11). Along the most posteromedial corner of the joint, the articular surface of the medial malleolus and the most distal portion of the medial gutter are inspected (Figs. 1-12 and 1-13).

Any recess of the ankle joint has the potential to lodge loose bodies. The most likely locations include the posterior aspect of the ankle joint and the distal portion of the medial and lateral gutters.

Anterolateral Portal

A spinal needled is used first to create the anterolateral portal. After the needle is placed into the joint, the tip of the needle should be carefully placed across the tibiotalar joint line. The direction of the needle is observed, and the portal location is moved proximal or distal according to the angle of the needle. If the needle is pointing proximally, the portal is moved superiorly,

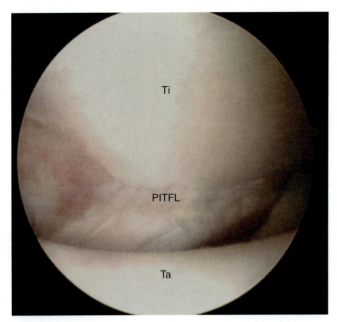

FIGURE 1-9 Posterolateral corner of the ankle joint visualized from the anteromedial portal. PITFL, posterior-inferior tibiofibular ligament; Ta, talus; Ti, tibia.

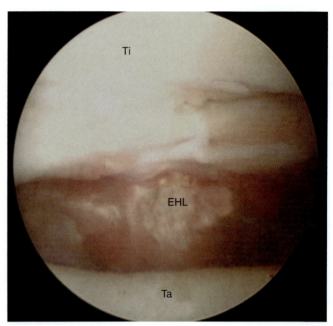

FIGURE 1-11 Posteromedial corner of the ankle joint visualized from the anteromedial portal. EHL, Intra-articular invagination of the extensor hallucis longus tendon; Ta, talus; Ti, tibia.

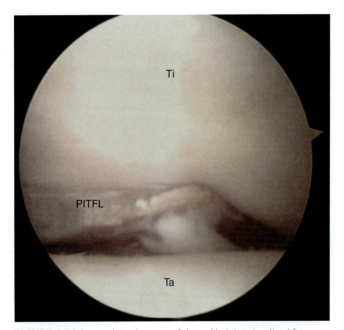

FIGURE 1-10 Posterolateral corner of the ankle joint visualized from the anteromedial portal. PITFL, posterior-inferior tibiofibular ligament; Ta, talus; Ti, tibia.

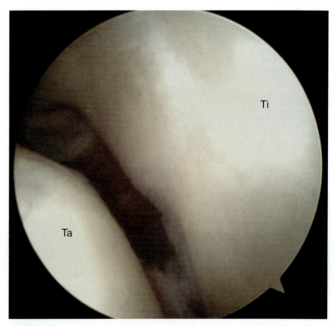

FIGURE 1-12 Medial gutter of the ankle joint visualized from the anteromedial portal. Ta, talus; Ti, tibia.

and if the needle is pointing distally, the portal is moved distally. The location of the dorsal cutaneous branch of the superficial peroneal nerve also determines the location of the portal. To address medially located pathology, the portal usually is positioned medial to the dorsal cutaneous branch of the superficial peroneal nerve and vice versa for laterally located pathology. After creation of the anterolateral portal, inspection of the anterior aspect of the lateral gutter is quite feasible, as is the most distal portion of the gutter itself (Fig. 1-14).

The syndesmosis is easier to visualize from this portal. Instability of the syndesmosis may be assessed by observing the presence of diastasis between the tibia and the fibula. The fibula and the tibia may be easily stressed from this approach with the use of a working instrument. An advantage of the anterolateral portal is to have a clear visualization of the anterior and medial portion of the tibia, especially the medial malleolus. This area offers the landmark to proceed with an adequate resection of the most distal and anterior tibial osteophytes.

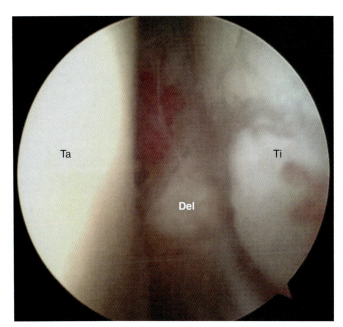

FIGURE 1-13 Medial gutter of the ankle joint visualized from the anteromedial portal. Del, Intra-articular portion of the deep fibers of the deltoid ligament; Ta, talus; Ti, tibia.

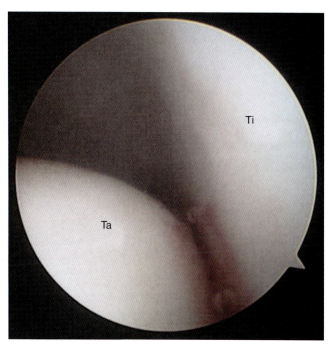

FIGURE 1-15 Anteromedial aspect of the ankle joint visualized from the anteromedial portal. Ta, talus; Ti, tibia.

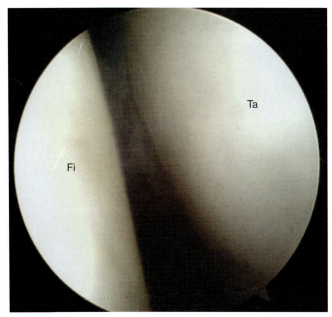

FIGURE 1-14 Lateral gutter of the ankle joint visualized from the anterolateral portal. Fi, fibula; Ta, talus.

Accessory Anterior Portals

An accessory anteromedial portal and an accessory anterolateral portal can be created to gain access to the medial and lateral aspects of the talus, respectively. The portals improve the potential for examination of those areas and for additional work along the medial and lateral gutters (i.e., resection of fracture fragments from the talus or loose bodies lodged along the gutters).

The accessory anteromedial portal is created 1 cm distal and medial to the anteromedial portal. Similarly, the accessory anterolateral portal is created 1 cm distal and lateral to the anterolateral portal. Some difficulties can be expected when simultaneously using the arthroscopic instruments along the anteromedial and accessory anteromedial portals because of the proximity of the portals and the angle required for placing the instruments in such a limited space. The same principle applies to the laterally located portals over the ankle joint (Figs. 1-15 to 1-18).

Posterior Access to the Ankle Joint

Posterior portals are best accessed with the patient in the prone position (Figs. 1-19 to 1-23). This approach can significantly facilitate visualization of the ankle joint, improve understanding of the topographic anatomy of the posterior aspect of the ankle, and decrease the chances for contamination of the surgical field.

Posterolateral Portal

The posterolateral portal is created first. It is located along the most superior aspect of the calcaneus tuberosity and is immediately adjacent to the Achilles tendon. Through this approach, the posterior aspect of the talus is visualized. Special attention is required to avoid any violation of the subtalar joint located immediately distal to the posterior process of the talus.

The posterior-inferior tibiofibular ligament fibers are located superior to the entry site to the ankle joint. Otherwise, visualization of the ankle would be significantly more difficult and demanding. At this point, the FHL tendon is visualized, and it is always kept medial to our working instruments.

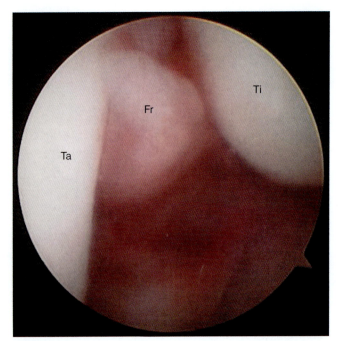

FIGURE 1-16 Anteromedial aspect of the ankle joint visualized from the accessory anteromedial portal. Fr, bony fragment from medial wall of the talus; Ta, talus; Ti, tibia.

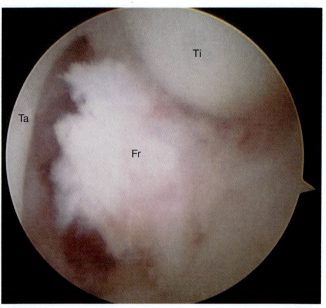

FIGURE 1-17 Anteromedial aspect of the ankle joint visualized from the accessory anteromedial portal. Fr, bony fragment from medial wall of the talus mobilized; Ta, talus; Ti, tibia.

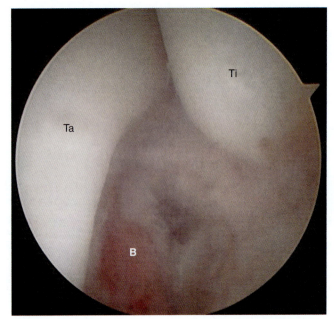

FIGURE 1-18 Anteromedial aspect of the ankle joint visualized from the accessory anteromedial portal. B, medial wall of talus after excision of fragment from medial wall; Ta, talus; Ti, tibia.

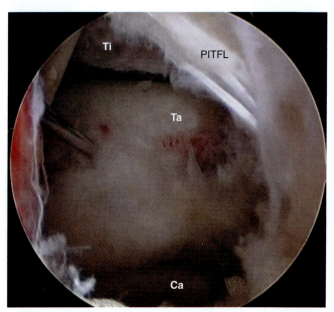

FIGURE 1-19 Posterior aspect of the ankle and subtalar joint visualized from the posterolateral portal. Ca, calcaneus; PITFL, posterior-inferior tibiofibular ligament; Ta, talus; Ti, tibia.

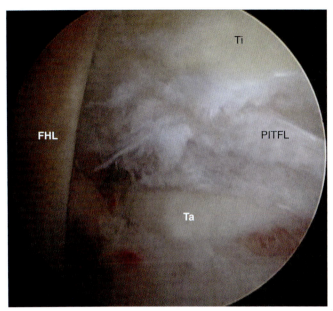

FIGURE 1-20 Posteromedial corner of the ankle visualized from the posterolateral portal. FHL, flexor hallucis longus tendon; PITFL, posterior-inferior tibiofibular ligament; Ta, talus.

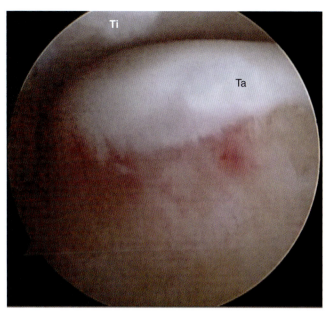

FIGURE 1-21 Posterolateral aspect of the ankle visualized from posteromedial portal. Ta, talus; Ti, tibia.

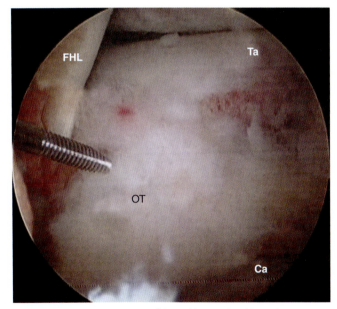

FIGURE 1-22 Posterior aspect of the ankle visualized from the posterolateral portal. Ca, calcaneus; FHL, flexor hallucis longus tendon; OT, os trigonum; Ta, talus.

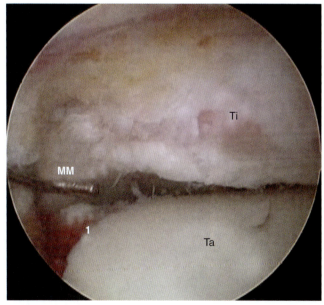

FIGURE 1-23 Posteromedial corner of the ankle. MM, medial malleolus; Ta, talus; Ti, tibia; 1, intra-articular split fracture of the posterior aspect of the talus.

Posteromedial Portal

The posteromedial portal is created immediately adjacent to the medial border of the Achilles tendon at the most superior aspect of the calcaneus tuberosity. The instruments must be placed perpendicular to the long axis of the foot when penetrating the portal site, and eventually, the instruments are swept into a more vertical position to penetrate the posterior aspect of the ankle joint. Under direct visualization, the location of the instruments is confirmed to be lateral to the FHL tendon to avoid any damage to the posteromedial neurovascular structures.

Through these portals, the posterior third of the tibiotalar joint is inspected, and any loose bodies or osteochondral lesions of the posterior aspect of the ankle joint are identified. Other indications for this approach include an arthroscopic resection of the os trigonum or assessment of the most superior and posterior aspects of the posterior facet of the subtalar joint.

The posterocentral portal has fallen out of favor for reasons similar to those affecting the anterocentral portal. With accurate placement of the posteromedial and posterolateral portals, most posterior ankle pathology can be addressed through the two portals and with a low risk of complications. The operator must be aware of the possibility of causing damage to the posterior neurovascular structures if the location of the FHL tendon is not clearly visualized and respected.

PEARLS & PITFALLS

1. The notch of Harty is an indentation on the distal medial tibial articular surface that creates an area of improved access for initial placement of the arthroscope during ankle arthroscopy.

2. The most common complication of ankle arthroscopy is nerve injury, which can be avoided by being aware of the variable anatomy of the cutaneous nerves, particularly the branches of the superficial peroneal nerve; by using the nick and spread technique for portal creation; and by avoiding the use of invasive skeletal distraction techniques.

3. The arthroscopic surgeon must be comfortable using both anterior and posterior portals to provide consistent access to the anterior and posterior compartments of the ankle joint.

4. The operator must avoid the anterocentral portal anteriorly and the trans-Achilles tendon portal posteriorly. The anterocentral portal places the anterior neurovascular structures at high risk for injury, and the trans-Achilles tendon portal has the potential to injure the tendon, causing postoperative symptoms. Neither is required for adequate visualization of the joint.

REFERENCES

1. Burman MS. Arthroscopy or the direct visualization of joints. *J Bone Joint Surg Am.* 1931;13:669-695.
2. Watanabe M. *Selfoc-Arthroscope. Watanabe No. 24 Arthroscope.* Tokyo, Japan: Teishin Hospital; 1972.
3. Ewing JW, Tasto JA, Tippert JW. Arthroscopic surgery of the ankle. *Instr Course Lect.* 1995;44:325-340.
4. Ferkel RD. *Arthroscopic Surgery: The Foot and Ankle.* Philadelphia, PA: Lippincott-Raven; 1996.85-103.
5. Sitler DF, Amendola A, Bailey CS, et al. Posterior ankle arthroscopy: an anatomic study. *J Bone Joint Surg Am.* 2002;84A:763-769.
6. Stephens MM, Kelly PM. Fourth toe flexion sign: a new clinical sign for identification of the superficial peroneal nerve. *Foot Ankle Int.* 2000;21:860-863.
7. Horwitz MT. Normal anatomy and variations of the peripheral nerves of the leg and foot. *Arch Surg.* 1938;36:626.
8. Feiwell LA, Frey CC. Anatomic study of arthroscopic protal sites of the ankle. *Foot Ankle.* 1993;14:142-147.
9. Voto SJ, Ewing JW, Fleissner PR Jr, et al. Ankle arthroscopy: neurovascular and arthroscopic anatomy of standard and trans-Achilles tendon portal placement. *Arthroscopy.* 1989;5:41-46.

SUGGESTED READINGS

Ferkel RD, Scranton PE. Current concepts review: arthroscopy of the ankle and foot. *J Bone Joint Surg Am.* 1993;75A:1223-1242.

Stetson WB, Ferkel RD. Ankle arthroscopy. I. Technique and complications. *J Am Acad Orthop Surg.* 1996;4:17-23.

Van Dijk CN, van Bergen CJA. Advancements in ankle arthroscopy. *J Am Acad Orthop Surg.* 2008;16:635-646.

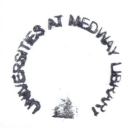

Gross Anatomy of the Subtalar Joint

Carol Frey

The subtalar joint is a complex and functionally important joint of the lower extremity that plays a major role in the movement of inversion and eversion of the foot.[1,2] The complex anatomy of the subtalar joint makes arthroscopic and radiographic evaluation difficult. However, advances in small joint arthroscopic techniques and instrumentation have expanded the use of arthroscopy in the subtalar joint. Arthroscopic visualization of the subtalar joint includes the posterior joint, anterior joint, and sinus tarsi. The tarsi sinus is extra-articular, but for practical purposes, it is included in the description of subtalar arthroscopy and the relevant anatomy.

The surgeon must comprehend the gross and arthroscopic anatomy of the subtalar joint to improve surgical performance and recognize abnormal pathology. Because the lateral and posterior anatomic approaches are used for performing subtalar joint arthroscopy,[3-6] knowledge of the superficial anatomy in these areas is important.

SUBTALAR JOINT ANATOMY

For arthroscopic purposes, the subtalar joint can be divided into anterior (talocalcaneonavicular) and posterior (talocalcaneal) articulations (Fig. 2-1).[3-7] The anterior and posterior articulations are separated by the tarsal canal and the lateral opening of this canal, called the sinus tarsi, which is a soft, palpable area approximately 2 cm anterior to the tip of the lateral malleolus. The medial root of the inferior extensor retinaculum, the cervical and talocalcaneal interosseous ligaments, fatty tissue, and blood vessels are found within the sinus tarsi and tarsal canal. The ligaments that support the subtalar joint on the lateral side consist of a superficial, intermediate, and deep layer (Fig. 2-2). The superficial layer consists of the lateral talocalcaneal ligament, the posterior talocalcaneal ligament, the medial talocalcaneal ligament, the lateral root of the inferior extensor retinaculum, and the calcaneofibular ligament. The intermediate layer is formed by the

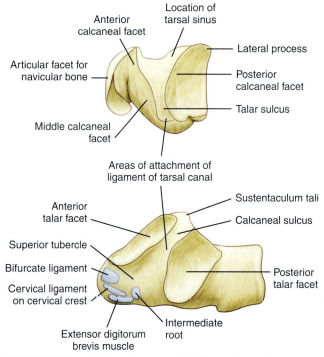

FIGURE 2-1 The subtalar joint can be divided into the anterior (talocalcaneonavicular) and posterior (talocalcaneal) articulations.

intermediate root of the inferior extensor retinaculum and the cervical ligament. The deep layer consists of the medial root of the inferior extensor retinaculum and the interosseous ligament (Fig. 2-3).[8-11]

The talocalcaneonavicular joint, or anterior subtalar joint, is composed of the talus, the posterior surface of the tarsal navicular, the anterior surface of the calcaneus, and the plantar calcaneonavicular (spring) ligament. The anterior portion of the subtalar joint includes the anterior and middle articulating facets.

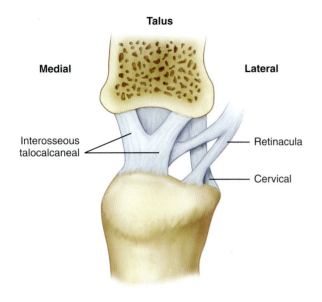

FIGURE 2-2 The ligaments that support the subtalar joint on the lateral side consist of superficial, intermediate, and deep layers.

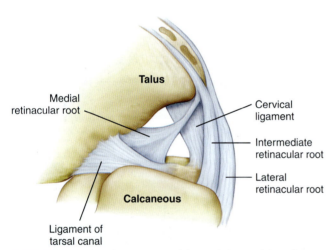

FIGURE 2-3 The deep layer consists of the medial root of the inferior extensor retinaculum and the interosseous ligament.

Compared with the posterior joint, the anterior subtalar joint is more difficult to examine with the arthroscope because the thick ligaments that fill the sinus tarsi and tarsal canal may block the initial view. The anterior joint normally has no connection to the posterior joint because the thick interosseous ligament fills the tarsal canal and separates the two anatomic areas (Fig. 2-4).

The posterior subtalar joint has a long axis oriented obliquely 40 degrees to the midline of the foot, facing laterally. It is a synovium-lined joint consisting of the convex posterior facet of the calcaneus and the concave posterior facet of the talus. The posterior subtalar joint consists of the posterior calcaneal facet of the undersurface of the talus and the posterior articular surface of the calcaneus. The joint capsule is reinforced on the lateral side by the lateral talocalcaneal ligament and the calcaneofibular ligament. The posterior joint has a posterior capsular pouch with small lateral, medial, and anterior recesses (Fig. 2-5).

ANATOMY OF PORTAL PLACEMENT AND SAFETY

Lateral Approach Anatomy

Arthroscopic evaluation of the subtalar joint has traditionally been performed using a lateral approach. Three portals are recommended for visualization and instrumentation of the subtalar joint using the lateral approach (Fig. 2-6). The anatomic landmarks for lateral portal placement include the lateral malleolus, the anterior process of the calcaneus, the sinus tarsi, and the Achilles tendon. The lateral malleolus and anterior process of the calcaneus are easy to palpate. The sinus tarsi is a palpable depression between the distal tip of the fibula and the anterior process of the calcaneus, although it can be filled with large amounts of adipose tissue. Inversion and eversion of the foot may be helpful in palpating the sinus tarsi.

The point of entry for the anterior portal is usually about 2 cm anterior and 1 cm distal to the tip of the distal fibula, directing the instrument slightly upward and about 40 degrees posteriorly. The location of the portal in cadaveric dissection studies is an average of 28 mm (range, 23 to 35 mm) anterior to the tip of the fibula (Fig. 2-7).[7] Structures at risk when placing the portal include the dorsal intermediate cutaneous branch of the superficial peroneal nerve, the dorsal lateral cutaneous branch of the sural nerve, the peroneus tertius tendon, and the small branch of the lesser saphenous vein. The dorsal intermediate cutaneous branch of the superficial peroneal nerve is located an average of 17 mm (range, 0 to 28 mm) anterior to the portal. The dorsal lateral cutaneous branch of the sural nerve (indentified in 8 of 15 specimens) was located an average of 8 mm (range, 2 to 12 mm) inferior to the anterior portal.[7] The peroneus tertius tendon was located an average distance of 21 mm (range, 8 to 33 mm) anterior to the portal. A small branch of the lesser saphenous vein consistently coursed along the anterolateral aspect of the foot in the vicinity of the anterior portal. It is located an average of 2 mm (range, 0 to 5 mm) from the anterior portal and was lacerated 20% of cases in one report of portal safety.[7] With use of the anterior portal, care must be taken to avoid injury to the dorsal intermediate cutaneous branch of the superficial peroneal nerve as it divides on the dorsum of the foot. A small branch of the lesser saphenous vein is also at risk, although damage to the structure is unlikely to cause significant problems.

Meticulous attention to proper portal creation technique minimizes the risk of injury to superficial nerve and vascular structures. The nick and spread technique is recommended; only the skin is incised with a no. 10 scalpel blade, the subcutaneous tissues are bluntly dissected using a mosquito forceps, and the capsule is penetrated with a blunt trocar.

The middle portal is located approximately 1 cm anterior to the tip of the fibula, directly over the sinus tarsi. It places no significant anatomic structures at risk.

The posterior portal is located an average of 25 mm (range, 20 to 28 mm) posterior and 6 mm (range, 0 to 10 mm) proximal to the tip of the fibula.[7] Compared with other subtalar portals, the posterior portal used for the lateral approach is more likely to cause nerve or vessel damage. Structures subject to injury with

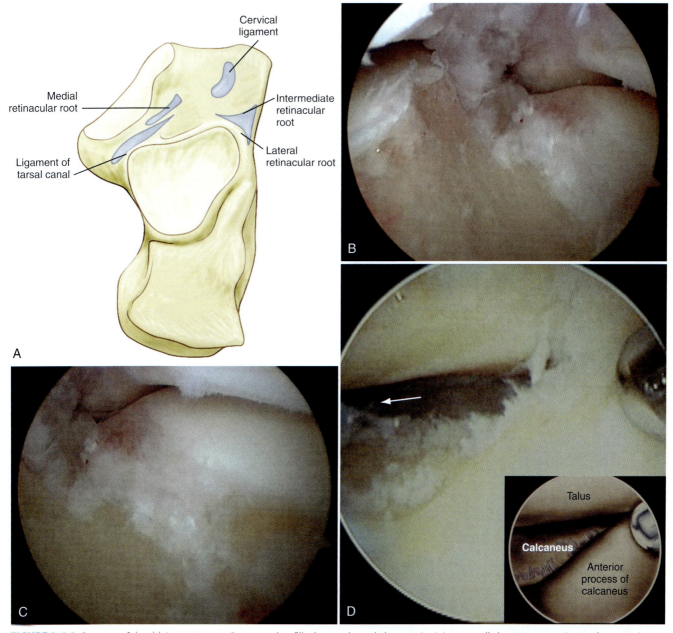

FIGURE 2-4 A, Because of the thick interosseous ligament that fills the tarsal canal, the anterior joint normally has no connection to the posterior joint. The interosseous ligaments that insert on the floor of the sinus tarsi have been cleared away. **B,** The anterior joint is seen to the right and the posterior joint to the left. **C,** The anterior joint is clearly seen with the floor of the sinus tarsi in the foreground. **D,** The anterior process of the calcaneus is seen under the tip of the shaver.

posterior portal placement include the sural nerve, lesser saphenous vein, peroneal tendons, and the Achilles tendon. Great care must be taken during posterior portal placement to avoid injury, especially to the sural nerve and lesser saphenous vein.

The sural nerve and lesser saphenous vein run parallel to each other along the posterolateral aspect of the ankle, with the nerve coursing posterior to the vein at the level of the ankle joint. In 7 of 10 cases reported by Frey,[7] the posterior portal was located posterior to the sural nerve, and in two cases, it was found to be anterior to the nerve. The average distance from the sural nerve to the posterior portal was 4 mm (range, 8 mm posterior to 6 mm anterior). In one case, the sural nerve was transected during portal placement, and in another, a small laceration was

made in the lesser saphenous vein. The peroneal tendon sheath was located an average of 11 mm (range, 6 to 16 mm) anterior to the portal, and the Achilles tendon was an average of 15 mm posterior (range, 10 to 20 mm) to the portal. Neither tendon was damaged in the series, but the tendons' proximity should be considered.

Accessory portals for posterior subtalar arthroscopy have been described in the literature. The accessory anterolateral and posterolateral portals are used as needed for viewing and instrumentation. The accessory anterolateral portal is usually slightly anterior and superior to the standard anterior portal. The accessory posterolateral portal is made behind the peroneal tendons, lateral to the standard posterior portal.[12-16]

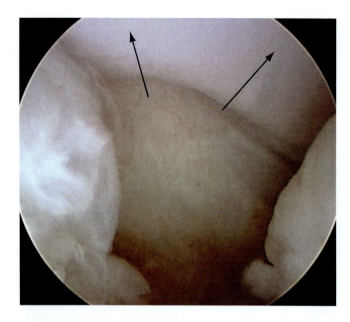

FIGURE 2-5 The posterior joint has a posterior capsular pouch with small lateral, medial, and anterior recesses. The calcaneus is seen to the right, and the *two arrows* point to the posteroinferior surface of the talus. The posterior pouch is seen to the left in this view.

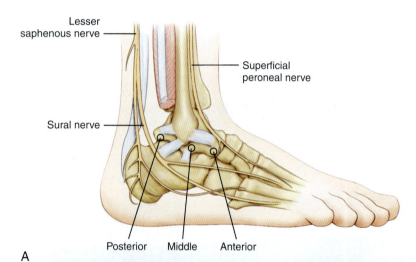

A

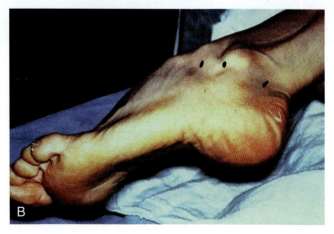

B

FIGURE 2-6 A, Three standard portals are used to approach the subtalar joint: anterior, middle, and posterior. **B,** Anatomic landmarks are used for placement of the lateral portals: the distal fibula, the anterior process of the calcaneus, and the sinus tarsi between the fibula and calcaneus. The patient is in the lateral decubitus position.

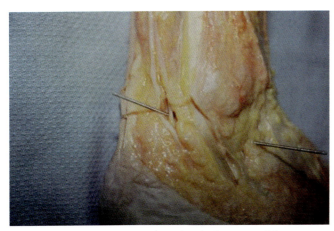

FIGURE 2-7 Some structures are at risk with placement of the anterior and posterior portals. The posterior portal is just in front of the sural nerve, and the anterior portal is near the branches of the superficial peroneal nerve.

Posterior Approach Anatomy

Posterior subtalar arthroscopy can be performed from a purely posterior approach using posterolateral and posteromedial portals (Fig. 2-8).[17,18] This is a two-portal endoscopic approach to the hindfoot, which becomes arthroscopic after it enters the subtalar joint. The posterior approach can be accomplished with the patient in the prone position. The posterior approach has been reported to provide better access to the medial and anterolateral aspects of the posterior subtalar joint,[17,18] but the posterolateral and posteromedial portals used to approach the subtalar joint are the same as those used to approach the posterior aspect of the ankle and the hindfoot.

The patient is placed in the prone position. The posterolateral portal usually is made at or slightly above the level of the tip of the lateral malleolus. The posterolateral portal is lateral to the Achilles tendon. The posteromedial portal is made just medial to the Achilles tendon. In the horizontal plane, the posteromedial portal is located at approximately the same level as the posterolateral portal. The important anatomic landmarks are the Achilles tendon and the lateral malleolus.

The medial aspect of the posterior subtalar joint is tighter than on the lateral side, possibly increasing the risk of iatrogenic cartilage damage. The tibial nerve, the posterior tibial artery, and the medial calcaneal nerve are in proximity and can be at risk when the posteromedial portal is used. Several investigators have studied the relative safety of the posterior portals for hindfoot endoscopy in anatomic specimens.[17-20] Mekhail and colleagues determined the average distance between the point of entry of the posteromedial arthroscope and the posterior tibial neurovascular bundle to be 1.0 cm. The closest distance was 8 mm.[19] Sitler evaluated the safety of posterior ankle arthroscopy in 13 cadaver specimens.[18] Posteromedial and posterolateral portals were established in each specimen, and after performing arthroscopy to determine how much of the talar dome could be visualized, plastic cannulas were placed into the portal locations. Magnetic resonance imaging (MRI) was used to document the distance of the cannulas to neurovascular structures, and these measurements were correlated with the results of anatomic dissections. The average distance between the posteromedial cannula and the tibial nerve was 6.4 mm (range, 0 to 16.2 mm). The distance between the posterior tibial artery and the cannula was on average 9.6 mm (range, 2.4 to 20.1 mm). The average distance between the cannula and the medial calcaneal nerve was 17.1 mm (range, 19 to 31 mm). The location of the posterolateral portal in relation to the tip of the lateral malleolus is an important measurement to determine the proximity of the portal to relevant anatomic structures. It appears that the posterolateral and posteromedial portals used for subtalar arthroscopy are relatively safe, are reproducible, and can be used for the treatment of intra-articular and extra-articular hindfoot pathology.

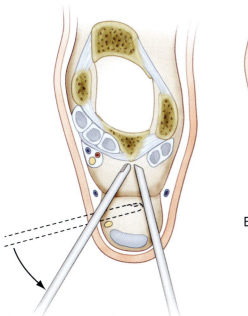

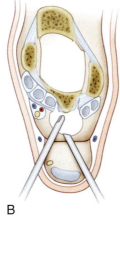

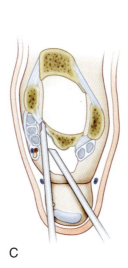

FIGURE 2-8 Posterior subtalar arthroscopy can be performed using posterolateral and posteromedial portals.

A

B

C

Os Trigonum Gross Anatomy

Because the os trigonum can be approached through the subtalar joint, it is included in the description of relevant gross anatomy (Fig. 2-9).[21-23] Terminology regarding the anatomy of the posterior aspect of the talus and the subtalar joint can be confusing. The posterior surface of the talus ("process posterior") consists of the posterior medial and the posterior lateral processes, also known as tubercles. Between these tubercles glides the flexor hallucis longus tendon in its small sulcus, which is directed obliquely, downward, and inward, angling anteriorly (Fig. 2-10).

The size of the posterolateral process of the talus, also called Stieda's process, can vary markedly. It courses in continuity inferiorly with the posterolateral aspect of the articular surface of the talus, making it a partially intra-articular structure, and it is therefore possible to examine it with the arthroscope. Its superior surface, however, is nonarticular and provides an insertion site for the posterior talofibular ligament and a portion of the fibulo-astragalocalcaneal ligament of Rouvière and Canela Lazaro. Occasionally, an accessory ossicle communicates with the posterolateral tubercle, and this is called the os trigonum. It also has multiple surfaces: anterior, inferior, and posterior. The anterior surface articulates with the posterolateral tubercle and the inferior surface with the os calcis. The posterior surface is nonarticular. When the os trigonum fuses, it is called a trigonal process and becomes essentially a large, lateral, articulating tubercle. It is

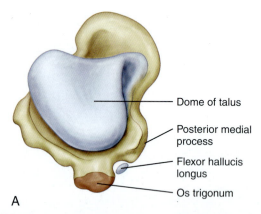

Dome of talus

Posterior medial process

Flexor hallucis longus

Os trigonum

A

FIGURE 2-10 Between the tubercles of the posterior talus, the flexor hallucis longus (FHL) tendon glides in a small sulcus. The FHL is directed obliquely, downward, and inward, angling anteriorly.

often difficult to discern a fracture of Stieda's process from an os trigonum based on radiographs alone. Computed tomography scans and views of the opposite foot are helpful.

The medial tubercle of the talus is an extension of the medial talar articular surface. It provides an attachment site for a portion of the deep and superficial deltoid ligament, the medial talocalcaneal ligament, and part of the fibrous tunnel overlying the flexor hallucis longus tendon.

None of these terms should be confused with the lateral process of the talus, which is a distinctly different structure located on the midlateral aspect of the talus. It provides an insertion site for the lateral talocalcaneal ligament. The lateral process of the talus is of arthroscopic importance because it is a palpable landmark and can be identified intra-articularly on the medial side of the lateral gutter of the subtalar joint. The lateral talocalcaneal ligament coming off the lateral process makes up a thick portion of the lateral capsule of the subtalar joint (Fig. 2-11).

CONCLUSIONS

Advances in small joint techniques and instrumentation have expanded the use of arthroscopic techniques in the subtalar joint. The surgeon must thoroughly understand the gross and arthroscopic anatomy of the subtalar joint. This knowledge can facilitate performance of arthroscopic techniques and recognition of abnormal pathology in the subtalar joint.

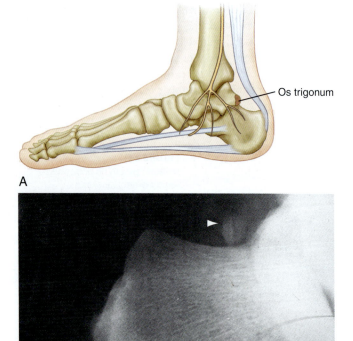

Os trigonum

A

B

FIGURE 2-9 A, The posterior lateral process, or tubercle, of the talus is called Stieda's process. Occasionally, an accessory ossicle communicates with the posterolateral tubercle, and it is called the os trigonum. **B,** A lateral radiograph of the foot shows the os trigonum.

REFERENCES

1. Inman VT. The subtalar joint. In: *The Joints of the Ankle*. Baltimore, MD: Williams & Wilkins; 1976.35-44.
2. Perry J. Anatomy and biomechanics of the hindfoot. *Clin Orthop.* 1983;(177):9-15.
3. Parisien JS. Arthroscopy of the posterior subtalar joint. In: *Current Techniques in Arthroscopy*. 3rd ed. New York, NY: Thieme; 1998:161-168.
4. Parisien JS. Posterior subtalar joint arthroscopy. In: Guhl JF, Parisien JS, Boynton MD, eds. *Foot and Ankle Arthroscopy*. 3rd ed. New York, NY: Springer-Verlag; 2004.175-182.
5. Frey C, Feder KS, DiGiovanni C. Arthroscopic evaluation of the subtalar joint: does sinus tarsi syndrome exist? *Foot Ankle Int.* 1999; 20: 185-191.
6. van Dijk CN, Scholten PE, Krips R. A 2-portal endoscopic approach for diagnosis and treatment of posterior ankle pathology. *Arthroscopy.* 2000; 16:871-876.

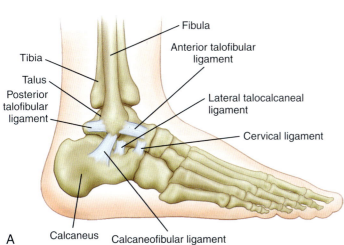

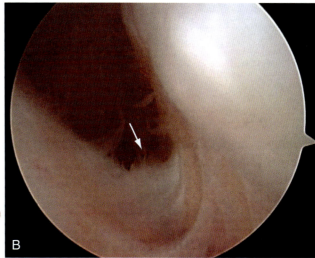

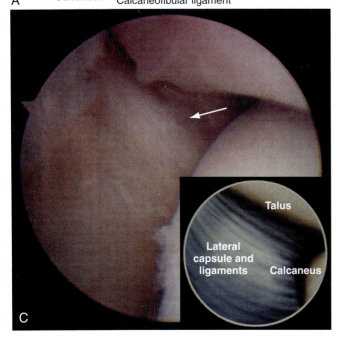

FIGURE 2-11 A, The lateral talocalcaneal ligament comes off the lateral process of the talus and makes up a thick portion of the lateral capsule of the subtalar joint. **B,** The capsule inserts on the lateral aspect of the calcaneus and makes up the floor of the lateral gutter of the subtalar joint. **C,** The lateral capsule of the subtalar joint can be seen, along with the location of the lateral talocalcaneal ligament fibers *(arrow).*

7. Frey C, Gasser S, Feder K. Arthroscopy of the subtalar joint. *Foot Ankle Int.* 1994; 15:424-428.
8. Lapidus PW. Subtalar joint: its anatomy and mechanics. *Bull Hosp Joint Dis.* 1955; 16:179-195.
9. Viladot A, Lorenzo JC, Salazar J, Rodriguez A. The subtalar joint: embryology and morphology. *Foot Ankle.* 1984; 5:54-66.
10. de Palma L, Santucci A, Ventura A, Marinelli M. Anatomy and embryology of the talocalcaneal joint. *Foot Ankle Surg.* 2003; 9:7-18.
11. Harper MC. The lateral ligamentous support of the subtalar joint. *Foot Ankle.* 1991; 11:354-358.
12. Beimers L, Frey C, van Dijk CN. Arthroscopy of the posterior subtalar joint. *Foot Ankle Clin.* 2006; 11:369-390.
13. Tasto JP. Arthroscopic subtalar arthrodesis. *Tech Foot Ankle Surg.* 2003; 2:122-128.
14. Gavlik JM, Rammelt S, Zwipp H. The use of subtalar arthroscopy in open reduction and internal fixation of intra-articular calcaneal fractures. *Injury.* 2002; 33:63-71.
15. Gavlik JM, Rammelt S, Zwipp H. Percutaneous, arthroscopically assisted osteosynthesis of calcaneus fractures. *Arch Orthop Trauma Surg.* 2002; 122:424-428.
16. Jerosch J. Subtalar arthroscopy—indications and surgical technique. *Knee Surg Sports Traumatol Arthrosc.* 1998; 6:122-128.
17. Lijoi F, Lughi M, Baccarani G. Posterior arthroscopic approach to the ankle: an anatomic study. *Arthroscopy.* 2003; 19:62-67.
18. Sitler DF, Amendola A, Bailey CS, et al. Posterior ankle arthroscopy: an anatomic study. *J Bone Joint Surg Am.* 2002;84A:763-769.
19. Mekhail AO, Heck BE, Ebraheim NA, Jackson WT. Arthroscopy of the subtalar joint: establishing a medial portal. *Foot Ankle Int.* 1995; 16: 427-432.
20. Feiwell LA, Frey C. Anatomic study of arthroscopic portal sites of the ankle. *Foot Ankle.* 1993; 14:142-147.
21. Chao W. Os trigonum. *Foot Ankle Clin.* 2004; 9:787-796, vii.
22. Marumoto JM, Ferkel RD. Arthroscopic excision of the os trigonum: a new technique with preliminary clinical results. *Foot Ankle Int.* 1997; 18:777-784.
23. Williams MM, Ferkel RD. Subtalar arthroscopy: indications, technique, and results. *Arthroscopy.* 1998; 14:373-381.

SUGGESTED READINGS

Ferkel RD. Subtalar arthroscopy. In: Whipple TL, ed. *Arthroscopic Surgery: The Foot and Ankle.* Philadelphia, PA: Lippincott-Raven; 1996.231-254.
Parisien JS, Vangsness T. Arthroscopy of the subtalar joint: an experimental approach. *Arthroscopy.* 1985;1:53-57.
Sarrafian S. Osteology. In: Sarrafian S. ed. *Anatomy of the Foot and Ankle.* Philadelphia, PA: Lippincott; 1983:35-106.

Instrumentation and Operative Setup for Ankle and Subtalar Arthroscopy

Bradley E. Slagel • Kevin R. Willits

Although ankle arthroscopy was described in the 1930s by Takagi in Japan and Burman in the United States, there was little interest due to limited joint space accessibility. Improvements in instrumentation during the 1970s resulted in renewed interest in ankle arthroscopy. This chapter explores operating room setup and instrumentation and describes our current practice with regard to anterior ankle arthroscopy and subtalar arthroscopy.

PREOPERATIVE CONSIDERATIONS

Diagnostic Assessment

Before planning operative management, an accurate and thorough preoperative assessment is required to come to a diagnosis or at least provide a limited differential diagnosis. The location and nature of the ankle pathology determine the appropriate position, distraction method, and instrumentation to be used to perform the operative procedure most effectively. A thorough history, physical examination, and basic imaging should be used to make the diagnosis.

If doubt remains after this assessment, more advanced imaging and possibly diagnostic injections may assist in determining the nature and location of the pathology[1]. Liberal use of preoperative diagnostic injections can pinpoint symptomatic pathology, which can aid in decision making for the operating room setup. A patient with anterior and posterior ankle pathology may have complete resolution of symptoms with an anterior ankle injection, obviating the need for posterior access and vice versa. For lesions on the talar dome, it is essential to assess the extent of ankle plantar flexion to determine whether an anterior approach alone is sufficient to access the lesion.

Operating Room Setup

The operating room must be large enough to accommodate all of the necessary personnel and equipment. Personnel usually include a surgeon and an assistant, a scrub nurse, a circulating nurse, and an anesthetist. The operating room must be large enough to allow each of these individuals to move around the room without contaminating the surgical field or instrumentation. The room must also contain an operating table, anesthesia equipment, an arthroscopy tower, an equipment table, and one or two Mayo stands.

Some surgeons may choose to use an arthroscopic pump. Occasionally, fluoroscopy is necessary, which requires a significant amount of space. The arthroscopy tower should be mobile to optimize its position for each case. The components of the arthroscopy tower are listed in Box 3-1 and shown in Figure 3-1. The equipment table is used for therapeutic instruments. The instruments routinely used during the diagnostic arthroscopy (e.g., scalpels, 18-gauge needle, trocars, cannulas, probes) are placed on a Mayo stand for easy accessibility (Fig. 3-2). Backup equipment should be readily available in the event that additional instrumentation is required.

Box 3-1 Arthroscopy Tower Components

- Video camera
- Video monitor
- Motorized shaver
- Light source
- Video recorder
- Printer

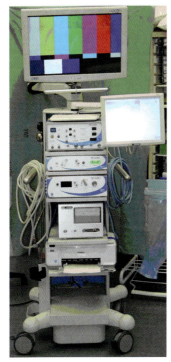

FIGURE 3-1 The components of the arthroscopy tower.

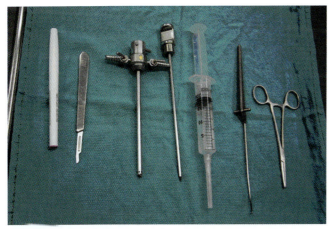

FIGURE 3-2 The instruments routinely used during diagnostic arthroscopy include scalpels, an 18-gauge needle, trocars, cannulas, and probes.

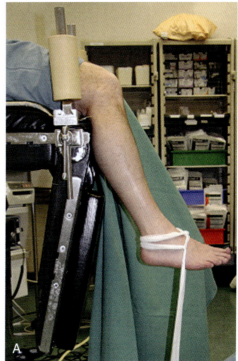

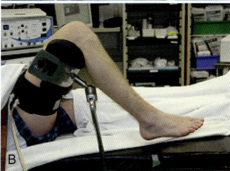

FIGURE 3-3 A and **B,** The two common variations of the supine position.

Anesthesia and Positioning

Ankle arthroscopy may be conducted under general, spinal, or local anesthesia. Use of general or spinal anesthesia is preferable, because both facilitate tourniquet use, if needed, and muscle relaxation that can facilitate ankle distraction. However, local anesthesia remains an option if required because of patient characteristics.

The most appropriate patient positioning for ankle arthroscopy is a matter of the surgeon's preference. Supine and lateral positions are well described. There are two common variations of the supine position (Fig. 3-3). In the first, the patient is placed supine with the operative leg placed in a knee holder.

The knee is placed just distal to the break in the operating room table, and the foot of the bed is lowered to allow the lower leg to rest unsupported.[2] A second option is to place the patient supine and use a well-padded thigh holder to position the operative leg such that the hip is flexed 45 degrees and the leg is allowed to hang, providing access to the ankle.[3] The lateral position has been described by Parisien (Fig. 3-4).[4] It involves placing the patient in a 45-degree lateral position with the operative side up. A platform (box or sheets) is placed underneath the operative leg to elevate it above the nonoperative leg. The hip is externally rotated to access the anterior aspect of the ankle. The leg can be returned to neutral position for access to the lateral or posterior aspects of the ankle. Harbach[5] modified the lateral position with the addition of a thigh holder, which allows the ankle to hang similar to the supine position described previously. Although all previously described positions may be used for subtalar arthroscopy, the most common approaches are from the lateral position or posteriorly with the patient in the prone position.

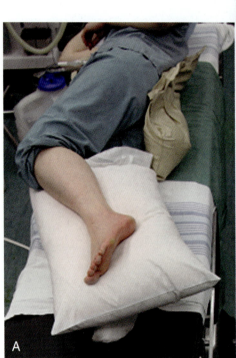
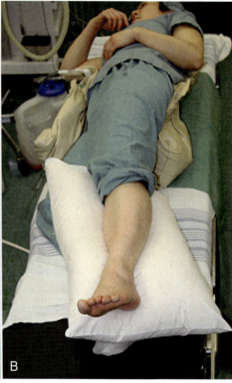

FIGURE 3-4 A and **B,** *The lateral position involves placing the patient in a 45-degree lateral position with the operative side up. A platform (box or sheets) is placed underneath the operative leg to elevate it above the nonoperative leg. The hip is externally rotated to access the anterior aspect of the ankle.*

ARTHROSCOPIC METHODS AND INSTRUMENTATION

Distraction

Interest in ankle arthroscopy resumed in the 1970s with the advent of smaller arthroscopes. Unfortunately, the smaller equipment provides less visibility and is susceptible to breaking. In the 1980s, ankle distraction was added to the procedure as a means of improving visibility and accessibility. Distraction can be classified as invasive or noninvasive. The noninvasive technique is further classified as controlled, semicontrolled, and uncontrolled traction.

Although several methods of invasive distraction exist, all involve drilling traction pins or wires into bone. The well-described Guhl technique uses two ³⁄₁₆-inch threaded Steinmann pins and an external distraction device containing a strain gauge and a pivoting distal end.[6] The proximal pin is placed into the distal tibia approximately 3 to 5 cm proximal to the ankle joint and 1 cm posterior to the anterior tibial crest. The distal pin is placed into the calcaneus 2 to 2.5 cm anterior to its posterior border and just beneath the peroneal tendons. Both pins are placed in unicortical fashion from lateral to medial aspects. The calcaneus pin should be aimed 20 degrees distally. Many other techniques have been described, including medial distraction with the distal pin in the talus[7]; medial and lateral distraction[8]; a single, smooth, 0.045-mm wire passed through the sinus tarsi and attached to weights[9]; and a single pin through the calcaneus attached to a fracture table.[10]

Noninvasive distraction techniques have largely replaced the need for invasive distraction. Uncontrolled techniques are simple to execute, but it is difficult to maintain a consistent amount of distraction. Gravity distraction achieved by hanging the leg with the knee flexed 90 degrees is the most basic form of uncontrolled distraction. Manual traction using the surgeon's free hand or an assistant's hand to grasp the foot and pull longitudinally is another method. Only small amounts of distraction are possible using these techniques.

Yates and Grana[11] described a means of applying semicontrolled distraction. A small loop is tied in the center of a Kerlix gauze roll. The free ends of the roll are wrapped around the ankle and then passed through the loop. The ends are tied together and then placed underneath the surgeon's foot. Traction can be added by stepping (similar to stepping on a gas pedal) on the loop underfoot (Fig. 3-5A). Cameron[12] modified this technique by passing the loop behind the surgeon's back, rather than underfoot (see Fig. 3-5B). To apply distraction, the surgeon leans backward.

Takao and colleagues[13] use a different bandage configuration to produce equal distraction anteriorly and posteriorly (see Fig. 3-5B). These methods of distraction require little equipment and are very cost effective. However, it is difficult to maintain consistent traction, and some operators may find the multitasking of operating and controlling distraction somewhat onerous. Another disadvantage is that placing the Kerlix roll underfoot or behind the back may compromise the sterility of the procedure.

Through controlled methods, specific amounts of distraction can be applied and maintained with ease. The most common means of controlled distraction is to use one of the many commercially available, sterile foot straps and attach the sling

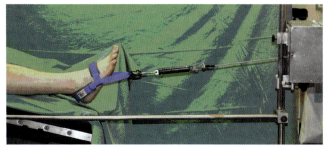

FIGURE 3-6 The most common means of controlled distraction uses one of the many commercially available sterile foot straps and attaches the sling to a tensioning device.

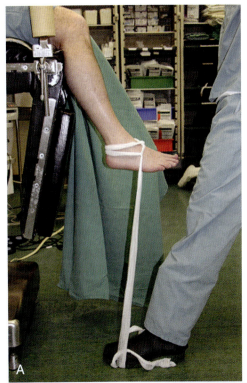

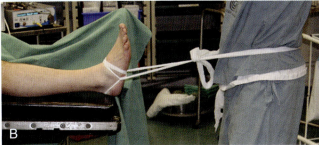

FIGURE 3-5 To achieve semicontrolled distraction, a small loop is tied in the center of a Kerlix gauze roll. The free ends of the roll are wrapped around the ankle and then passed through the loop. The ends are tied together and placed underneath the surgeon's foot. **A,** Traction can be added by stepping (similar to stepping on a gas pedal) on the loop underfoot. **B,** The technique can be modified by passing the loop behind the surgeon's back, rather than underfoot.

to a tensioning device (Fig. 3-6). This system allows the surgeon to keep both hands free. The foot may be placed into various degrees of plantar flexion by modifying the position of the straps. In many of these systems, the entire apparatus is sterile, which avoids contamination concerns that exist with the semicontrolled techniques. Waseem and coworkers[14] routinely use the foot strap technique. However, for tight arthritic ankles, they advocate using a clamp from the AO pinless fixator applied to the patient's heel and attached to a traction setup. Aydin[15] described a distraction technique in which a kyphoplasty balloon is inserted through an arthroscopic portal and is inflated to distract the joint. The entire joint can be visualized, but it is necessary to move the balloon to different positions within the ankle. The controlled techniques are more costly than the uncontrolled and semicontrolled methods.

The acceptable amount of weight and duration of traction depend on the technique used. Guhl[6] recommends 7 to 8 mm of distraction with his invasive technique.

Distraction should not be increased after slight bending of the pins has been noticed. The distraction force required usually is 30 to 50 pounds, and it should not continue longer than 45 to 60 minutes to avoid excessive stretching of the ligament. Using cadaveric ankles, Albert and associates[16] found that complications were avoided if less than 135 N of distraction force was used. Beyond 135 N, they encountered pin bending and bony destruction of the calcaneus. Takao and colleagues[13] compared the bandage distraction technique described by Yates and Grana[11] with their own and found better distraction (90% anterior and posterior opening) using the Takao technique with 8 kg of force. They recommended a maximum of 8 to10 kg of force be used because the test subjects felt pain at greater than 10 kg of force. Dowdy and coworkers[17] advise that foot straps be used for less than 1 hour at a maximum distractive force of 30 pounds because the subjects in their study developed reversible nerve conduction changes above this threshold.

Invasive distraction is now rarely used. Although it provides greater distraction,[17] the risk of complications is also much greater. Box 3-2 lists the potential complications of invasive and noninvasive distraction. Despite the potential for complications with invasive distraction, studies have not shown a significant difference in morbidity for invasive or noninvasive distraction. Ferkel and associates[3] found no difference in complication rates between invasive and noninvasive distraction. Guhl[6] reported a 10% complication rate in his series using invasive distraction, but ultimately, only three complications were related to distraction and only one (i.e., scarred nodule adjacent to the peroneal sheath) resulted in patient morbidity. Tibial stress fractures through the pin site have been reported.[20,21] Stone and Guhl[21] recommend avoidance of stressful activities for 6 to 12 weeks postoperatively after the use of invasive distraction.

The contraindications to distraction are found in Box 3-3. Several investigators have found that distraction is rarely necessary.[1,22,23] The need for distraction can be minimized or eliminated by using smaller arthroscopic instruments or by a more accurate preoperative diagnosis. Distraction may make some portions of ankle arthroscopy more difficult. The space available deep to the anterior capsule is decreased with traction.[1] Because most therapeutic ankle arthroscopy procedures occur within the anterior

Box 3-2 Potential Complications of Invasive and Noninvasive Distraction in Ankle Arthroscopy

INVASIVE DISTRACTION

- Vascular complications
  Deep peroneal artery injury
  Lesser saphenous vein injury
- Neurologic complications
  Deep peroneal nerve injury
  Sural nerve injury
- Tendinous complications
  Peroneal tendon injury
- Ligament stretching or disruption
- Infection (soft tissue or bone)
- Pin breakage
- Fractures
  Acute pull-out
  Delayed second degree to stress riser
- Pain at the insertion site
- Subtalar joint injury
- Hypertrophic scar
- Sharp injury to surgeon or patient

NONINVASIVE DISTRACTION

- Neuropraxia
- Skin abrasion

Data from references 3, 6, 14, 17, 18, and 19.

Box 3-3 Contraindications to Invasive and Noninvasive Distraction in Ankle Arthroscopy

INVASIVE DISTRACTION

- Reflex sympathetic dystrophy
- Open physis
- Osteopenia
- Infection

NONINVASIVE DISTRACTION

- Impaired circulation
- Diabetes
- Ankle edema
- Fragile skin

Adapted from Boynton MD, Parisien JS, Guhl JF, Vetter CS. Setup, distraction, and instrumentation. In: Guhl JF, Parisien JS, Boynton MD, eds. *Foot and Ankle Arthroscopy*. 3rd ed. New York, NY: Springer-Verlag; 2004.

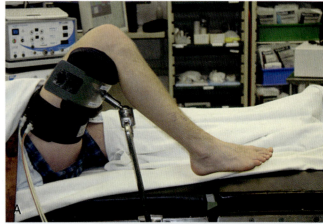

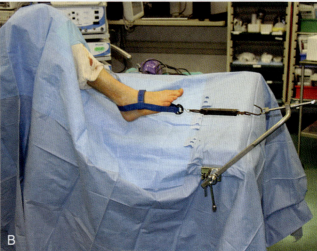

FIGURE 3-7 Ankle arthroscopy with local anesthetic alone. **A,** The patient is positioned supine with the hip flexed 45 degrees and the thigh supported by a well-padded thigh holder. **B,** The foot is attached to a sterile foot strap, which is fixed to a sterile tensioning device.

compartment, many surgeons find distraction unnecessary. Distraction usually is not employed in subtalar arthroscopy.

Preferred Method: Anesthesia, Position, and Distraction

Most ankle arthroscopies at our center are performed under general anesthesia. Spinal anesthesia is used if there is a contraindication to general anesthesia.

Ankle arthroscopy with local anesthesia alone has been used only in rare circumstances. We prefer to position the patient supine with the hip flexed 45 degrees and the patient's thigh supported by a well-padded thigh holder (Fig. 3-7A). The foot is attached to a sterile foot strap, which is fixed to a sterile tensioning device (see Fig. 3-7B). Although the posterolateral portal is

accessible, we prefer to use this position for anterior ankle arthroscopy alone. Preoperatively, we determine the need or potential need for posterior ankle arthroscopy. Patients who have posterior ankle pathology are placed in the prone position after an anterior ankle arthroscopy is performed or as a solitary procedure (see Chapter 7). Two separate setups are used for the rare patient who requires anterior and posterior ankle arthroscopies rather than trying to accomplish the anterior and posterior arthroscopies in the supine or lateral position. Noninvasive foot strap distraction is routinely used at 20 to 30 pounds of distraction to facilitate joint visualization. We decrease or remove the traction if increased space is needed for procedures in the anterior compartment beneath the anterior capsule.

Instrumentation

Arthroscopes

Arthroscopes are available in a variety of lengths, diameters, and lens angles. The most commonly used arthroscopes for ankle arthroscopy are the 4.0-mm, 30-degree arthroscope and the 2.7-mm, 30-degree arthroscope (Fig. 3-8). Occasionally a 70-degree arthroscope may be beneficial to improve visualization of the posterior

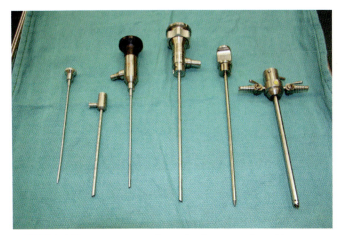

FIGURE 3-8 The most commonly used arthroscopes for ankle arthroscopy are the 4.0-mm, 30-degree arthroscope and the 2.7-mm, 30-degree arthroscope.

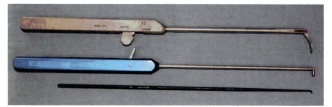

FIGURE 3-9 Probes come in various curvatures, lengths, and diameters.

aspect of the joint. We have found the 4.0-mm, 30-degree arthroscope is effective for most anterior ankle arthroscopies. This arthroscope has the advantage of a greater field of view and increased intra-articular flow compared with the 2.7-mm arthroscope. Subtalar arthroscopy is better and more safely performed with the 2.7-mm arthroscope because of increased joint congruency.

Video Cameras, Monitors, and Light Source

Standard arthroscopic video equipment is adequate for ankle arthroscopy. Although high-definition video equipment provides greater detail and picture quality, no direct effect on patient outcomes has been reported.

Inflow System

Gravity inflow from 3-L bags of saline is used for all ankle arthroscopies. The bags are routinely elevated to maximum vertical height of 3 m, and a tourniquet is inflated to 300 mm Hg during the arthroscopy. This method of inflow provides more consistent flow with less turbulence and a simplified operating room setup. No difficulties with visualization have been encountered using this technique. In our experience, gravity inflow has been superior to inflow by means of pump systems.

Handheld Instruments

Ankle arthroscopy instruments usually are smaller in length and diameter than those used in the knee and shoulder. Their decreased size improves accessibility to all areas of the ankle but increases the likelihood of instrument breakage.

Probes. The probe is the most basic of instruments, and it the most frequently used. It acts as an extension of the surgeon's hand, allowing mobilization and palpation of structures. It is also a useful tool for measuring the size of chondral lesions.

Calibrated probes can increase the accuracy of measurement. Calibrations are preferably marked in ink rather than scored into the metal, because scoring creates stress risers that can lead to instrument breakage.[18] Probes come in various curvatures, lengths, and diameters (Fig. 3-9). Articulating probes are commercially available (Arthrex) and allow the probe to enter the joint straight and then articulate and lock at 90 degrees. Shorter probes are more useful in ankle arthroscopy because they have a shorter lever arm and are easier to control.

Basket Forceps. Basket forceps (i.e., punches) are used for débridement. Wide tips are available for greater efficiency, and narrow tips are available for improved control. A variety of angulations exist to facilitate maneuverability (Fig. 3-10).

Curettes. Curettes are available in ring or cup formation. Ring curettes are often helpful for débriding osteochondritis dissecans lesions. Straight and angled versions are available (Fig. 3-11).

Rasps. Small rasps are occasionally useful for smoothing bony edges after débridement.

Graspers. Graspers are used to remove loose bodies or broken instruments from the joint. They are available in straight or curved shafts and in a variety of tip angles (Fig. 3-12).

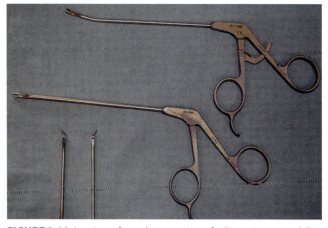

FIGURE 3-10 A variety of angulations exist to facilitate maneuverability of basket forceps.

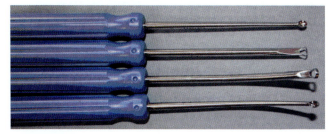

FIGURE 3-11 Ring curettes are often helpful for débriding OCD lesions. Straight and angled versions are available.

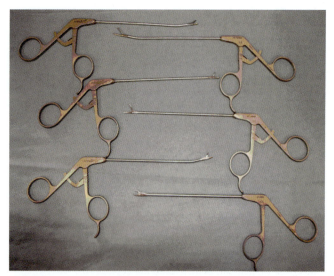

FIGURE 3-12 Graspers are used to remove loose bodies or broken instruments from the joint. They are available in straight or curved shafts and in a variety of tip angles.

Osteotomes. Small osteotomes are useful for osteophyte removal (Fig. 3-13).

Aiming Devices. Aiming devices are useful for accurate drilling when a transosseous approach is required. The aiming devices used for cruciate reconstruction in the knee are usually sufficient, but small joint devices can assist in tight joints.

Awls. Awls are useful for microfracture of chondral lesions. A variety of tip angulations exist to facilitate appropriate access within the confined space of the ankle joint (Fig. 3-14).

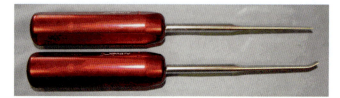

FIGURE 3-13 Small osteotomes are useful for osteophyte removal.

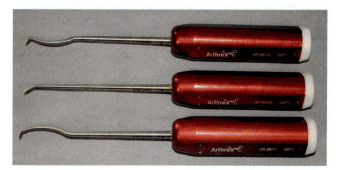

FIGURE 3-14 Awls are useful for microfracture of chondral lesions. A variety of tip angulations exist to facilitate appropriate access within the confined space of the ankle joint.

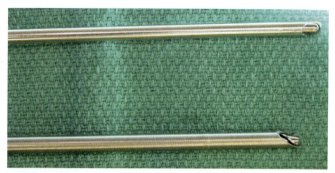

FIGURE 3-15 Motorized instruments often enable the surgeon to execute the procedure more efficiently. Shavers and burrs of various sizes, angles, and degrees of aggressiveness are available.

Motorized Instruments

Motorized instruments frequently enable the surgeon to execute the procedure more efficiently. Shavers and burrs of various sizes, angles, and degrees of aggressiveness are available (Fig. 3-15). The larger instruments enable the procedure to be performed quickly; however, the amount of joint space available ultimately determines the size that is used. Less aggressive instruments should be used near vulnerable structures or when learning a new procedure. Conceptually, the instruments are constructed similarly, with a rotating blade or burr housed in a sheath that is attached to suction. The surgeon is able to adjust the direction of rotation and the amount of suction.

Retrieving Instruments

Suction instruments with magnetic tips can be useful for retrieval of broken instruments. Their use may avoid the need for extra portals or an arthrotomy.

PEARLS & PITFALLS

PEARLS

1. Preoperative assessment determines the pain-generating lesion. Preoperative diagnostic injections can pinpoint symptomatic pathology aiding in decision making for operating room setup.
2. Noninvasive consistent traction improves accessibility of intra-articular and periarticular pathology.

PITFALLS

1. Preoperative assessment should include extent of ankle plantar flexion, because this may directly impact the accessibility of lesions from an anterior approach.
2. Pathology is assessed from medial and lateral viewing portals to ensure the adequacy of treatment.

REFERENCES

1. Van Dijk CN, Scholte D. Arthroscopy of the ankle joint. *Arthroscopy.* 1997;13:90-96.
2. Andrews JR, Previte WJ, Carson WG. Arthroscopy of the ankle: technique and normal anatomy. *Foot Ankle.* 198;6:29-33.
3. Ferkel RD, Dalton DH, Guhl JF. Neurological complications of ankle arthroscopy. *Arthroscopy.* 1996;12:200-208.
4. Parisien JS, Vangsness T. Operative arthroscopy of the ankle. Three years' experience. *Clin Orthop Relat Res.* 1985;(199):46-53.
5. Harbach GP, Stewart JD, Lambert EW, Anderson C. Ankle arthroscopy in the lateral decubitus position. *Foot Ankle Int.* 2003;24:597-599.

6. Guhl JF. New concepts (distraction) in ankle arthroscopy. *Arthroscopy.* 1988;4:160-167.

7. Baker CL, Graham JM. Current concepts in ankle arthroscopy. *Orthopedics.* 1993;16:1027-1035.

8. Brazytis KE, Hergenroeder PT. Arthroscopic ankle surgery. Overcoming anatomic difficulties with improved techniques. *AORN J.* 1992;55:492-502.

9. Wright G. Technique tips. Skeletal traction for ankle arthroscopy. *Foot Ankle Int.* 1996;17:119.

10. Casteleyn PP, Handelberg F. Technical note. Distraction for ankle arthroscopy. *Arthroscopy.* 1995;11:633-634.

11. Yates CK, Grana WA. A simple distraction technique for ankle arthroscopy. *Arthroscopy.* 1988;4:103-105.

12. Cameron SE. Technical note. Noninvasive distraction for ankle arthroscopy. *Arthroscopy.* 1997;13:366-369.

13. Takao M, Ochi M, Shu N, et al. Bandage distraction technique for ankle arthroscopy. *Foot Ankle Int.* 1999;20:389-391.

14. Waseem M, Barrie JL. A new distraction method in difficult ankle arthroscopy. *J Foot Ankle Surg.* 2002;41:412-413.

15. Aydin AT, Ozcanli H, Soyuncu Y, Dabak TK. Technical note. A new noninvasive controlled intra-articular ankle distraction technique on a cadaver model. *Arthroscopy.* 2006;22:905.e1-905.e3.

16. Albert J, Reiman P, Njus G, et al. Ligament strain and ankle joint opening during ankle distraction. *Arthroscopy.* 1992;8:469-473.

17. Dowdy PA, Watson BV, Amendola A, Brown JD. Noninvasive ankle distraction: relationship between force, magnitude of distraction, and nerve conduction abnormalities. *Arthroscopy.* 1996;12:64-69.

18. Boynton MD, Parisien JS, Guhl JF, Vetter CS. Setup, distraction, and instrumentation. In: Guhl JF, Parisien JS, Boynton MD, eds. *Foot and Ankle Arthroscopy.* 3rd ed. New York, NY: Springer-Verlag; 2004.

19. Palladino SJ. Distraction systems for ankle arthroscopy. *Clin Podiatr Med Surg.* 1994;11:499-511.

20. Ferkel RD, Guhl JF, Van Beucken K, et al. Complications in ankle arthroscopy: analysis of the first 518 cases [abstract]. *Orthop Trans.* 1993;16:726.

21. Stone JW, Guhl JF. Ankle arthroscopy. In: Pfeffer GB, Frey CC, Anderson RB, Mizel MS, eds. *Current Practice in Foot and Ankle Surgery.* Vol 1. New York, NY: McGraw-Hill; 1993.

22. Sandmeier RH, Renstrom PAFH. Ankle Arthroscopy. *Scand J Med Sci Sports.* 1995;5:64-70.

23. Sun YQ, Slesarenko YA. Joint distraction may be unnecessary in ankle arthroscopy. *Orthopedics.* 2006;29:118-120.

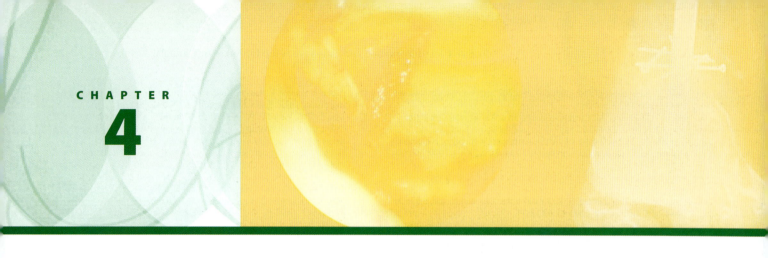

Diagnostic Arthroscopy for the Ankle and Subtalar Joints

James W. Stone

The ankle is a highly constrained joint composed of complex, curved articular surfaces that are stabilized by ligaments with various degrees of laxity. These anatomic constraints make arthroscopy of the ankle joint more difficult than in larger joints such as the knee and shoulder. Early attempts to perform arthroscopy of the ankle joint were met with various degrees of success. In a 1931 cadaver study, Burman suggested that the ankle joint "… is not suitable for arthroscopy."[1]

Arthroscopists in the 1980s began to apply modern techniques to instrumentation of the ankle and defined the basic portals with which to approach the joint.[2-4] Since then, two technical advances have facilitated routine performance of ankle arthroscopy for diagnosis and surgical procedures. First, the development of high-quality, small-diameter arthroscopes has allowed instrumentation of the ankle with increased ability to visualize the entire joint while decreasing the likelihood of iatrogenic articular cartilage injury. Second, techniques have been developed for noninvasive joint distraction to facilitate instrument passage and decrease joint injury.[5] Without distraction, it is often impossible to visualize the central and posterior compartments of the joint from the anterior portals. Early attempts to distract the joint used pins placed into the tibia and calcaneus that were connected to a distractor device similar to an external fixator. The use of these devices was associated with significant complications, including pin tract infection and neurovascular injury.[6] Elimination of these complications while effectively distracting the joint with noninvasive strap distraction is a major advantage, and invasive ankle joint distraction is no longer recommended.

PATIENT POSITIONING

The patient is placed supine on the operating table with the hip and knee flexed and supported by a well-padded leg holder (Fig. 4-1). I prefer a leg holder with a long thigh segment and

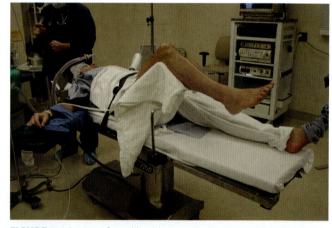

FIGURE 4-1 Position for ankle arthroscopy. The patient is supine, and the hip and knee are supported by a well-padded leg holder. The leg holder has a broad thigh support so that as distraction force is applied to the ankle, it is dissipated over a wide area of the thigh rather than concentrated in the popliteal fossa.

short knee segment to diffuse the distraction force over the wide area of the thigh rather than concentrating the force in the popliteal space and potentially causing obstruction to venous outflow. Sterile drapes are applied after skin preparation.

A sterile clamp is attached to the operating table side rail over the sheets, and a bar is fixed to the clamp. The noninvasive ankle distractor strap is placed around the hindfoot and midfoot and connected to the bar using a segment of sterile two-sided Velcro. This distraction setup allows the ankle and foot to rest in a plantigrade position while retaining the ability to move the ankle in dorsiflexion and plantar flexion intraoperatively (Fig. 4-2).

Invasive distraction is not required for standard ankle arthroscopy. It poses unnecessary risks to neurovascular structures, along with risks of infection and stress fracture.

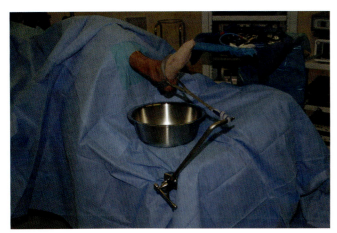

FIGURE 4-2 The leg is prepared and draped with sterile sheets, and the noninvasive distractor is applied to the ankle. The strap that is placed around the hindfoot and midfoot is attached to the bar using a strip of Velcro, with which the distraction force can be varied.

Anatomic landmarks are then marked with a sterile marking pen. I outline the medial malleolus and the anterior joint line along with the contour of the distal fibula. Also marked are the position of the tibialis anterior tendon medially, the peroneus tertius tendon laterally, and the lateral border of the Achilles tendon posteriorly. The position of the superficial peroneal nerve branch passing over the anterolateral ankle can often be appreciated by plantar flexing and inverting the ankle.

PORTAL CREATION

Careful attention to portal creation technique can minimize the incidence of iatrogenic injury to neurovascular structures. The nick and spread technique is advised. Each portal is created by incising only the skin, avoiding penetration of the subcutaneous tissues with the knife blade. A small hemostat clamp is used to spread the subcutaneous tissues down to the level of the capsule. The capsule is penetrated using a blunt trocar to minimize the risk of iatrogenic articular cartilage injury.

The three standard working portals for ankle arthroscopy are the anteromedial portal, the anterolateral portal, and the posterolateral portal (Fig. 4-3). The anterocentral portal was used in the early days of ankle arthroscopy because of the purported benefit of increased visualization in the central compartment. However, this portal placement poses significant risk of injury to the deep peroneal nerve and the dorsalis pedis artery. The use of small joint arthroscopes and noninvasive joint distraction obviates the use of this portal for ankle arthroscopy.

The first portal created should be the anteromedial portal. In most patients, there is an indentation in the anteromedial articular surface of the distal tibia, known as the notch of Harty, that facilitates passage of instruments across the ankle joint from medial to lateral aspects. The surgeon palpates the tibialis anterior tendon and inserts an 18-gauge needle into the joint immediately adjacent to the tendon's medial border (Fig. 4-4). As the needle enters the joint, the surgeon notices the sound of air entering the joint, which also allows the ankle to be distracted more easily. Needle placement is adjusted proximally or distally until the position that allows easiest passage across the joint is identified as the optimal location for the portal. The cannula is introduced through this portal, and the 2.7-mm arthroscope is introduced into the joint.

With the arthroscope in the anteromedial portal, the posterolateral portal is created under direct visualization. The portal is located adjacent to the lateral border of the Achilles tendon and approximately 1 to 2 cm distal to the anterior portal so that an upwardly angled 18 gauge needle passes into the joint beneath the posterior syndesmotic ligament complex and accommodates the posterior curvature of the talar dome (Fig. 4-5). Another 2.7-mm cannula is placed and functions as a dedicated inflow cannula attached to an arthroscopic fluid pump.

Although inflow can be performed by gravity, the arthroscopic pump allows control over the inflow pressure and the maximum flow rate allowed by the pump. The surgeon must monitor the condition of the soft tissue of the calf frequently during the case to ensure that fluid extravasation does not result in excessive swelling.

The anterolateral portal is placed in a manner similar to placement of the anteromedial portal adjacent to the lateral border of the peroneus tertius. Careful attention to portal creation technique minimizes the risk of injury to branches of the superficial peroneal nerve, the most commonly injured nerve in ankle arthroscopy, which is always located close to the anterolateral portal. The arthroscopic view is directed laterally to visualize entry of the 18-gauge needle, ensuring optimal position as the needle is passed across the joint.

Accessory portals medially or laterally may be required in some circumstances, particularly if surgery is being performed deep in the medial or lateral gutters. Optimal location for these portals is identified using a needle, and as long as there is approximately 1 cm between the standard portal and the accessory portal, wound-healing problems should be minimal. The trans-Achilles tendon portal described in the early days of ankle arthroscopy is not necessary and poses unnecessary risks of injury to the tendon.

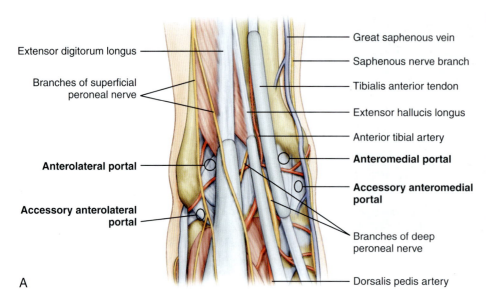

Extensor digitorum longus

Branches of superficial peroneal nerve

Anterolateral portal

Accessory anterolateral portal

Great saphenous vein

Saphenous nerve branch

Tibialis anterior tendon

Extensor hallucis longus

Anterior tibial artery

Anteromedial portal

Accessory anteromedial portal

Branches of deep peroneal nerve

Dorsalis pedis artery

A

FIGURE 4-3 Sketch showing the anatomy of the ankle in relation to the standard portals. **A,** The anteromedial portal is located immediately adjacent to the medial border of the tibialis anterior tendon at the level of the joint line. The anterolateral portal is located lateral to the lateral border or the peroneus tertius tendon. Accessory medial or lateral portals may be placed to approach the particular pathology found at surgery, and the location is guided using an 18-gauge needle intraoperatively. **B,** Posterolateral and posteromedial portal positions are shown in relation to significant anatomic structures.

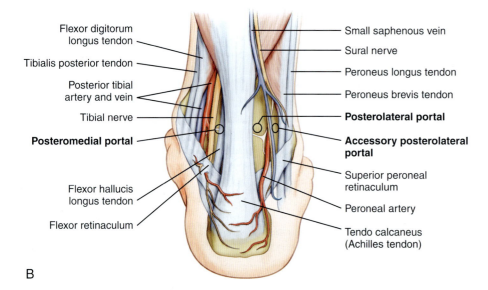

Flexor digitorum longus tendon

Tibialis posterior tendon

Posterior tibial artery and vein

Tibial nerve

Posteromedial portal

Flexor hallucis longus tendon

Flexor retinaculum

Small saphenous vein

Sural nerve

Peroneus longus tendon

Peroneus brevis tendon

Posterolateral portal

Accessory posterolateral portal

Superior peroneal retinaculum

Peroneal artery

Tendo calcaneus (Achilles tendon)

B

PITFALLS
- Avoid injury to superficial neurovascular structures using the nick and spread technique for portal creation:
  1. Incise only the skin with a no. 11 blade.
  2. Spread subcutaneous tissue with mosquito forceps.
  3. Penetrate the joint capsule with a blunt trocar.
- Avoid portal complications such as sinus formation:
  1. Make the portal large enough to easily pass instruments without causing soft tissue damage.
  2. Use simple sutures at the conclusion of the case.
  3. Impose a brief period of postoperative immobilization (about 1 week) in a splint to allow soft tissue healing.

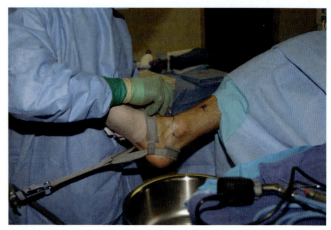

FIGURE 4-4 Each portal is located using an 18-gauge needle to determine the optimal position that allows easy passage of the instruments across the joint.

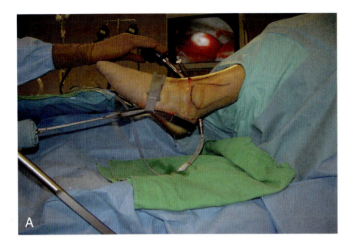

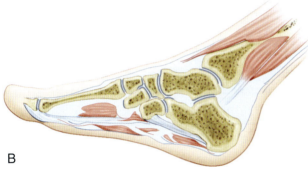

FIGURE 4-5 A, Intraoperative photograph shows the relative position of the posterolateral portal to the anterior portal. The posterolateral portal is approximately 1 to 2 cm distal to the level of the anterior portals and angled upward to accommodate the curvature of the talar dome. **B,** Cross-sectional sketch shows the anatomy of the ankle joint, which dictates the angle at which the posterior portal must be placed to accommodate the curvature of the talar dome.

DIAGNOSTIC ARTHROSCOPY

Diagnostic ankle arthroscopy is initiated from the medial portal using a 2.7-mm, 30-degree arthroscope. A 70-degree arthroscope should be available to enhance visualization in the medial and lateral gutters or in the posterior joint when viewing from the anterior aspect. Almost all ankles can be instrumented using the 2.7-mm arthroscope, but a 1.9-mm backup arthroscope may be useful in a particularly tight joint.

Ferkel has emphasized the importance of an organized approach to diagnostic ankle arthroscopy with a 21-point examination that starts with the anteromedial approach, then uses the anterolateral approach, and concludes with direct posterior viewing from the posterolateral portal.[7] Depending on the pathology, initial visualization of the joint may be impaired by hypertrophic synovium or bony exostoses, and limited débridement may be required at the start of the case. It is important to débride any hypertrophic synovium with a mechanical shaver, keeping the blade directed away from the relatively thin capsule of the anterior joint to avoid inadvertent injury to the anterior neurovascular structures while also avoiding injury to the joint surfaces. Bipolar intra-articular cautery facilitates hemostasis when performing the procedure without tourniquet inflation.

The tip of the medial malleolus is visualized from the anteromedial portal along with the deep deltoid ligament spanning the space between the malleolus and the talus (Fig. 4-6). A probe is introduced from the anterolateral portal to palpate structures with the arthroscope in the anteromedial portal. The surgeon then directs the arthroscope up the medial gutter (Fig. 4-7) and into the tibiotalar joint through the notch of Harty (Fig. 4-8). At this point, the arthroscope usually can be maneuvered in a posterolateral direction across the dome of the talus, affording visualization of the entire dome of the talus and the posterior joint structures (Fig. 4-9).

The interosseous ligament complex is identified posteriorly (Fig. 4-10). These ligaments display a variable anatomy and have been described differently in anatomic dissection studies. Ferkel has described three major ligament components.[8] Superiorly, the broad posterior-inferior tibiofibular ligament represents the most distal end of the syndesmosis and its most distal fibers can be seen intra-articularly as the most superior component of the complex coursing from superior and medial to inferior and lateral aspects. Beneath this ligament is the less robust transverse tibiofibular ligament,

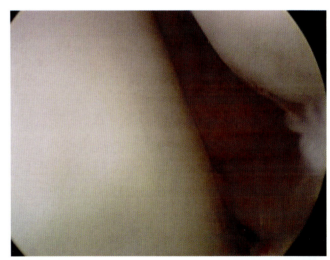

FIGURE 4-6 Arthroscopic view from the anteromedial portal shows the tip of the medial malleolus, the talus, and the fibers of the deltoid ligament.

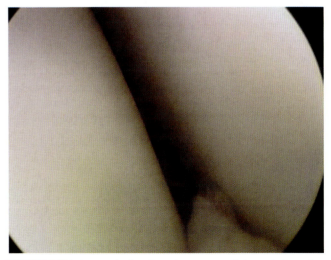

FIGURE 4-7 Arthroscopic view from the anteromedial portal shows the medial gutter of the right ankle.

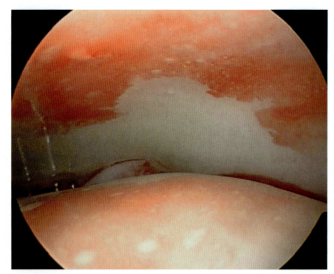

FIGURE 4-8 Arthroscopic view from the anteromedial portal shows the anteromedial dome of the talus in the foreground and the articular surface of the medial malleolus in a right ankle (dry joint).

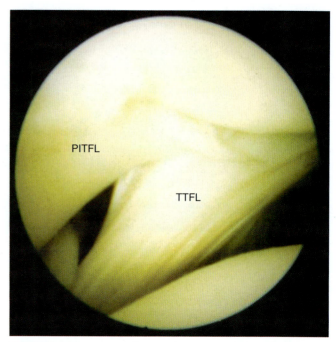

FIGURE 4-10 Posterior syndesmotic ligaments include the posterior-inferior tibiofibular ligament (PITFL) and the transverse tibiofibular ligament (TTFL) of the right ankle.

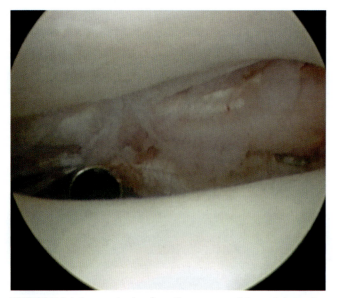

FIGURE 4-9 Arthroscopic view from the anteromedial portal shows the midportion of the talar dome, the distal tibial articular surface above, and in the background, the inflow cannula entering the joint beneath the posterior syndesmotic ligaments.

by directing the arthroscope's viewing angle laterally (Fig. 4-11). The structures to be identified are the lateral dome of the talus, the distal tibiofibular joint, and the soft tissues of the syndesmosis. The arthroscope is then gently withdrawn, revealing the anterior tibia, which should be carefully examined for the presence of bony exostosis (Fig. 4-12). The view of the anterior joint may be facilitated by decreasing the amount of joint distraction while dorsiflexing the ankle to allow the anterior capsule to distend. The arthroscope's viewing angle is then directed along the neck of the talus to evaluate the capsular insertion on the talar neck (Fig. 4-13). As the arthroscope is directed laterally, the well-defined inferior fascicle of the

which attaches to the posterior fibular tubercle on the fibula and to the posterior portion of the distal tibial articular surface, spanning to the medial malleolus. The tibial slip is the most inferior of the posterior interosseous structures. Golano and colleagues have described the posterior ligament anatomy to include the posterior-inferior tibiofibular ligament, which is also called the tibial slip.[9] The transverse ligament was defined as the deep component of the posterior-inferior tibiofibular ligament. The flexor hallucis longus tendon may be seen as a vertically oriented structure in the posterior ankle compartment when the capsule is thin, and this structure is made more prominent by flexing and extending the great toe.

Depending on the degree of inherent joint laxity, it may not be possible to maneuver the arthroscope directly across to the lateral side of the joint, but the lateral joint structures can be visualized

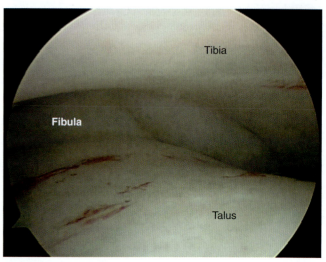

FIGURE 4-11 Lateral view from the anteromedial portal across the talar dome of the right ankle. The distal fibula is visible in the background, as is soft tissue in the tibiofibular syndesmosis.

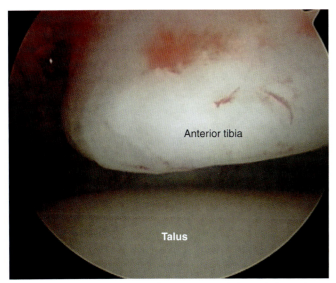

FIGURE 4-12 Arthroscopic view from anteromedial portal shows the distal tibial articular surface of the right ankle.

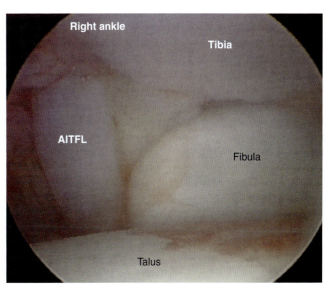

FIGURE 4-14 Arthroscopic view from the anteromedial portal in the right ankle shows the distal tibiofibular articulation and the vertically oriented fibers of the anterior-inferior tibiofibular ligament (AITFL).

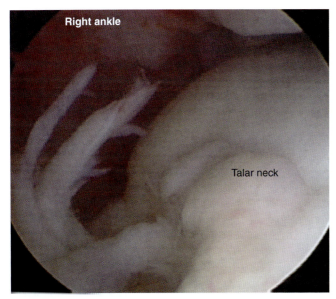

FIGURE 4-13 Arthroscopic view from the anteromedial portal shows the talar neck of the right ankle.

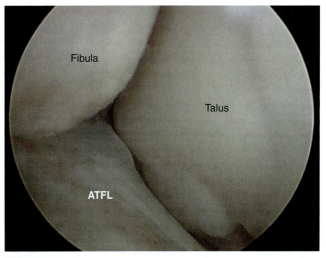

FIGURE 4-15 Arthroscopic view from the anteromedial portal in the right ankle. The distal fibula and the adjacent articular surface of the talus are seen, along with the arching fibers of the anterior talofibular ligament (ATFL).

anterior-inferior tibiofibular ligament is identified as a vertically oriented structure connecting the tibia and fibula (Fig. 4-14).

The arthroscope is directed into the lateral gutter and then down to the level of the tip of the lateral malleolus (Fig. 4-15). The anterior talofibular ligament can usually be defined starting from its origin on the anterior-inferior fibula and curving to insert on the talus.

The arthroscope is then switched to the anterolateral portal, and a diagnostic examination is performed from this approach starting at the tip of the lateral malleolus, which can usually be viewed more completely from this approach. In addition to the anterior talofibular ligament, the entire articular surface of the lateral gutter is evaluated from this viewpoint, and the posterior

talofibular ligament often can be seen at the posterior extent of the gutter. The arthroscope is then directed up the lateral gutter and into the anterolateral joint to visualize the syndesmosis, distal fibula, lateral tibia, and lateral dome of the talus. All structures visualized from the anteromedial portal are evaluated from the anterolateral perspective for complete assessment.

The final assessment of the joint is from the posterolateral approach, with the inflow and arthroscopic probe placed in one of the anterior portals. This view optimizes visualization of the posteromedial talar dome and may be especially useful for treatment of osteochondral lesions of the posteromedial talar dome, which may be difficult to appreciate fully from anterior approaches. In this circumstance, the lesion is viewed from the posterior portal, and instruments are introduced from the anterior portal. The posterior portal also affords excellent visualization of the deep deltoid ligament as the arthroscope is advanced from the posterior tip of the medial malleolus, up the medial gutter, and over the talar dome. The arthroscope is then directed horizontally along the posterior talar dome and beneath the posterior tibiofibular ligament complex. The more lateral aspect of the talar dome and the posterior talofibular articulation may be difficult to appreciate from the posterolateral portal, depending on the patient's anatomy and area of penetration of the posterior cannula beneath the syndesmotic ligaments. A complete inspection of the posterior recess completes the examination.

SUBTALAR JOINT ARTHROSCOPY

Practical applications of arthroscopic techniques to the subtalar joint have been facilitated by the development of small-diameter, high-quality optics. Initial efforts to visualize this small, highly constrained joint with standard 4-mm arthroscopes had little success. However, the joint can be approached reliably using the 2.7- or 1.9-mm arthroscopes for diagnostic arthroscopy, along with an expanding list of indicated procedures that are outlined in later chapters. Refinement of the technique for posterior ankle and subtalar joint arthroscopy has expanded our ability to visualize the subtalar joint.

As in the ankle joint, the subtalar joint presents a complex, curved articular surface that is even more tightly held in position by ligaments, especially the stout talocalcaneal interosseous ligament. Application of mechanical distraction adds little to our ability to separate the articular surfaces because of these ligaments, and the procedure usually is performed without the distractor.

Standard subtalar arthroscopy is performed with the patient positioned supine on the operating table with a bump placed beneath the hip to create a semilateral position. There are three basic lateral portals for subtalar joint instrumentation. Alternatively, a patient undergoing ankle and subtalar joint arthroscopy may remain in the supine position with the hip and knee flexed and supported by the leg holder, as described for standard ankle arthroscopy.

The anterolateral portal is placed approximately in the soft spot of the sinus tarsi, about 2 cm anterior and 1 cm distal to the tip of the fibula (Fig. 4-16). The posterolateral portal is placed approximately 2 cm posterior and 1 cm proximal to the tip of the fibula, which is lateral to the border of the Achilles tendon. If the subtalar arthroscopy is performed after ankle joint arthroscopy, the posterolateral portal used for the ankle can be redirected into the subtalar joint. The central portal is located just distal and inferior to the lateral malleolus tip. This portal is immediately anterior to the peroneal tendon sheath.

I find that arthroscopy of the subtalar joint is more reproducible if the portal locations are first confirmed using 18-gauge needles. A needle is introduced into the presumptive anterolateral portal. When correctly placed, this needle should pass easily in a posteromedial direction and is located just posterior to the talocalcaneal interosseous ligament. Another needle is placed into the posterolateral position, and saline is injected into one of the needles. Outflow of the saline through the other needle confirms appropriate position for the two portals.

The nick and spread technique is used to place 2.7-mm cannulas into the portals, and the arthroscope is introduced into the anterior portal to initiate diagnostic arthroscopy. The talocalcaneal interosseous ligament is identified by turning the viewing angle of the arthroscope to point in an anterior direction. After that ligament is identified, the arthroscope is turned to view posteriorly, and the joint line is followed into the lateral gutter. The central portal is then established under direct visualization by introducing an 18-gauge needle and confirming that the needle location affords optimal access to the joint surfaces.

The joint is examined from the anterior view while placing a probe into the central portal. The arthroscope is introduced posterior to the interosseous ligament and advanced as far medial as possible to visualize the deep portion of the ligament and medial articular surface of the posterior subtalar joint (Fig. 4-17). As the arthroscope is slowly withdrawn, the more superficial portion of the ligament and the anterolateral margin of the posterior subtalar joint are examined (Fig. 4-18). As the arthroscope is manipulated into the lateral gutter, rotating it for viewing and keeping the joint line visible as the corner is rounded, the lateral talocalcaneal ligament is the first ligament capsular condensation observed (Fig. 4-19). Proceeding slightly more posteriorly, the operator can see the location of the calcaneofibular ligament.

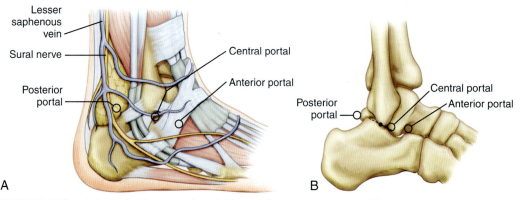

FIGURE 4-16 Sketch shows the placement of standard portals for subtalar arthroscopy. The anteromedial portal is approximately 1 cm distal and 2 cm anterior to the tip of the fibula in the palpable sinus tarsi. The posterolateral portal is located approximately 1 cm proximal and 2 cm proximal to the tip of the fibula. The central portal is placed just anterior to the tip of the fibula and just anterior to the peroneal tendon sheath.

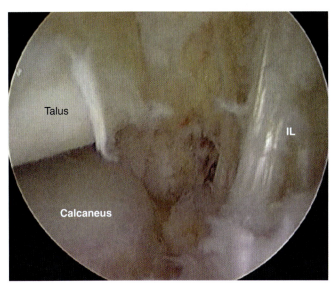

FIGURE 4-17 Arthroscopic view of right subtalar joint from anterolateral portal shows the talocalcaneal interosseus ligament (IL) on the right and the anterior portion of the posterior subtalar joint to the left.

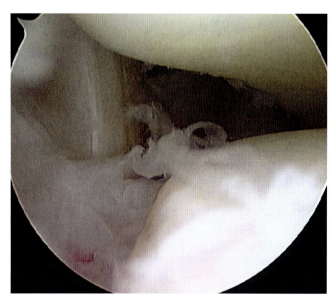

FIGURE 4-19 Arthroscopic view of the right subtalar joint from the anterolateral portal shows the lateral gutter with the lateral talocalcaneal ligaments on the left.

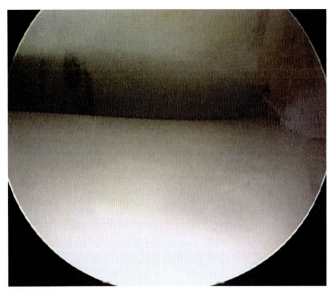

FIGURE 4-18 Arthroscopic view of the right subtalar joint from the anterolateral portal.

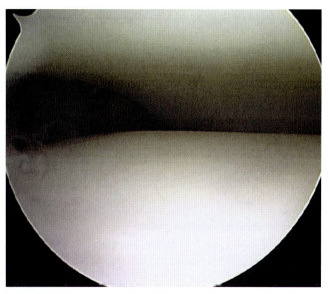

FIGURE 4-20 Arthroscopic view of the posterior extent of the right subtalar joint.

In some joints, the arthroscope can be advanced from the anterolateral portal further into the lateral gutter to the posterolateral recess (Fig. 4-20). As the viewing angle is turned toward the joint, the articular surface of the posterior process of the talus, or the os trigonum if present, can be seen. Turning the viewing angle toward the capsule laterally reveals the posterior talocalcaneal ligament.

If the arthroscope cannot be advanced into the posterolateral recess from the anterolateral portal, the arthroscope is switched to the posterior portal to achieve visualization of the structures previously described. In a relatively lax ankle, the arthroscope can be advanced across the joint, and the interosseous ligament can be examined from this posterior view. The examination should start in the lateral gutter. The arthroscope then is withdrawn carefully as the posterolateral corner is rounded and the central and the medial aspects of the posterior subtalar joint are examined. If feasible, the arthroscope is advanced into the posteromedial gutter and then anteriorly to visualize as much of the medial articular surface as possible.

PEARLS &PITFALLS

PEARLS
- Subtalar arthroscopy can be performed reliably without joint distraction in most cases and with 2.7- or 1.9-mm-diameter arthroscopes with 30- and 70-degree viewing angles
- Portal creation should be performed using the nick and spread technique to avoid injury to superficial neurovascular structures.

POSTERIOR ANKLE AND SUBTALAR ARTHROSCOPY

When the anticipated ankle or subtalar pathology is definitively localized to the posterior compartment, the joints may be assessed using a posterior approach. This approach was pioneered by van Dijk in the Netherlands. The procedure described subsequently is based on his report of posterior ankle arthroscopy.

The patient is placed prone on the operating table with the foot and ankle extended slightly past the end of the table and supported with a small bolster (Fig. 4-21). If distraction is necessary, a soft tissue distractor may be placed as for routine anterior arthroscopy and attached to the surgeon, who can apply traction when necessary by leaning backward. However, much posterior pathology can be approached without distraction, including os trigonum, posterior bony or soft tissue impingement, pathology of the flexor hallucis longus tendon, and posterior articular pathology of the talus or calcaneus.

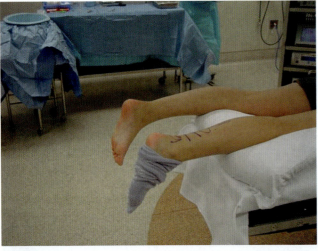

FIGURE 4-21 Patient placement position for prone posterior ankle and subtalar joint arthroscopy.

Portals are placed immediately adjacent to the medial and lateral borders of the Achilles tendon at approximately the level of the tip of the fibula (Fig. 4-22). The nick and spread technique is used to avoid injury to superficial neurovascular structures. The standard 4-mm arthroscope can be used for posterior ankle arthroscopy.

To visualize the posterior ankle joint, a space must be created in the area just posterior to the joint. Soft tissue (i.e., fatty tissue) must be débrided to create the space without causing injury to any other structures. The goal is to create a space and to visualize the flexor hallucis longus tendon. After the great toe flexor is visualized, safe dissection can be performed lateral to this tendon, avoiding injury to the posteromedial neurovascular structures that lie medial to the tendon. It is essential to use proper technique in the initial exposure.

The arthroscope cannula with a blunt trocar is introduced into the lateral portal and directed toward the great toe until bone is palpated. The arthroscope is introduced into this cannula. Inflow is placed under low-pressure and low-flow parameters, but there is no actual space in which to see; only the fat is visible immediately posterior to the joint. The 3.5-mm shaver is introduced from the medial portal at a perpendicular angle to the arthroscope, and it is advanced until it makes contact with the arthroscope's cannula. The shaver is then directed along the cannula until it reaches the level of the arthroscope's tip (Fig. 4-23). Initial shaving is performed with the open end of the shaver directed laterally and the viewing angle of the arthroscope directed medially. In this fashion, the blade is less likely to be directed toward the flexor hallucis longus tendon and the neurovascular structures medial to it. With minimal shaving, a space is created, and the flexor hallucis longus is identified.

After the tendon is identified, it is protected from the surgical instruments, and all dissection is directed lateral to the tendon (Fig. 4-24). A capsulectomy is performed, revealing the ankle joint above and the subtalar joint below. The posterior process of the talus, or the os trigonum if present, is identified along with the attachment of the posterior talofibular ligament (Fig. 4-25). A bipolar electrocautery device is useful to achieve hemostasis and to perform accurate dissection of soft tissue from bone. Pa-

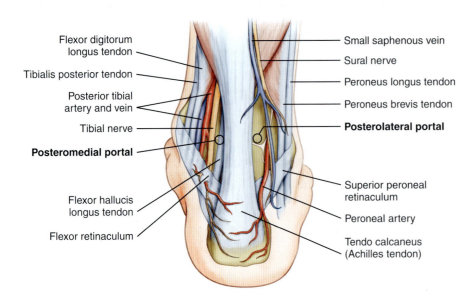

Flexor digitorum longus tendon

Tibialis posterior tendon

Posterior tibial artery and vein

Tibial nerve

Posteromedial portal

Flexor hallucis longus tendon

Flexor retinaculum

Small saphenous vein

Sural nerve

Peroneus longus tendon

Peroneus brevis tendon

Posterolateral portal

Superior peroneal retinaculum

Peroneal artery

Tendo calcaneus (Achilles tendon)

FIGURE 4-22 Sketch shows the placement of standard posteromedial and posterolateral portals for posterior ankle and subtalar joint arthroscopy. The portals are placed approximately at the level of the tip of the fibula.

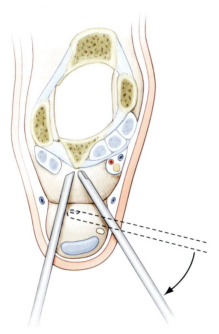

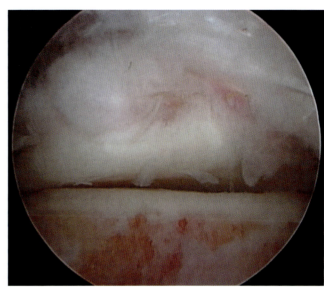

FIGURE 4-25 Posterior ankle arthroscopy shows the subtalar joint.

FIGURE 4-23 Sketch shows a cross-sectional view of the ankle, with the arthroscope in the posterolateral portal and the shaver in the posteromedial portal. The arthroscope cannula is placed in the direction of the first web space, and the shaver is directed perpendicular to the arthroscope cannula until it makes contact with it. The shaver is then guided along the shaft of the arthroscope cannula to the tip. A space is created by resecting posterior fat with the shaver blade pointed laterally and the arthroscope angled medially. Dissection proceeds laterally after identifying the flexor hallucis longus tendon medially.

thology in both joints can be addressed from this approach, and operative arthroscopy is described in Chapter ••.

PEARLS&PITFALLS

- Carefully create space for visualization using a shaver with the blade pointing laterally until the flexor hallucis longus tendon is identified and protected.
- Do not dissect in the soft tissues medial to the flexor hallucis longus tendon
- Avoid portal complications such as sinus formation by placing simple sutures to approximate skin edges at the conclusion of the case and by a period of postoperative immobilization in a splint of approximately 1 week.

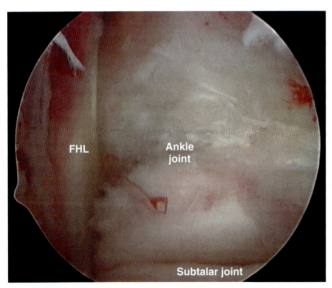

FIGURE 4-24 Posterior ankle arthroscopy of the right ankle shows the flexor hallucis longus tendon (FHL) on the left and the ankle and subtalar joints on the right.

CONCLUSIONS

Diagnostic arthroscopy of the ankle joint can be routinely performed using small joint arthroscopes with noninvasive distraction. Standard portals include anteromedial, anterolateral, and posterolateral portals. A systematic process using each of the portals affords complete visualization of the joint and approaches for instrumentation and surgical procedures.

The subtalar joint can be examined from a lateral approach using three standard portals or from the direct posterior approach. Only the posterior subtalar joint is visualized in standard subtalar arthroscopy.

The posterior ankle and subtalar joints can be viewed from the direct posterior approach using the technique of van Dijk. This approach is particularly useful for the treatment of posterior ankle impingement, os trigonum syndrome, posterior osteochondral defects of the ankle and subtalar joint, and pathology involving the flexor hallucis longus tendon.

REFERENCES

1. Burman MS. Arthroscopy or the direct visualization of joints: an experimental cadaver study. *J Bone Joint Surg Am.* 1931; 13:669-695.
2. Andrews JR, Previte WJ, Carson WG. Arthroscopy of the ankle: technique and normal anatomy. *Foot Ankle.* 1985; 6:29-33.
3. Parisien JS. Diagnostic and operative arthroscopy of the ankle: technique and indications. *Bull Hosp Jt Dis Orthop Inst.* 1985; 45:38-47.
4. Parisien JS, Vangsness T, Feldman R. Diagnostic and operative arthroscopy of the ankle. An experimental approach. *Clin Orthop Relat Res.* 1987; 224:228-236.
5. Stetson WB, Ferkel RD. Ankle arthroscopy. I. Technique and complications. *J Am Acad Orthop Surg.* 1996; 4:17-23.
6. Ferkel RD, Small HN, Gittins JE. Complications in foot and ankle arthroscopy. *Clin Orthop Rerlat Res.* 2001; 391:89-104.
7. Ferkel RD, Scranton PE. Current concepts review: arthroscopy of the ankle and foot. *J Bone Joint Surg Am.* 1993; 75:1233-1242.
8. Ferkel RD, Weiss RA. Correlative surgical anatomy. In: Ferkel RD, ed. *Arthroscopic Surgery. The Foot and Ankle.* Philadelphia, PA: Lippincott-Raven; 1996.85-102.
9. Golano P, Mariani PP, Rodrigues-Niedenfuhr M, et al. Arthroscopic anatomy of the posterior ankle ligaments. *Arthroscopy.* 2002; 18:353-358.
10. Van Dijk CN, Scholten PE, Krips R. A 2-portal endoscopic approach for diagnosis and treatment of posterior ankle pathology. *Arthroscopy.* 2000; 16:871-876.
11. Scholten PE, Sierevelt IN, van Dijk CN. Hindfoot endoscopy for posterior ankle impingement. *J Bone Joint Surg Am.* 2008; 90:2665-2672.
12. Van Dijk CN, van Bergen CJA. Advancements in ankle arthroscopy. *J Am Acad Orthop Surg.* 2008; 16:635-646.

SUGGESTED READINGS

Ferkel RD, ed. *Arthroscopic Surgery: The Foot and Ankle.* Philadelphia, PA: Lippincott-Raven; 1996.

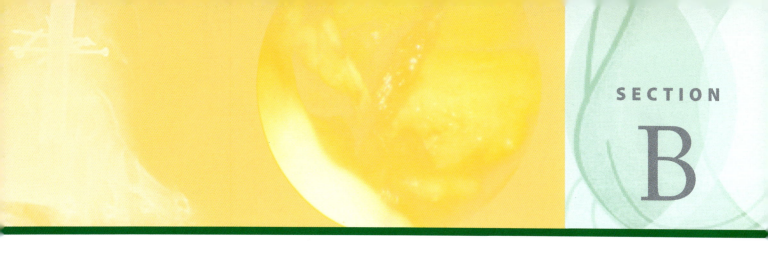

Techniques for the Foot and Ankle

Bony Impingement of the Ankle and Subtalar Joints

Tanawat Vaseenon ● Annunziato Amendola

Ankle sprains are one of the most common injuries seen in sports medicine, and most heal without persistent pain or chronic disability.[1,2] However, some patients with ankle sprains continue to have persistent pain and dysfunction.[2,3] Two common sources of chronic pain and disability—persistent ankle instability and impingement—may occur separately or concomitantly. Impingement, which is entrapment of an anatomic structure that leads to pain and decreased range of motion of the ankle, can be classified as soft tissue or osseous.[4]

Osseous or bony impingement most commonly results from spur formation along the anterior margin of the distal tibia and talus or from a prominent posterolateral talar process (i.e., os trigonum). Soft tissue impingement usually results from scarring and fibrosis associated with synovial, capsular, or ligamentous injury, and it most often occurs in the anterolateral gutter, medial ankle, or region of the syndesmosis.[5]

Of the first few ankle impingement syndromes reported in the English literature, all involved bone. They usually have occurred in athletes whose sports necessitated sudden acceleration, jumping, and extremes of dorsiflexion or plantar flexion. The so-called athlete's ankle was first mentioned in the orthopedic literature by Morris[6] and was subsequently reported by McMurray,[7] who called it footballer's ankle. McMurray stated that the footballer's ankle was peculiar to the professional soccer player, especially those older than 25 years who have played for many years. In later studies, this entity was described in many other athletic activities, including rugby players, football players, ballet dancers, jumpers, and runners, and it can occur in any sport.

BONY IMPINGEMENT

Etiology

Osteophytes are protrusions of bone and cartilage around the joint space. Osteophytic formations occur with weight-bearing articular cartilage damage, such as osteoarthritis of the hip and knee, and occur without weight-bearing articular cartilage damage, such as bony impingement lesions.[8]

Controversy exists about the cause of bony osteophytes around the ankle with normal articular cartilage. Adjacent or articulating bones that are repetitively in contact can stimulate the cambium layer, the deep layer of periosteum that has osteogenic potential, to form osteophytes. The osteophytic prominence causes bony impingement, often increases in size, and eventually may break off, forming a loose body. After the spur is formed, it may alter normal mechanics or motion of the ankle. Morris[6] and McMurray[7] described osseous exostoses of the anterior rim of the tibia and the sulcus of the talus, and they believed these to result from a traction injury of the joint capsule of the anterior aspect of the ankle that occurred when the foot was in extreme plantar flexion (i.e., capsule-ligament traction). However, the capsule of the ankle attaches above the location of the tibial osteophytes and distal to the talar ones. In later studies, anatomic observations during arthroscopic surgery confirmed that tibial osteophytes were located at the joint level and talar osteophytes were found proximal to the talar neck notch, away from the capsular attachment sites (Fig. 5-1); the osteophytes were intra-articular.[9,10] O'Donoghue[11] attributed these exostoses to direct osseous impingement during forced dorsiflexion or to post-traumatic calcification. Van Dijk and colleagues[12] attributed the osteophytes to medial impingement from inversion of the talus onto the medial tibia and thought they might be related to instability

(Fig. 5-2). The osteophytes were related to direct trauma associated with the impingement of the anterior articular border of the tibia in the talar neck during forced dorsiflexion of the ankle joint.

Classification

In 1992, Scranton and McDermott[8] classified four types of anterior ankle impingement by the radiographic appearance of bony spurs (Table 5-1). The classification system grades the degree of spur formation and assists in predicting the length of recovery time. Van Dijk's 1997 radiographic classification (Table 5-2) was based on osteoarthrosis of the ankle on plain radiographs (Fig. 5-3).[10] The degree of osteoarthritic change is a better prognostic indicator for the outcome of arthroscopic surgery for anterior ankle impingement than size and location of spurs.

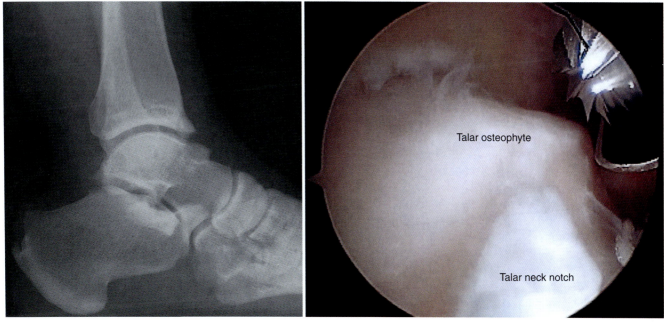

FIGURE 5-1 Talar osteophyte lies away from the capsular attachment.

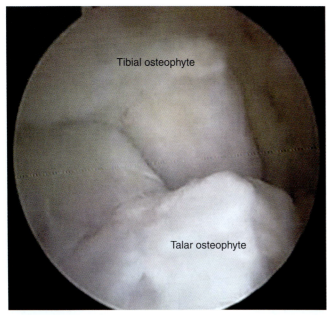

FIGURE 5-2 Anteromedial osteophytes of the tibia and the talus.

TABLE 5-1 Classification of Anterior Ankle Impingement

Type	Characteristics
I	Synovial impingement; radiographs show inflammatory reaction, up to 3-mm spur formation
II	Osteochondral reaction exostosis; radiographs show osseous spur formation greater than 3 mm; no talar spur is present
III	Significant exostosis with or without fragmentation, with secondary spur formation on the dorsum of the talus seen; often with fragmentation osteophytes
IV	Pantalocrural arthritic destruction; radiographs suggest medial, lateral, or posterior degenerative arthritic changes

From Scranton PE Jr, McDermott JE. Anterior tibiotalar spurs: a comparison of open versus arthroscopic débridement. Foot Ankle. *1992;13:125-139.*

TABLE 5-2 Classification of Osteoarthritic Changes of the Ankle Joint

Grade	Characteristics
0	Normal joint or subchondral sclerosis
I	Osteophytes without joint space narrowing
II	Joint space narrowing with or without osteophytes
III	Total disappearance or deformation of the joint space

From van Dijk CN, Tol JL, Verheyen CC. A prospective study of prognostic factors concerning the outcome of arthroscopic surgery for anterior ankle impingement. Am J Sports Med. 1997;25:737-745.

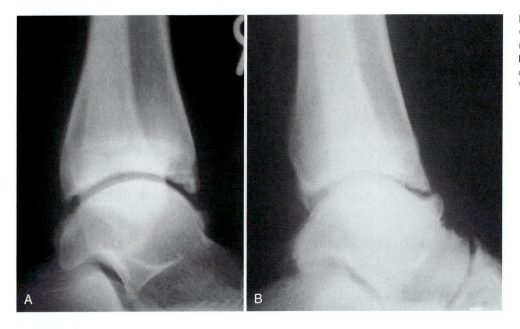

FIGURE 5-3 A, Osteophytes without joint space narrowing (Scranton type III, Van Dijk grade I). **B,** Joint space narrowing with osteophytes (Scranton type IV, Van Dijk grade II).

THE ANKLE JOINT

Anatomy

The talus articulates with the os calcis so that the axis of the talus is roughly in line with the first web space of the foot and the axis of the os calcis is in line with the fourth web space. In dorsiflexion, bony impingement occurs anteromedially between the neck of the talus and the anterior lip of the tibia. In plantar flexion, bony impingement occurs posterolaterally between the os calcis and the posterior lip of the tibia. The impingement can be found in all quadrants around the ankle: anterior, lateral, posterior, and medial. Bony impingement most often occurs anteromedially and posterolaterally, whereas soft tissue impingement occurs anterolaterally and posteromedially.

The Anterior Ankle

Anterior impingement syndrome of the ankle is the most common cause of anterior ankle pain in many sports participants. Repetitive forced dorsiflexion also can result in impaction-related microtrauma of the anterior chondral margin of the tibiotalar joint. Over time, attempted repair with resultant fibrosis and fibrocartilage proliferation leads to the formation of osteophytes.[7] When osteophytes form, they limit dorsiflexion, facilitate further impingement, and result in more periosteal stimulation, creating a repetitive cycle. Careful inspection of the pathologic anatomy shows that osteophytes do not form in the capsular insertion but instead where bones come together.[11] Osteophytes can break off and become loose bodies (Fig. 5-4).

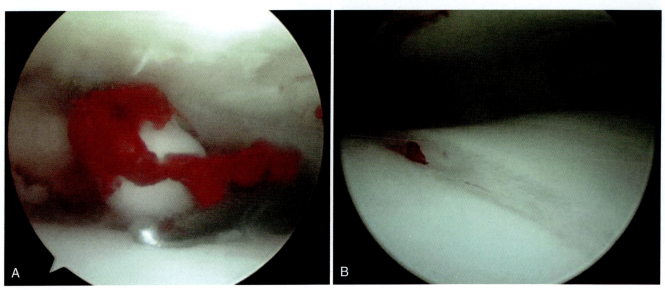

FIGURE 5-4 A, Loose body in a female basketball player with recurrent ankle sprains. **B,** Articular grooving from the loose body.

In supination injury, damage to the anterior non–weight-bearing cartilage rim occurs.[12] The cartilage proliferation, scar tissue formation, and calcification that may result from attempted repair depend on the degree of initial damage and on chondral and bone cell stimulation. Recurrent forced dorsiflexion of the ankle is the main factor in the development of spurs.[13,14] Another factor is recurrent microtrauma, and it has been demonstrated that spur formation is related to recurrent ball impacts in soccer players.[15] The entire process of spur formation and hypertrophied synovium or fibrosis is exacerbated by recurrent ankle sprains and persistent ankle instability. Synovial changes may result from chronic inflammation of the soft tissue (e.g., synovial fold, subsynovial fat, collagen tissue) that was crushed during forced dorsiflexion movements between spurs.[16]

The common history of patients with anterior ankle impingement is recurrent inversion sprain. The typical patient is a young athlete presenting with chronic anterior ankle pain.[17] Pain likely results from entrapment of hypertrophied synovial tissue between the talus and the anterior tibia, which is exacerbated by the presence of anterior spurs. Patient usually present with swelling after activity and with limited ankle dorsiflexion movement.

Physical examination reveals anterior tenderness and thickening of the synovium, often with an effusion, palpable osteophytes with the ankle in slight plantar flexion, limited dorsiflexion when compared with the opposite ankle, and a positive dorsiflexion impingement sign (i.e., pain with forced dorsiflexion of the ankle when the knee is flexed).

Standard lateral radiographs of the ankle usually show spurs. The weight-bearing lateral view with the ankle in maximal dorsiflexion (i.e., plié view) demonstrates anterior impingement, and this view commonly is used in evaluating dancers. Conventional magnetic resonance imaging (MRI) accurately detects and localizes anterior tibiotalar spurs, adjacent reactive synovitis and fibrosis, subchondral bone edema, and other coexisting lesions, such as collateral ligament complex injury, osteochondral lesions of the talus, or intra-articular bodies. There is little or no additional information gained through indirect magnetic resonance (MR) arthrography for evaluating anteromedial impingement compared with conventional MRI.[18]

Several conditions can mimic the anterior impingement syndrome, including osteochondritis dissecans of the talus, a "high" ankle sprain involving the anterior tibiofibular ligament,[19] impingement by Bassett's ligament,[1] an aberrant distal insertion of the anterior tibiofibular ligament that can cause persistent symptoms, Ferkel's disease,[16] an accumulation of debris and synovitis in the anterolateral gutter, degenerative joint disease of the tibiotalar or talonavicular joints (especially in the early phases when the radiographic findings are subtle), and a stress fracture or an osteoid osteoma in the tarsal navicular.

Conservative treatment with rest, physical therapy, shoe modification, or local injection constitutes first-line therapy for most cases of anterior ankle impingement. If all modalities of conservative treatment are unsuccessful, operative treatment may be indicated. The goal of surgery is removal the osteophytes to restore the anterior space and to reduce the chance of symptoms recurring. Numerous investigators have reported good results with open ar-

throtomy, but it can be complicated by cutaneous nerve entrapment, wound dehiscence, damage of the long extensor tendons, and formation of hypertrophic scar tissue.[7,11,17] In recent years, the arthroscopic treatment of anterior ankle impingement has had a high success rate. The first series reported by Biedert[3] had a success rate of approximately 67%. Ferkel and colleagues[16] reported a success rate of approximately 84% for 31 patients with soft tissue impingement of the ankle. Ogilvie-Harris and colleagues[20] described an average of 39 months' follow-up for patients who were treated for anterior ankle impingement by arthroscopic removal of bony spurs. The good and excellent results were obtained for 88% of 17 patients.[20] In a prospective study, Amendola and coworkers[21] treated 79 cases of ankle impingement by arthroscopic débridement. Fifteen cases of soft tissue impingement and 14 cases of anterior bony impingement were included in the study. There were statistically significant decreases in subjective analog scores. Eighty percent of the soft tissue impingement lesions and 86% of the bony impingement lesions benefited from the procedure. Eighteen percent of patients had neurologic complications, including partial deep peroneal nerve neurapraxia and superficial peroneal nerve irritation.[21]

Scranton and colleagues[8] reported the comparative open and arthroscopic treatment of ankle impingement. The recovery time of the arthroscopic treatment patients was approximately one half of the time of open treatment patients. The patients treated arthroscopically returned to full athletic training 1 month faster than the other group.[8]

Tol and associates[9] described the results for 5 to 8 years of follow-up for the arthroscopic treatment of anterior impingement in the ankle. Excellent or good results were obtained for 100% of patients without osteoarthritis, 77% of patients with grade I disease, and 53% of patients with grade II diseases according to the classification for osteoarthritis of the ankle (see Table 5-2).[22] Osteophytes recurred in two thirds of the ankles with grade I osteoarthritis, but the recurrence of osteophytes did not correlate statistically with the return of symptoms. Narrowing of the joint space increased in 47% of patients with grade II osteoarthritis.[9]

Anteromedial Ankle Impingement

Anteromedial ankle pain is caused by impingement of the anterior portion of the medial malleolus on a spur on the medial shoulder of the talus. Spurs often occur on both sides of the joint. They result from injury to the deltoid ligament complex, leading to scar formation and synovitis along the anteromedial joint line. Patients complain of pain along the anteromedial joint line that is aggravated by walking or sporting activities. Patients often report a clicking sensation and painful limited dorsiflexion of the ankle. On physical examination, the anteromedial aspect of the ankle appears swollen and is tender to palpation over the anterior tibiotalar fascicle of the deltoid ligament. The anteromedial spur often can be palpated on physical examination but usually cannot be visualized on standard anteroposterior and lateral radiographs of the ankle. In a cadaver study, Tol and colleagues[15] described medially located talar osteophytes and anteromedial tibial osteophytes that were up to 7.3 mm in diameter,

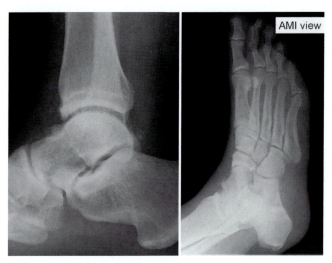

FIGURE 5-5 A special oblique anteromedial impingement view.

originated from the anteromedial border, and could remain undetected due to overprojection or superposition of the lateral part of the talar neck and body and the prominent anterolateral border of the distal tibia, respectively.[15]

These osteophytes are easy to miss (i.e., "hidden spurs"). A special oblique anteromedial impingement view (Fig. 5-5) has been developed to aid in the detection of anteromedial spurs, and it is obtained with the beam tilted in a 45-degree craniocaudal direction with the leg in 30 degrees of external rotation and the foot in plantar flexion in relation to the standard lateral radiograph position.[23] The sensitivity of lateral radiographs for detecting anterior tibial and talar osteophytes is 40% and 32%, and their specificity is 70% and 82%, respectively. The combination of lateral and oblique anteromedial impingement radiographs of the ankle increase the sensitivity to 85% for tibial osteophytes and 73% for talar osteophytes.[24]

Conventional MRI has not been useful in detecting anteromedial impingement syndrome. Robinson and associates[25] demonstrated that the cross-sectional MR arthrography could confirm anteromedial ankle impingement. Their findings included capsular and synovial soft tissue thickening anterior to the tibiotalar ligaments and associated osseous abnormalities such as anteromedial osteophytes.[25] The impingement is thought to be soft tissue entrapment associated with previous injury to the anterior tibiotalar fascicle of the deltoid ligament complex. A thickened anterior tibiotalar ligament can impinge on the anteromedial corner of the talus, often resulting in adjacent fibrosis or a meniscoid lesion and synovitis that may lead to adjacent spur formation.

Anterocentral Ankle Impingement

The anterocentral site is the classic location of anterior ankle impingement. There are four possible locations of spurs:

1. Some spurs occur primarily on the lip of the tibia. This type of spur is ideal for arthroscopic treatment. Under direct vision, the tibial lip can be removed easily with a burr, holding the ankle in maximal dorsiflexion or using an osteotome with blunt edges to prevent damage the dome of the talus, as described by Scranton and McDermott.[8]

2. Some spurs occur primarily on the neck of the talus. This type is more difficult to treat with the arthroscopy alone because osteophytes often are within the capsular insertion on the neck of the talus. Stripping off the capsule distally is necessary to visualize the pathology. Intraoperative imaging may be needed to ensure adequate removal.

3. Some spurs occur on the tip of the tibia and the neck of the talus. This type is common and is the most difficult to deal with. Mini-arthrotomy may be needed for treatment. Sometimes, loose bodies have broken off the osteophytes.

4. Multiple anterior osteophytes can occur with severe osteoarthritis of the ankle. Anterior débridement is of questionable effectiveness.

Anterolateral Ankle Impingement

Anterolateral ankle pain usually is not caused by bony impingement, because the tibia and talus do not come together in this location. Almost anterolateral ankle impingement is caused by soft tissues. The two common causes of impingement are Bassett's ligament and synovial impingement.

Bassett's Ligament. Bassett's ligament impingement is caused the distal fascicle of the anteroinferior tibiofibular ligament.[1] It is a thickened distal fascicle of the anteroinferior tibiofibular ligament (AITFL) that extends far distally on the lateral malleolus. Nikolopoulos and coworkers[26] considered this fascicle to be an independent accessory ligament. This anatomic structure represents a separate ligament rather than a distal component of the AITFL. A fibrofatty septum separated the AITFL from the accessory fascicle, similar to the one that covered the intermediate space between the interosseous and the anterior tibiofibular ligament.[26] The lateral shoulder of the talus impinges against the distal fascicle of the AITFL when the ankle is plantar flexed. Patients had a history an inversion sprain of the ankle followed by chronic pain in the anterior aspect of the ankle, but they had no gross ligamentous instability. The post-traumatic anterolateral hyperlaxity due to an injured ATFL resulted in anterior extrusion of the talar dome with dorsiflexion, which contacted the distal fascicle of the AITFL with more pressure and friction.[1]

On physical examination, patients had isolated point tenderness on the anterolateral aspect of the talar dome and in the AITFL, a popping sensation, and aggravation of pain with dorsiflexion and eversion, all of which suggest the diagnosis. Bassett's ligament impingement is difficult to clinically diagnose, but it can be assessed with the arthroscope when patients present without loss of stability of the ankle.

Conservative treatment is preferred for at least 6 months before operative intervention is considered. There are four indications for AITFL resection:

1. Contact between the AITFL and the talus is prominent at the beginning of plantar flexion and inversion of the ankle.
2. Increased contact between the talus and the ligament continues until maximum dorsiflexion with abrasion of the articular cartilage.
3. The fascicle is bent on the anterolateral edge of the talus with dorsiflexion and dorsiflexion-inversion.

4. A distally inserting fascicle is identified on the fibula, close to the origin of the ATFL on the fibula.[4]

Temporarily relieving distraction is advised when resecting the AITFL because the AITFL lesion may be missed during distraction.[26] Numerous surgeons have reported good to excellent results (89% to 100%)with arthroscopic resection.

Synovial Impingement. Synovial impingement is a chronic, painful condition in which an accumulation of scar tissue and synovitis are trapped in the anterolateral gutter of the ankle, usually after inversion injuries.[16] Wolin and associates[27] were the first to describe synovial hypertrophy in the anterolateral aspect of the ankle. They called this, perhaps misleadingly, a *meniscoid lesion*, and histologic examination demonstrated that it was hyalinized connective tissue. Ankle arthroscopists have since recognized that there is a spectrum of sites where impingement can occur and that the condition is characterized by a range of histologic findings. The meniscoid appearance is unusual and is a pathologic rather than an anatomic variant.

Symptoms of synovial impingement are similar to those of Bassett's ligament impingement. On physical examination, pain is elicited by thumb pressure over the anterolateral aspect of the plantar flexion position of the ankle, and the ankle impingement sign is positive. Pain also can be caused by continued thumb pressure over the lateral gutter of the ankle in plantar flexion and when the foot is moved from a plantar flexed position to a fully dorsiflexed position. Synovial impingement is amenable to arthroscopic débridement.

Imaging may be of value, but the condition is usually a diagnosis based on clinical findings. Radiographs demonstrate no specific abnormality associated with anterolateral soft tissue impingement but are useful in excluding coexisting osseous abnormalities, such as fracture, osteochondral lesion of the talus, or anterior tibial spur formation. Computed tomography (CT) arthrography may provide evidence of anterolateral impingement, including intra-articular oblique linear formation, nodular thickening of the capsule, or irregularity of the edges of the anterolateral groove of the ankle.[28] Conventional MRI of the ankle has a wide range of sensitivities (39% to 100%) and specificities (50% to 100%) with regard to establishing the diagnosis of anterolateral impingement.[29-31] Factors associated with increased sensitivity and specificity of conventional MRI for confirming anterolateral impingement include the presence of a joint effusion and the experience level of the radiologist.[31,32] The diagnosis can be suggested by MRI when fluid in the lateral gutter outlines an abnormal soft tissue structure separate from the anterior talofibular ligament.[31] MR arthrography is highly accurate in the assessment of anterolateral impingement, with a sensitivity of 96%, specificity of 100%, and accuracy of 100% when clinical signs of anterolateral impingement are present.[33]

DeBerardino and coworkers[34] reported a 96% rate of good or excellent results for arthroscopic treatment of soft tissue impingement of the ankle in athletes after an average follow-up of 27 months. Kim SH and colleagues[35] reported good or excellent results (94% to 96%) with arthroscopic débridement for impingement of the anterolateral soft tissues of the ankle.

The Lateral Ankle

The lateral ankle can be a complex site of pain and discomfort, and an accurate diagnosis can be difficult. Symptoms often begin after ankle sprains.

The "meniscoid" of the ankle is the soft tissue trapped between the lateral shoulder of the talus and the lateral malleolus. McCarroll and associates[36] described this lesion in four soccer players who had a history of frequent ankle sprains, and after failing conservative treatment, they underwent arthroscopic débridement of the lesion. After appropriate rehabilitation, all four returned to competition with cessation of the symptoms; only one player rarely had pain.

Fracture of the lateral process of the talus[37] causes impingement beneath the lateral malleolus. *Snow-boarder's fracture* is a synonym for this fracture because of the increased incidence in this patient population. The fracture is often misdiagnosed as an ankle sprain, and routine plain radiographs often are read as normal. CT is the investigation of choice. Treatment is surgical excision or open reduction and internal fixation.[38]

The os subfibulare is an accessory ossicle that may be asymptomatic. It can be loosened by injury and become symptomatic.

An avulsion fracture of the tip of fibula can remain mobile or become trapped in or under the lateral ankle joint and become symptomatic. It also can occur in the insertion of the calcaneofibular ligament. Treatment depends on the size of the avulsion fragment. If it is small, it should be excised, and the stump of the ligament should be sutured into the tip of the lateral malleolus.

The pain of chronic, healed os calcis fractures may be difficult to differentiate from subtalar joint impingement pain. A small injection of local anesthetic beneath the tip of the lateral malleolus can help to differentiate impingement from an os calcis fracture.

The Medial Ankle

Medial ankle pain usually is not caused by bony impingement. Medial ankle sprains are rare because the medial structures are strong and rigid compared with lateral sprains, but after medial ankle instability occurs, medial osteophytes may cause bony medial impingement (Fig. 5-6). The medial ankle pain common in athletes typically is caused by posterior tibial tendonitis. Flexor hallucis longus (FHL) tendonitis often is found in dancers (i.e., dancer's tendonitis), and it causes posteromedial pain. In dancers, the most common cause of pain around the medial malleolus comes from "rolling in" (i.e., pronating) to obtain proper turnout. This is one of many overuse syndromes causing chronic strain on the deltoid ligament. The lesion results from the chronic strain on the deep posterior fibers of the deltoid ligament complex between the medial talus and the medial malleolus. Injury leads to the formation of scar tissue and fibrosis located along the posteromedial joint line that becomes entrapped between the posterior talus and medial malleolus, resulting in persistent medial ankle pain. This lesion may be isolated, but it most often coexists with symptoms of anterolateral ankle pain and instability. If the lesion remains unrecognized and untreated, medial ankle impingement may result in persistent pain after lateral ankle reconstruction.[39,40]

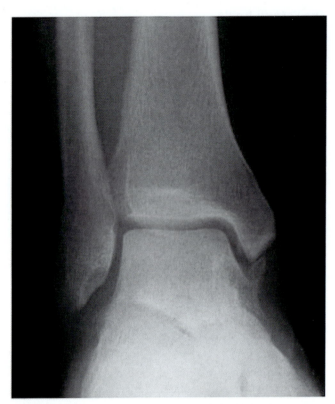

FIGURE 5-6 Osteophytes are causing medial ankle impingement.

The Posterior Ankle

Posterior ankle impingement, or talar compression syndrome,[13] is natural result of full weight bearing in maximal plantar flexion of the ankle in full pointe position. It is also referred to as os trigonum syndrome, posterior triangle pain, and posterior tibiofibular impingement. Posterior ankle pain is common in athletes, dancers, gymnasts, swimmers, divers, figure skaters, and soccer players who require repetitive and extreme plantar flexion.

The key structures involved in posterior ankle impingement syndrome can be divided into osseous and soft tissue components. The osseous components include the posterior tibia and talus and the superior calcaneum. Posterior talar anatomy variations are the principal predisposing osseous factors in posterior ankle impingement syndrome. The posterior aspect of the talus has two tubercles: the medial tubercle and lateral tubercle. The lateral tubercle is the origin of the posterior tibiofibular ligament. If it is large, it is referred to as the posterior process of the talus, or Stieda's process. The os trigonum is the ununited lateral tubercle on the posterior aspect of the talus. It is present in 7% to 14% of people, and it is often bilateral.[41,42] The os trigonum is the second most common accessory bone in the foot; the accessory navicular is the most common.

The key soft tissue structures involved in posterior ankle impingement syndrome include the FHL tendon, the posterior ankle ligaments, and the joint capsule and synovium. The FHL tendon forms a groove on the posterior tibial plafond before passing between the medial and lateral tubercles. This groove is converted into a fibro-osseous tunnel by condensations of fibrous connective tissue between two tubercles. The FHL tendon runs from its origin on the fibula laterally to its insertion in the distal phalanx of the hallux medially. The posterior talofibular ligament (PTFL) passes horizontally from the posteroinferior tip of the fibular malleolus to the lateral tubercle of the posterior process of the talus. The tibial slip connects the PTFL to the medial malleolus and is located just inferior to the intermalleolar (transverse tibiofibular) ligament, which runs from the medial posterior tibial plafond to the posteroinferior tip of the fibular malleolus. If the intermalleolar ligament is thickened, it may be caused by posterior ankle impingement syndrome.

Pain may result from osseous structures of the posterior ankle impacting one another or from compression of the soft tissue between the two opposing osseous structures. FHL tendon irritation is often caused by the adjacent impingement. Pain also can result from acute trauma to the posterolateral talar process or as a result of chronic repetitive microtrauma, causing direct injury to Stieda's process or the os trigonum.[43]

Clinical diagnosis of posterior impingement can be difficult compared with anterior impingement. It is much less common, and the affected structures of the posterior ankle are much deeper, with numerous overlying soft tissue support structures that may be the source of posterior ankle pain, such as the Achilles tendon, FHL tendon, tarsal tunnel, and retrocalcaneal bursa. A lateral radiograph of the ankle may demonstrate a prominent Stieda process or os trigonum, but radiographs usually are unremarkable in patients who have posterior ankle impingement. An underexposed 25-degree lateral rotation radiograph usually reveals more calcified deposits than does the conventional view.

Conventional MRI is the most beneficial investigation for suspected posterior ankle impingement because of various types of ankle impingement. MRI can delineate the anatomic site of the abnormality accurately and demonstrate evidence of posterior ankle impingement and coexisting pathology. The MRI features can be divided into osseous and soft tissue abnormalities. Positive MRI findings include edema within or surrounding the os trigonum or posterolateral tubercle of the talus, FHL tenosynovitis, posterior capsular synovitis, and thickening or tears of the PTFL, posteroinferior tibiofibular ligament, and intermalleolar ligament. Hindfoot CT scans are extremely useful and are superior to MRI for demonstrating the lesion's location and size in osteochondral ankle pathology. The differential diagnoses of posterior ankle impingement are talar or calcaneal stress fractures and osteochondral injuries.

Most patients with posterior ankle impingement respond to conservative treatment, such as rest, shoe modification, and physical therapy. Image-guided steroid and local anesthetic injection into areas of focal inflammation provides diagnostic confirmation and long-lasting symptomatic relief in most patients, and this approach avoids the need for surgery.[44]

Posterolateral Ankle Impingement

Posterolateral ankle impingement manifests as posterolateral pain in the back of the ankle when the posterior lip of the tibia closes against the superior border of the os calcis. Posterolateral ankle impingement is the natural result of full weight bearing in maximal plantar flexion of the ankle in the demi-pointe or full pointe position (Fig. 5-7).

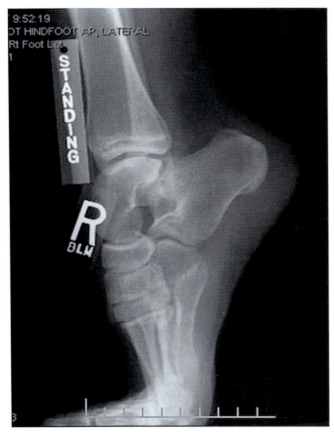

FIGURE 5-7 The demi-pointe position of the ankle is causing posterior ankle pain.

Posterolateral ankle impingement is often associated with an os trigonum or trigonal process in the back of the ankle. It is rare in most athletes. Chronic repetitive microtrauma can lead to inflammation of the os trigonum. Sometimes, acute trauma in plantar flexion may result in a contusion, compression, or fracture of the posterior process of the talus. People who have an os trigonum may or may not be symptomatic, and the degree of symptoms is not always related to its size. Occasionally, symptoms can be caused by soft tissue entrapment between the posterior lip of the talus and the os calcis. Entrapment manifests as posterior lateral pain of the ankle when the posterior lip of the tibia closes against the superior border of the os calcis. It can be confirmed on physical examination by tenderness behind the peroneal tendons in the back of the lateral malleolus (often mistaken for peroneal tendinitis) and pain with forced passive hyperplantar flexion of the ankle (i.e., plantar flexion sign), causing the posterior talar process or the os trigonum to be compressed between the posterior rim of the tibia and the calcaneus. The examiner can apply a rotational movement on the point of maximal plantar flexion, thereby "grinding" the posterior talar process or os trigonum between tibia and calcaneus. A negative test result can rule out a posterior ankle impingement. A positive test result in combination with pain on posterolateral palpation indicates posterior ankle impingement.

Posterior ankle impingement is seen best on a lateral view of the ankle en pointe or in full plantar flexion. The MRI findings include bone marrow edema located within the posterior talus or within the posterolateral talar process or os trigonum, a prominent posterior calcaneal process, and the posterior tibia a with downward sloping signal. Common soft tissue abnormalities include posterior capsule thickening, a fluid-distended posterior joint space, increased T2-weighted signal, or postcontrast enhancement along the posterior margin of the ankle that indicates synovitis and FHL tenosynovitis.[45-47]

The combined presence of bone marrow edema and posterior ankle synovitis may suggest the diagnosis of posterolateral ankle impingement (Fig. 5-8). The diagnosis can be confirmed by injection of 0.5 mL of a local anesthetic into the posterior soft tissue behind the peroneal tendon. If the pain is relieved by this small injection, the diagnosis is almost certain. The most common cause of posterolateral ankle pain is os trigonum syndrome. The differential diagnosis includes acute ankle injury causes, such as PTFL avulsion, fracture of the trigonal process (i.e., Shepherd's fracture), and acute disruption of the os trigonum

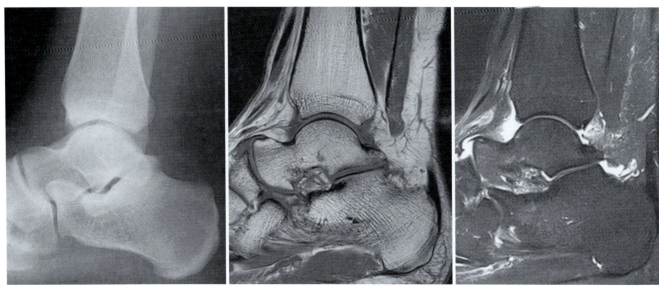

FIGURE 5-8 Magnetic resonance imaging shows bone marrow edema and posterior ankle synovitis.

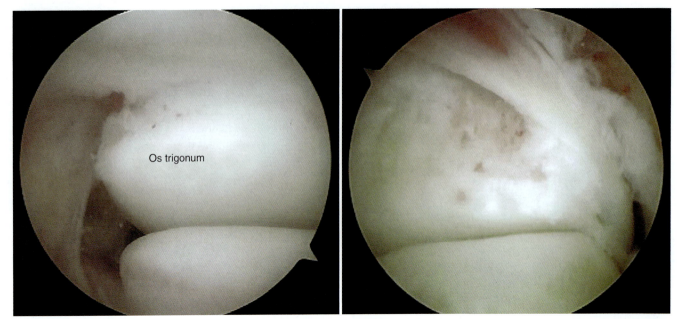

FIGURE 5-9 The os trigonum is causing posterior ankle impingement.

synchondrosis, and chronic injury causes, such as posterior capsule and adjacent soft tissue thickening, peroneal tendonitis, loose avulsion fragments of the posterolateral ankle ligament, and loose bodies. The talus is relatively plantar flexed and adducted, which causes further stress on the trigonal process by means of tension in the posterior talocalcaneal ligament in the pes planus foot. In cavus foot, the talus is supinated, moving the posterior surface medially and inferiorly and causing stress on the trigonal process by means of a tense PTFL.

Best and colleagues[48] reported anomalous muscles caused posterolateral impingement. The peroneus quartus, which originated on the fibula separate from the peroneal muscles, extended distal to the level of the ankle joint and inserted onto the peroneal tubercle of the calcaneus. The peroneocalcaneus internus muscles arose from the posterolateral aspect of the FHL muscle, coursing along the lateral margin of the FHL tendon within the tendon sheath and inserting onto the distal aspect of the medial margin of the sustentaculum tali.[48]

Treatment should follow an orderly sequence. The first step, similar to the treatment for tendonitis, is activity modification (i.e., following the injunction to first do no harm), avoidance of an equinus position, physical therapy (not to force the foot into equinus to achieve further plantar flexion), and nonsteroidal anti-inflammatory drugs (NSAIDs). Symptoms usually subside without further intervention. If this approach fails or the symptoms recur, an injection of 0.25 to 0.5 mL of a mixture of a long-acting and a short-acting corticosteroid often can give dramatic and permanent relief of symptoms.

When local anesthesia does not relieve symptoms, the lesion should be treated by surgical excision. It should be stressed that the presence of an os trigonum usually is not a surgical problem; most athletes with os trigonum do not need to have them removed surgically. Surgical excision is indicated only after failure of conservative treatment. Abramowitz and colleagues[49] reported the outcomes for resection of a symptomatic os trigonum with an

open posterolateral approach. The postoperative American Orthopaedic Foot and Ankle Society (AOFAS) score averaged 87.6 points. Complications included a 19% rate of sural nerve sensory loss, which was temporary in four and permanent in four patients; a 2% rate of the superficial wound infection; and a 2% rate of reflex sympathetic dystrophy.[49] The two posterior portal techniques provide excellent visualization of the posterior ankle structures, and the views obtained are superior to those in open procedures. The os trigonum may be separated and removed from the posterior talar process. Loose bodies and fragments of bone may be removed easily. The FHL tendon sheath may be released (Fig. 5-9).[50]

Posteromedial Ankle Impingement

Bony impingement does not commonly occur at the posteromedial aspect of the ankle because the tibia and talus do not come together in this location. Most posteromedial ankle impingement is caused by soft tissues. The key soft tissue structures are the posteromedial flexor tendons, joint capsule, and posterior fibers of the tibiotalar ligament (PTTL). The osseous structures affecting posteromedial ankle impingement include the posteromedial talar process, the posterior aspect of the medial malleolus, and an isolated accessory ossicle.

Tendonitis of the FHL tendon behind the medial malleolus of the ankle is common in dancers (i.e., dancer's tendonitis), but it also occurs in sports participants. It is often misdiagnosed as posterior tibial or Achilles tendonitis. The FHL passes through a fibro-osseous tunnel behind the talus between the medial and lateral tubercles to the level of the sustentaculum tali like a rope through a pulley. As it passes through this pulley, it is easily strained. The positions of en pointe and demi-pointe in ballet require the FHL tendon to function through an extreme range of motion while passing through its fibro-osseous tunnel.[13]

Frequent, prolonged repetitive motion of dance movements can lead to irritation and swelling of the FHL tendon. Chronic

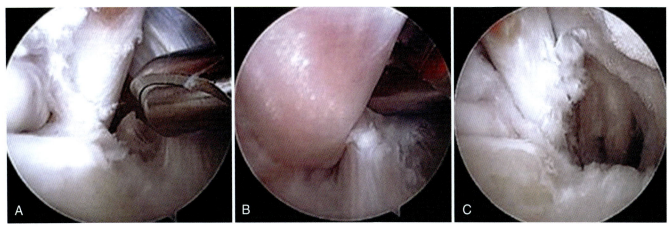

FIGURE 5-10 Tendonitis of the flexor hallucis longus tendon in a young girl. Excursion often causes impingement of the muscle belly within the fibro-osseous tunnel. **A,** Before release. **B,** Metatarsophalangeal joint dorsiflexion. **C,** After release.

inflammation and hypertrophy of the musculotendinous unit within this tunnel can lead to painful stenosing tenosynovitis, analogous to de Quervain disease in the wrist. If a nodule or partial tear is present, triggering of the big toe may occur. This condition is known as *hallux saltans*. In severe case, the tendon may become completely frozen in the sheath, causing pseudohallux rigidus.

Physical examination findings include localized tenderness and swelling over the FHL sheath behind and lateral to the medial malleolus. Palpation of the sheath during active and passive motion of the hallux elicits the patient's symptoms. Dorsiflexion of the first metatarsophalangeal joint can be reduced or absent when the ankle is in maximum dorsiflexion and the muscle fibers of the FHL are drawn into the FHL tunnel, producing a functional hallux rigidus (i.e., Thomasen's sign) (Fig. 5-10). This finding is not always pathologic, and it may be present in asymptomatic patients. Usually, there is no pain with forced plantar flexion of the ankle. The differential diagnoses of posteromedial ankle pain are FHL tendonitis, soleus syndrome, posterior tibial tendonitis, and posteromedial fibrous tarsal coalition (Table 5-3). The muscles that adhere to the neurovascular bundles behind the medial malleolus arise from the gastrocnemius-soleus complex and insert onto the quadrates plantae muscle.[48]

Nonoperative treatment is typically useful for posteromedial ankle impingement. Rest and modified activities (e.g., no pointe work) are important components of therapy to break the chronic cycle of repetitive trauma, and NSAIDs can help. Steroid injections into the sheath of the tendon may be done infrequently but usually should be avoided. Injection of an anesthetic to confirm the diagnosis is easy to perform but is usually not needed. Operative release of the fibro-osseous tunnel is indicated when conservative treatment has failed.

The insidious onset of posteromedial ankle pain 4 to 6 weeks after a supination injury and tenderness in the posteromedial ankle in forced plantar flexion and inversion are diagnostic of posteromedial ankle impingement. The MRI findings include posteromedial capsular thickening, loss of striation of the PTTL, and posteromedial synovitis (Fig. 5-11).[51] Injection of a steroid and long-acting anesthetic along with dry needling of the capsular abnormality allows most patients return to activity rapidly. Surgical resection of capsular thickening is successful in resistant cases.[52]

Posterior ankle impingement can be treated by open or arthroscopic techniques. The open technique has a success rate of 73% to 90% and mean time to return to sporting activities or dancing of 3 to 6 months, but it has a complication rate of 12% to 24%.[49,53] Arthroscopic treatment improves the success rate (good or excellent results for 80% of cases) and has a shortened recovery time (return to sport activities at 9 weeks) and a decreased complication rate (1% to 9%).[54,55] The overall results for bony impingement appear to be better than those for soft tissue impingement.

Van Dijk and associates[56] described the two-portal posterior endoscopic approach to the hindfoot with the patient in the prone position. It offered excellent access to the posterior compartment of the ankle joint, the posterior subtalar joint, the FHL tendon, and the os trigonum. It caused less morbidity and facilitated a quick recovery.[56] Lijoi and coworkers[57] verified the safety of a posteromedial portal in the arthroscopic treatment of the hindfoot.[57] Phisitkul and colleagues[58] showed the potential to increase the arthroscopic working area in the posterior subtalar joint. Horibe and associates[59] described the posterolateral portal for arthroscopic visualization and the accessory posterolateral

TABLE 5-3 Differentiating Posterior Impingement Syndrome from Flexor Hallucis Longus Tendonitis

Posterior Impingement Syndrome	Flexor Hallucis Longus Tendonitis
Posterior lateral	Posterior medial
Tenderness behind fibula	Tenderness over flexor hallucis longus tendon
Pain with plantar flexion of the ankle	Pain or triggering with motion of the hallux
Positive plantar flexion sign	Positive Thomasen's sign
Mistaken for peroneal tendonitis	Mistaken for posterior tibial tendonitis

From Hamilton WG, Chao W. Posterior ankle pain in athletes and dancers. Foot Ankle Clin. *1999;4:811-832.*

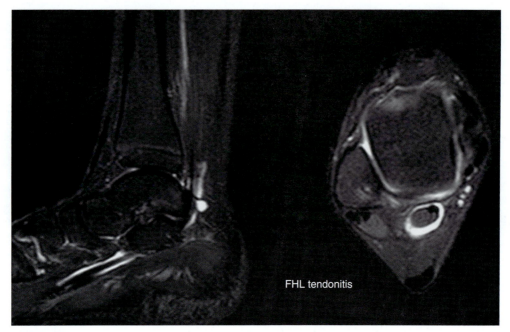

FIGURE 5-11 Magnetic resonance imaging shows posteromedial synovitis and flexor hallucis longus tendonitis.

portal for insertion of instruments to excise a symptomatic os trigonum without any complications. Willits and coworkers reported the short-term clinical outcome for posterior ankle arthroscopy in the treatment of posterior ankle impingement. The excellent or good results were obtained for 93% of patients. The mean score on the AOFAS Ankle and Hindfoot Scale was 91, and the score on the AOFAS Lower Extremity Functional Scale was 75. Complications included temporary numbness in the region of the scar and temporary ankle stiffness.[50]

THE SUBTALAR JOINT

Sinus Tarsi Syndrome

Sinus tarsi syndrome (STS) was first described by Denis O'Connor. STS is a rare condition characterized by pain in the sinus tarsi that usually occurs after a sprain.[60] STS has been associated with previous trauma, most commonly inversion ankle sprains.[61] Clinically, it manifests as pain or tenderness over the sinus tarsi laterally. The diagnosis is confirmed by complete relief of pain by injection of a local anesthetic in the sinus tarsi. Subtalar pain often is present, and some investigators have confirmed a high incidence of STS on imaging studies.[62]

Several theories have been proposed to explain the cause of STS, including interosseous talocalcaneal ligament scarring or injury, synovial inflammation with impingement, and sensory nerve traction injury, but the true cause is not clear. Different diagnostic techniques have been proposed for the evaluation of STS, including arthrography, MRI, and local injection of anesthetic.[63,64] However, the anatomy of the sinus tarsi, inconsistent inflammatory tissue and fibrosis, and chronicity of the problem make the diagnosis difficult.

Arthroscopy of the subtalar joint and sinus tarsi has provided another method of evaluation and treatment of this difficult problem. Investigators have described the results of arthroscopic

débridement of the sinus tarsi for chronic pain in this area. Frey and colleagues[65] reviewed subtalar arthroscopies, and of the 14 feet that had a preoperative diagnosis of STS, all the diagnoses were changed at the time of arthroscopy. The postoperative diagnoses included 10 cases of interosseous ligament tears, 2 cases of arthrofibrosis, and 2 cases of degenerative joints. The investigators thought that STS was an inaccurate term that should be replaced with a specific diagnosis.[65]

Lee and coworkers[66] reported a rate of 88% for good or excellent results with arthroscopic treatment for STS. The mean score on the AOFAS Ankle and Hindfoot Scale improved from 43 preoperatively to 86 points postoperatively.[66]

Lateral Bony Impingement of the Subtalar Joint

The accessory anterolateral facet was first described in a study of the astragalus by Sewell.[67] The accessory anterolateral facet is associated with painful talocalcaneal impingement in cases of flatfoot deformity. The accessory anterolateral talar facet causes lateral bony impingement of the subtalar joint, as reported by Martus and colleagues.[68] Sarrafian reported that a large accessory talar facet was found in 4% of 100 tali specimens. An accessory anterolateral talar facet was present in 34% of the specimens in a pediatric bone study.[68] It was associated with male sex, a smaller angle of Gissane, and dorsal talar beaking. When subtalar eversion is removed, narrowing of the sinus tarsi is accentuated by the presence of a large accessory facet.[68] Malicky and associates[69] described CT imaging performed with the foot positioned in frames that simulated weight bearing in 19 patients with lateral talocalcaneal impingement. Impingement occurred between the lateral talar process and the calcaneal neck (Fig. 5-12).

Injection of an anesthetic to confirm the diagnosis is useful and easily performed. Arthroscopic resection is indicated when conservative treatment has failed (Fig. 5-13).

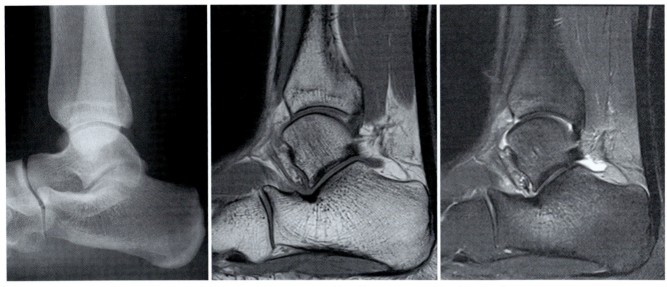

FIGURE 5-12 The accessory facet is causing lateral bony impingement of the subtalar joint.

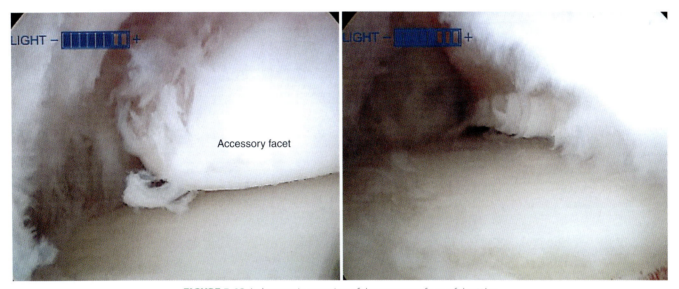

FIGURE 5-13 Arthroscopic resection of the accessory facet of the talus.

PEARLS & PITFALLS

PEARLS

1. A history of recurrent inversion sprain and chronic anterior ankle pain and a positive dorsiflexion impingement sign are keys to the diagnosis of anterior ankle impingement syndrome.
2. The oblique anteromedial impingement view can detect an anteromedial spur, which often cannot be visualized on standard anteroposterior and lateral radiographs of the ankle.
3. MR arthrography and injection of an anesthetic are highly accurate in the assessment of ankle impingement.
4. The key to achieving adequate bony and soft tissue decompression is repeated range-of-motion examination during arthroscopic visualization.
5. Decompression of impingement lesions in patients without evidence of joint osteoarthritis produces good results.

PITFALLS

1. Treatment of ankle impingement associated with ankle osteoarthritis may yield unpredictable results.
2. In the diagnosis of FHL impingement, tendon sheath injection usually is diagnostic, but fluoroscopy or ultrasound should be used to ensure accurate placement of the needle.
3. Injury to the superficial peroneal nerve and sural nerve from portal placement is the most common complication of ankle arthroscopy. Knowledge of the anatomy and blunt dissection are essential in preventing injury.
4. The posteromedial portal may be used in treating posterior impingement lesions, but care must be taken to avoid the posteromedial neurovascular bundle by always visualizing the FHL tendon.

REFERENCES

1. Bassett FH 3rd, Gates HS 3rd, Billys JB, et al. Talar impingement by the anteroinferior tibiofibular ligament. A cause of chronic pain in the ankle after inversion sprain. *J Bone Joint Surg Am*. 1990; 72:55-59.

2. Ogilvie-Harris DJ, Gilbart MK, Chorney K. Chronic pain following ankle sprains in athletes: the role of arthroscopic surgery. *Arthroscopy*. 1997; 13:564-574.

3. Biedert R. Anterior ankle pain in sports medicine: aetiology and indications for arthroscopy. *Arch Orthop Trauma Surg*. 1991; 110:293-297.

4. van den Bekerom MP, Raven EE. The distal fascicle of the anterior inferior tibiofibular ligament as a cause of tibiotalar impingement syndrome: a current concepts review. *Knee Surg Sports Traumatol Arthrosc*. 2007; 15:465-71.

5. Watson AD. Ankle instability and impingement. *Foot Ankle Clin*. 2007; 12:177-195.

6. Morris LH. Athlete's ankle. *J Bone Joint Surg Am*. 1943; 25:220.

7. McMurray TP. Footballer's ankle. *J Bone Joint Surg Br*. 1950;32B:68-69.

8. Scranton PE Jr, McDermott JE. Anterior tibiotalar spurs: a comparison of open versus arthroscopic débridement. *Foot Ankle*. 1992; 13:125-129.

9. Tol JL, Verheyen CP, van Dijk CN. Arthroscopic treatment of anterior impingement in the ankle. *J Bone Joint Surg Br*. 2001; 83:9-13.

10. van Dijk CN, Tol JL, Verheyen CC. A prospective study of prognostic factors concerning the outcome of arthroscopic surgery for anterior ankle impingement. *Am J Sports Med*. 1997; 25:737-745.

11. O'Donoghue DH. Impingement exostoses of the talus and tibia. *J Bone Joint Surg Am*. 1957;39A:835-852; discussion, 852.

12. van Dijk CN, Bossuyt PM, Marti RK. Medial ankle pain after lateral ligament rupture. *J Bone Joint Surg Br*. 1996; 78:562-567.

13. Hamilton WG. Foot and ankle injuries in dancers. *Clin Sports Med*. 1988; 7:143-173.

14. Parkes JC 2nd, Hamilton WG, Patterson AH, Rawles JG Jr. The anterior impingement syndrome of the ankle. *J Trauma*. 1980; 20:895-898.

15. Tol JL, Slim E, van Soest AJ, van Dijk CN. The relationship of the kicking action in soccer and anterior ankle impingement syndrome. A biomechanical analysis. *Am J Sports Med*. 2002; 30:45-50.

16. Ferkel RD, Karzel RP, Del Pizzo W, et al. Arthroscopic treatment of anterolateral impingement of the ankle. *Am J Sports Med*. 1991; 19: 440-446.

17. Cutsuries AM, Saltrick Kr, Wagner J, Catanzarti AR. Arthroscopic arthroplasty of the ankle joint. *Clin Podiatr Med Surg*. 1994; 11:449-467.

18. Haller J, Bernt R, Seeger T, et al. MR-imaging of anterior tibiotalar impingement syndrome: agreement, sensitivity and specificity of MR-imaging and indirect MR-arthrography. *Eur J Radiol*. 2006; 58:450-460.

19. Hamilton WG. Sprained ankles in ballet dancers. *Foot Ankle*. 1982; 3:99-102.

20. Ogilvie-Harris DJ, Mahomed N, Demaziere A. Anterior impingement of the ankle treated by arthroscopic removal of bony spurs. *J Bone Joint Surg Br*. 1993; 75:437-440.

21. Amendola A, Petrik J, Webster-Bogaert S. Ankle arthroscopy: outcome in 79 consecutive patients. *Arthroscopy*. 1996; 12:565-573.

22. van Dijk CN, Verhagen RA, Tol JL. Arthroscopy for problems after ankle fracture. *J Bone Joint Surg Br*. 1997; 79:280-284.

23. van Dijk CN, Wessel RN, Tol JL, Maas M. Oblique radiograph for the detection of bone spurs in anterior ankle impingement. *Skeletal Radiol*. 2002; 31:214-221.

24. Tol JL, Verhagen RA, Krips R, et al. The anterior ankle impingement syndrome: diagnostic value of oblique radiographs. *Foot Ankle Int*. 2004; 25:63-68.

25. Robinson P, White LM, Salonen D, Ogilvie-Harris D. Anteromedial impingement of the ankle: using MR arthrography to assess the anteromedial recess. *AJR Am J Roentgenol*. 2002; 178:601-604.

26. Nikolopoulos CE, Tsirikos AI, Sourmelis S, Papachristou G. The accessory anteroinferior tibiofibular ligament as a cause of talar impingement: a cadaveric study. *Am J Sports Med*. 2004; 32:389-395.

27. Wolin I, Classman F, Sideman S, Levinthal DH. Internal derangement of the talofibular component of the ankle. *Surg Gynecol Obstet*. 1950; 91:193-200.

28. Hauger O, Moinard M, Lasalarie JC, et al. Anterolateral compartment of the ankle in the lateral impingement syndrome: appearance on CT arthrography. *AJR Am J Roentgenol*. 1999; 173:685-690.

29. Farooki S, Yao L, Seeger LL. Anterolateral impingement of the ankle: effectiveness of MR imaging. *Radiology*. 1998; 207:357-360.

30. Liu SH, Nuccion SL, Finerman G. Diagnosis of anterolateral ankle impingement. Comparison between magnetic resonance imaging and clinical examination. *Am J Sports Med*. 1997; 25:389-393.

31. Rubin DA, Tishkoff NW, Britton CA, et al. Anterolateral soft-tissue impingement in the ankle: diagnosis using MR imaging. *AJR Am J Roentgenol*. 1997; 169:829-835.

32. Duncan D, Mologne T, Hildebrand H, et al. The usefulness of magnetic resonance imaging in the diagnosis of anterolateral impingement of the ankle. *J Foot Ankle Surg*. 2006; 45:304-307.

33. Robinson P, White LM, Salonen DC, et al. Anterolateral ankle impingement: MR arthrographic assessment of the anterolateral recess. *Radiology*. 2001; 221:186-190.

34. DeBerardino TM, Arciero RA, Taylor DC. Arthroscopic treatment of soft-tissue impingement of the ankle in athletes. *Arthroscopy*. 1997; 13:492-498.

35. Kim SH, Ha KI. Arthroscopic treatment for impingement of the anterolateral soft tissues of the ankle. *J Bone Joint Surg Br*. 2000; 82:1019-1021.

36. McCarroll JR, Schrader JW, Shelbourne KD, et al. Meniscoid lesions of the ankle in soccer players. *Am J Sports Med*. 1987; 15:255-257.

37. Hawkins LG. Fractures of the neck of the talus. *J Bone Joint Surg Am*. 1970; 52:991-1002.

38. Valderrabano V, Perren T, Ryc C, et al. Snowboarder's talus fracture: treatment outcome of 20 cases after 3.5 years. *Am J Sports Med*. 2005; 33:871-880.

39. Liu SH, Mirzayan R. Posteromedial ankle impingement. *Arthroscopy*. 1993; 9:709-11.

40. Paterson RS, Brown JN. The posteromedial impingement lesion of the ankle. A series of six cases. *Am J Sports Med*. 2001; 29:550-557.

41. Lawson JP. International Skeletal Society Lecture in honor of Howard D. Dorfman. Clinically significant radiologic anatomic variants of the skeleton. *AJR Am J Roentgenol*. 1994; 163:249-255.

42. Karasick D, Schweitzer ME. The os trigonum syndrome: imaging features. *AJR Am J Roentgenol*. 1996; 166:125-129.

43. Maquirriain J. Posterior ankle impingement syndrome. *J Am Acad Orthop Surg*. 2005; 13:365-371.

44. Robinson P, Bollen SR. Posterior ankle impingement in professional soccer players: effectiveness of sonographically guided therapy. *AJR Am J Roentgenol*. 2006; 187:W53-W58.

45. Bureau NJ, Cardinal E, Hobden R, Aubin B. Posterior ankle impingement syndrome: MR imaging findings in seven patients. *Radiology*. 2000; 215:497-503.

46. Peace KA, Hillier C, Hulme A, Healy JC. MRI features of posterior ankle impingement syndrome in ballet dancers: a review of 25 cases. *Clin Radiol*. 2004; 59:1025-1033.

47. Wakeley CJ, Johnson DP, Watt I. The value of MR imaging in the diagnosis of the os trigonum syndrome. *Skeletal Radiol*. 1996; 25:133-136.

48. Best A, Giza E, Linklater J, Sullivan M. Posterior impingement of the ankle caused by anomalous muscles. A report of four cases. *J Bone Joint Surg Am*. 2005; 87:2075-2079.

49. Abramowitz Y, Wollstein R, Barzilay Y, et al. Outcome of resection of a symptomatic os trigonum. *J Bone Joint Surg Am*. 2003; 85:1051-1057.

50. Willits K, Sonneveld H, Amendola A, et al. Outcome of posterior ankle arthroscopy for hindfoot impingement. *Arthroscopy*. 2008; 24:196-202.

51. Messiou C, Robinson P, O'Connor PJ, Grainger A.. Subacute posteromedial impingement of the ankle in athletes: MR imaging evaluation and ultrasound guided therapy. *Skeletal Radiol*. 2006; 35:88-94.

52. Koulouris G, Connell D, Schneider T, Edwards W. Posterior tibiotalar ligament injury resulting in posteromedial impingement. *Foot Ankle Int*. 2003; 24:575-583.

53. Hamilton WG, Geppert MJ, Thompson FM. Pain in the posterior aspect of the ankle in dancers. Differential diagnosis and operative treatment. *J Bone Joint Surg Am*. 1996; 78:1491-1500.

54. van Dijk CN. Hindfoot endoscopy. *Foot Ankle Clin*. 2006; 11: 391-414, vii.

55. Ferkel RD, Small HN, Gittins JE. Complications in foot and ankle arthroscopy. *Clin Orthop Relat Res*. 2001;(391):89-104.

56. van Dijk CN, Scholten PE, Krips R. A 2-portal endoscopic approach for diagnosis and treatment of posterior ankle pathology. *Arthroscopy*. 2000; 16:871-876.

57. Lijoi F, Lughi M, Baccarani G. Posterior arthroscopic approach to the ankle: an anatomic study. *Arthroscopy*. 2003; 19:62-67.

58. Phisitkul P, Tochigi Y, Saltzman CL, Amendola A. Arthroscopic visualization of the posterior subtalar joint in the prone position: a cadaver study. *Arthroscopy*. 2006; 22:511-515.

59. Horibe S, Kita K, Natsu-ume T, et al. A novel technique of arthroscopic excision of a symptomatic os trigonum. *Arthroscopy*. 2008; 24: 121e1-e4.

60. The American Academy of Orthopaedic Surgeons. OConnor, D. A new entity: sinus tarsi syndrome. *J Bone Joint Surg Am*. 1958; 40:715-731.

61. Williams MM, Ferkel RD. Subtalar arthroscopy: indications, technique, and results. *Arthroscopy*. 1998; 14:373-381.

62. Meyer JM, Garcia J, Hoffmeyer P, Fritschy D. The subtalar sprain. A roentgenographic study. *Clin Orthop Relat Res*. 1988(226):169-173.

63. Klein MA, Spreitzer AM. MR imaging of the tarsal sinus and canal: normal anatomy, pathologic findings, and features of the sinus tarsi syndrome. *Radiology*. 1993; 186:233-240.

64. Taillard W, Meyer JM, Garcia J, Blanc Y. The sinus tarsi syndrome. *Int Orthop*. 1981; 5:117-130.

65. Frey C, Feder KS, DiGiovanni C. Arthroscopic evaluation of the subtalar joint: does sinus tarsi syndrome exist? *Foot Ankle Int*. 1999; 20:185-191.

66. Lee KB, Bai LB, Song EK, et al. Subtalar arthroscopy for sinus Tarsi syndrome: arthroscopic findings and clinical outcomes of 33 consecutive cases. *Arthroscopy*. 2008; 24:1130-1134.

67. Sewell RB. A study of the astragalus. *J Anat Physiol*. 1904;38(Pt 4): 423-434.

68. Martus JE, Femino JE, et al. *Iowa Orthop J*. 2008; 28:1-8.

69. Malicky ES, Crary JL, Houghton MJ, et al. Talocalcaneal and subfibular impingement in symptomatic flatfoot in adults. *J Bone Joint Surg Am*. 2002; 84:2005-2009.

Soft Tissue Impingement of the Ankle Joint

Michael Tucker ● Champ L. Baker, Jr.

Lateral ligament sprains of the ankle joint are the most common musculoskeletal injury. They are especially common in sports such as ballet dancing, cross-country running, soccer, and basketball. Ankle sprains account for 45% of all injuries in basketball and 31% of all injuries in soccer.[1-3]

After an ankle sprain, anterolateral impingement syndrome is a common cause of continued lateral ankle pain and disability. This syndrome, which has been well documented, occurs in 20% to 40% of patients.[1] The diagnosis is often elusive, especially in ankles that are stable on examination. Morris, who called the condition *athlete's ankle*, first described impingement in the ankle in the literature in 1943.[4] It was later called *footballer's ankle* in a report by McMurray.[5]

The pathologic anatomy was first described as soft tissue pathology by Wolin and coworkers in 1950.[6] They described nine patients with continued pain and swelling of the lateral aspect of the ankle after an inversion injury. Arthrotomy of the ankle in these patients revealed a dense mass of hyalinized connective tissue that extended into the joint from the anteroinferior portion of the anterior talofibular ligament (ATFL). Wolin called this a *meniscoid lesion* because of its resemblance to a torn meniscus in the knee (Fig. 6-1). He believed pain and disability resulted from entrapment of this tissue between the fibula and talus with dorsiflexion of the ankle. Excision of this tissue resulted in pain relief in all nine patients.

Waller[7] later described an *anterolateral corner compression syndrome* that resulted in pain along the anteroinferior fibula and the anterolateral talus. Patients typically had a pronated foot with a valgus heel. This mechanism resulted in a synovial compression and chondromalacia of the lateral aspect of the talar dome. Guhl[8] described this condition as *anterolateral synovial impingement* when there is no evidence of ligamentous tissue and only hypertrophied synovium in the pathologic

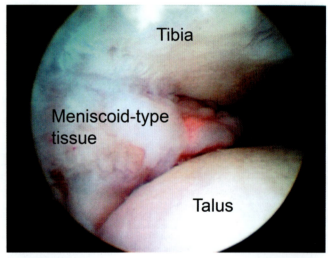

FIGURE 6-1 Partial tearing of the anterior talofibular ligament creates a meniscoid-type lesion that can become trapped in the joint.

specimen. Andrews and colleagues[9] emphasized the meniscoid lesion and hypothesized that it was caused by partial tearing of the ATFL. They thought the partially torn ligament became entrapped in the anterolateral gutter. Pain relief was reported with excision of this tissue.

Based on histopathologic analysis, Ferkel and associates[10] thought the impingement was caused by hypertrophied synovium. Later, Bassett and colleagues[11] described a distal fascicle of the anterior-inferior tibiofibular (syndesmotic) ligament (Fig. 6-2). During dorsiflexion of the ankle, this ligament was shown to come into contact with the anterolateral aspect of the talar dome. Presence of this fascicle was confirmed in 10 of 11 cadaveric specimens.

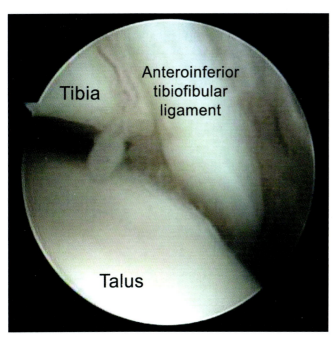

FIGURE 6-2 A Bassett lesion, or distal fascicle of the anteroinferior tibiofibular ligament, comes in contact with the talar dome during dorsiflexion of the ankle.

NORMAL AND PATHOLOGIC ANATOMY

The lateral ligamentous complex consists of the ATFL, the calcaneofibular ligament (CFL), and the posterior talofibular ligament (PTFL). The ATFL arises from the anterior aspect of the distal fibula and inserts on the body of the talus just anterior to the articular facet. It is usually 1.5 to 2 cm long and spans the anterior aspect of the ankle joint. It is confluent with the anterior lateral capsule. The CFL arises just distal to the origin of the ATFL; it does not arise from the tip of the fibula. The ligament runs posterior, medial, and inferior to its origin to insert on the calcaneus. It becomes confluent with the peroneal tendon sheath near its insertion. The PTFL arises from the posteromedial aspect of the lateral malleolus and runs medially to insert on the posterior aspect of the talus. The insertion is broad and involves almost the entire lip of the talus. The PTFL, like the ATFL, is confluent with the joint capsule.[1,12]

The borders of the lateral gutter include the fibula laterally, the talus medially, and the tibia with the anterior and posterior tibiofibular ligaments superiorly. The anteroinferior portion of the lateral gutter is bordered by the ATFL, the CFL, and the anteroinferior tibiofibular ligament (AITFL). Posteriorly, the gutter is bordered by the PTFL, the CFL, and the posterior tibiofibular ligament.

The classic sequence of ligament tears during a lateral ankle sprain begins with tearing of the ATFL. It proceeds to the CFL and AITFL, and the last ligament damaged is the PTFL. The ATFL is more vertically oriented and placed under tension with the ankle plantar flexed, making the ATFL function as a collateral ligament in this position. The CFL is more vertically oriented with the ankle in dorsiflexion, making the CFL a collateral in this position. The ATFL therefore resists inversion with the ankle

plantar flexed, and the CFL resists inversion wi siflexed. The PTFL inserts on the lateral aspec process of the talus and is injured only in the most sever ligament injuries.

There are three sites of impingement in anterolateral ankle impingement.[1] The first involves the ATFL and the area of the lateral gutter and lateral talar dome. The second involves the inferior fascicle of the AITFL, known as Bassett's ligament. The third is the superior portion of the AITFL.

The anterolateral impingement process begins with an inversion sprain, which tears the ATFL and AITFL, with occasional injury to the CFL. The injury is not severe enough to cause chronic instability. Repetitive motion leads to incomplete healing and inflammation in the areas of the healing ligaments, which leads to synovitis and formation of scar tissue. As the synovium and scar tissue increase in size, the mass may become impinged on by the tibia, fibula, and talus, leading to further irritation and pain. This mechanism can increase inflammation and result in chronic lateral ankle pain.

PATIENT EVALUATION

History and Physical Examination

Patients with anterolateral impingement typically present with a history of multiple ankle sprains followed by chronic, persistent ankle pain, especially with ambulation. Other complaints include ankle weakness and a feeling of the ankle giving way. It is not uncommon to have persistent catching and swelling in the anterolateral aspect of the ankle. Pain often is vague and poorly localized. It may involve the sinus tarsi and the syndesmotic region, depending on the location of the impingement. Pain is usually absent at rest and commences with weight bearing.[13,14]

Physical examination begins with observing the patient walk into the room. Because of marked inflammation and pain, the patient may have an antalgic gait. Inspection of the ankle frequently reveals swelling in the anterolateral aspect of the ankle and the lateral gutter. Palpation may elicit pain along the ATFL, along the lateral gutter, and occasionally along the CFL and the syndesmosis (Fig. 6-3). Pain over the ATFL and syndesmosis increases with dorsiflexion of the ankle during palpation. Tenderness depends on the location of the impingement. Determining the origin of the pain is important. Range of motion is typically normal with plantar flexion, but dorsiflexion may be limited because of the impingement. Excessive foot pronation, pes planus, and posterior tibial tendonitis can aggravate the condition. Patients usually do not have increased laxity with anterior drawer or varus stress testing. The examiner must be careful in differentiating pain in the anterolateral gutter from pain in the sinus tarsi. If injection of local anesthetic into the sinus tarsi eliminates the pain, the diagnosis is not anterolateral impingement.[1,13,14]

Diagnostic Imaging

Imaging modalities include radiography, tomography, computed tomography (CT), and magnetic resonance imaging (MRI). Radiographs are typically negative. They show absence of fractures, no widening of the ankle mortise, and no significant degenerative changes. Anterior tibial osteophytes and a shallow talar neck may

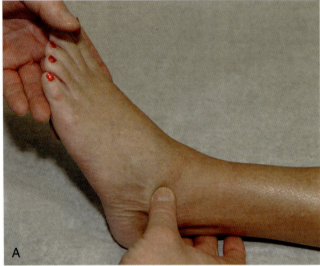

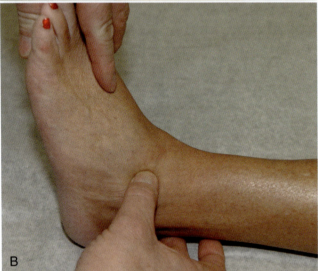

FIGURE 6-3 A, Palpation over the syndesmosis, lateral gutter, and anterior talofibular ligament. **B,** Dorsiflexion of the ankle may increase pain.

be present. Stress radiographs are negative because no instability is present.

Tomography and CT findings are typically negative. Hauger and colleagues[15] performed CT arthrography for patients with symptoms of anterolateral impingement. The investigators concluded that CT arthrography was a valid test if there was a nodular formation in the lateral gutter or if there was an irregular appearance of the edges of the lateral gutter. These findings corresponded to a meniscoid lesion or an abundant fibrous reaction on arthroscopy. These findings were also statistically associated with a chondropathy.

MRI has a sensitivity of 83.3%, a specificity of 78.6%, and a diagnostic accuracy of 78.8%.[1] Sagittal, T1-weighted and short tau inversion recovery (STIR) images can delineate edema or a soft tissue mass that has caused displacement of the subcutaneous fat normally found immediately adjacent to the lateral gutter. Rubin and coworkers[16] described the use of T2-weighted and fast-spin or STIR images in at least two orthogonal planes to study soft tissue anterolateral impingement. They found that ac-

curate assessment of the anterolateral gutter could be made only when fluid was distending the compartment. They also found that if the ATFL was not visualized, they could not differentiate whether the offending soft tissue was synovial tissue or the ligament. In such cases, they recommended physical examination and stress radiographs to help determine the cause of the impingement. They concluded that an MRI finding of an abnormal soft tissue mass in the lateral gutter distinct from the ATFL suggested the diagnosis of soft tissue impingement. Huh and associates[17] showed that contrast-enhanced, three-dimensional, fast-gradient recalled acquisition in steady state with radiofrequency spoiling MRI revealed high specificity of soft tissue impingement evaluation in patients with chronic post-traumatic ankle pain. Kinematic MRI has also been used to evaluate soft tissue impingement with some success.

TREATMENT

Indications and Contraindications

Failure of conservative treatment, including a short period of immobilization, progressive weight bearing, physical therapy, nonsteroidal anti-inflammatory medications, and selective injections for 3 to 6 months, is an indication for arthroscopic evaluation and treatment. Contraindications are limited and include functional instability and complex regional pain syndrome.[1]

Conservative Management

Initial treatment should include a period of at least 3 months of conservative care. Initial treatment methods are varied and include a period of immobilization. This may be a period of absolute immobilization in a cast or relative immobilization in a boot. Progressive weight bearing after immobilization is a good idea, especially if there was a recent ankle sprain. Beneficial physical therapy includes Achilles tendon stretching and anterior tibial and peroneal tendon strengthening. Ankle stabilization bracing or taping during athletic activities may alleviate some pain. Nonsteroidal anti-inflammatory medications for a short period may decrease some of the inflammation. Local steroid injections can help to decrease inflammation. Selective anesthetic injections may help differentiate anterolateral impingement from other diagnoses, such as sinus tarsi syndrome.[1,13,14]

Arthroscopic Technique

Ankle arthroscopy can be performed using a 1.9-mm, 2.7-mm, or 4.0-mm arthroscope. The 2.7-mm arthroscope is helpful for smaller joints and tight spaces and for subtalar joint arthroscopy. It is somewhat delicate, and for normal ankle arthroscopy, we prefer the 4.0-mm arthroscope because it is sturdier, provides an excellent picture, and allows inflow on the arthroscope. The 30-degree, 4.0-mm arthroscope is our first choice for ankle procedures, but the 2.7-mm arthroscope should be available, particularly for posterior viewing and for tight joints. Most companies manufacture sets of small joint instruments for the elbow and ankle.

Curettes, picks, and elevators of appropriate size for ankle instrumentation should be available. Many small shavers can be used for soft tissue and bone to facilitate access to the ankle joint

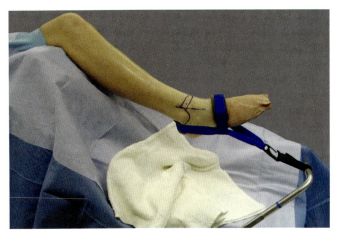

FIGURE 6-4 Noninvasive distraction. A strap around the ankle is attached to a bar off the end of the operating table. The surgeon can pull the bar distally to increase or decrease distraction.

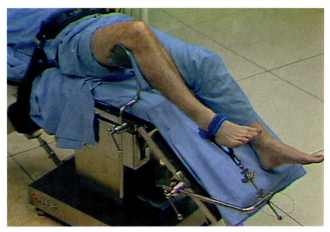

FIGURE 6-5 A well-padded thigh holder is used to elevate the leg, and the foot of the table can be lowered for distraction.

to remove pathologic tissue. Monopolar or bipolar, 2.0-mm radiofrequency probes are also helpful.

Ankle distraction has evolved considerably from the time when invasive distraction was always used. For arthroscopic procedures, particularly in the anterior compartment, several commercial products are available that enable soft tissue distraction. Noninvasive distraction can be gravity distraction or manual distraction, in which the operating surgeon uses a strap around the ankle to open the joint (Fig. 6-4). We prefer a Velcro strap to a metallic distractor because it allows easier on and off positioning and greater control of the amount of tension applied.

Invasive distraction involves placing pins in the tibia and talus or calcaneus to distract the ankle joint. Contraindications to invasive distraction are open physes, use in athletes who plan to return to their sport quickly, and complex regional pain syndrome. Invasive distraction has been associated with complications, including stress fracture, infection, and neurovascular injury. The use of small joint arthroscopes along with noninvasive distraction techniques has obviated invasive distraction for ankle arthroscopy in most situations. Noninvasive distraction can be used in most any patient as long as there are no skin problems with the application of the harness.

Arthroscopy of the ankle is usually performed with the patient in the supine position and the knee level or flexed. The lateral decubitus position with the patient supported on a beanbag or the prone position can be used for subtalar and hindfoot arthroscopy. We use a special thigh holder that is located inferior to the thigh tourniquet to elevate the leg and avoid pressure to the popliteal area (Fig. 6-5). The holder should be well padded to avoid neurovascular injury. The hip is flexed 40 to 90 degrees. The entire table is raised, and the head is elevated so the foot of the table can be lowered. This position allows the surgeon to stand or sit. It also provides posterior access to the ankle.

Ankle arthroscopy is usually performed through the anterolateral and the anteromedial portals (Table 6-1). Use of a central portal has been discontinued because of the potential for neurovascular injury.

After the patient is prepared and draped, anatomic landmarks are outlined on the skin. These landmarks include the medial

TABLE 6-1   Portal Anatomy

Portal Site	Landmarks	Structures at Risk
Anteromedial	Medial to anterior tibialis tendon	Saphenous vein and nerve Anterior tibialis tendon Extensor hallucis longus tendon
Anterolateral	Lateral to peroneus tertius tendon	Superficial peroneal nerve Extensor digitorum communis tendon Peroneus tertius tendon

malleolus, lateral malleolus, distal tibia, and talus. The procedure can be performed with or without a tourniquet; however, we prefer application of a tourniquet and exsanguination. Using an 18-gauge needle, 30 mL of normal saline is injected through the medial portal to distend the joint. An incision is made through the skin, and using the nick and spread technique to protect the cutaneous nerve, a hemostat is used to create the portal. Next, we introduce the blunt cannula and observe for extravasation of fluid to ensure entry into the joint. The arthroscope is then introduced to visualize the joint.

The anterolateral portal is then established using an outside in technique. An 18-gauge needle is used for correct localization of the portal. The skin is incised horizontally, it is spread with a hemostat, and a cannula and trocar are inserted.

The examination portion of the procedure begins in the lateral aspect of the ankle and includes visualization of the tibiotalar articulation and soft tissue in that area, the AITFL, the ATFL, and the inferior aspect of the fibula. The inferior fibular space should be inspected, particularly if preoperative symptoms include lateral ankle pain.

With proper distraction, the arthroscope can swing across the midportion of the joint. There is a sulcus between the tibia and talus that allows the arthroscope to be pushed posteriorly. From this position, the operator should be able to see the posterior capsule. The arthroscope is then moved to the medial portal, allowing the surgeon to look down the medial gutter. If after diag-

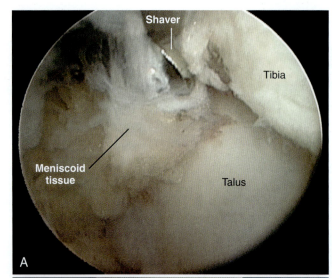

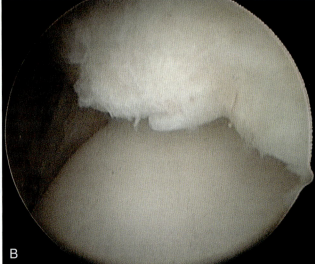

FIGURE 6-6 A, A shaver is used to clear meniscoid-type tissue from the joint. **B,** After the trapped tissue has been removed, the ankle should be flexed and extended to check joint motion.

nostic examination of the joint the diagnosis of soft tissue impingement is made, the arthroscope is placed medially, and a motorized shaver is brought into the lateral portal. The soft tissue entrapped between the tibia and talus that can be seen with forced dorsiflexion is then removed. Care is taken to visualize the AITFL. If the ligament is thought to be causing part of the impingement or it is partly frayed, a portion of it can be removed with the shaver or the radiofrequency probe (Fig. 6-6).

After decompression of the lateral compartment is complete, the arthroscope is placed laterally, and all soft tissue is removed from the medial compartment. The ankle joint is flexed and extended to ensure that all trapped tissue has been removed. If spurs are seen on the tibia or talus, they are removed at this time. Care must be taken with the shaver to avoid cutting anterior to the capsule, where the neurovascular structures lie. With proper distraction and fluid distention, arthroscopic removal of soft tissue is a very safe procedure. The radiofrequency probe is used to cauterize any residual bleeding, and the arthroscope is removed.

We prefer to close the portals postoperatively to prevent excess fluid leakage that can cross-contaminate and cause infection. We inject the joint with bupivacaine for postoperative pain relief, and a bulky wrap is applied. The tourniquet is then deflated.

The patient usually returns home the same day. He or she does not bear weight until the office visit in 4 to 5 days for evaluation and suture removal.

When soft tissue impingement is caused by mild ankle instability, ankle reconstruction is seldom indicated. However, if the ankle impingement is related to a chronically unstable ankle, we often perform arthroscopy before completing a modified Broström reconstruction procedure.

PEARLS & PITFALLS

- If the ankle joint space is tight in a smaller individual, a smaller arthroscope may be helpful.
- When using distraction, be sure there is ample room behind the ankle to allow for a posterior portal if needed.
- The nick and spread technique should be used for all incisions to avoid sensory nerve problems.
- Always use cannulas without side portals to prevent extravasation of fluid.
- Use the outside-in technique for establishing the operative portal to avoid scuffing articular cartilage.
- A monopolar or bipolar radiofrequency probe for tissue resection is helpful in limited space.
- After the diagnosis has been made, temporarily release the traction and flex and extend the ankle to detect soft tissue entrapment. Although most entrapment is in the lateral joint, both sides of the joint should be decompressed.
- Always close the portals to prevent oozing and possible secondary contamination.
- Rehabilitation must include exercises to restore proprioception to the ankle.

Postoperative Rehabilitation Protocol

Sutures are removed at 4 to 5 days after surgery.[14] At that time, the patient is allowed to start active assisted range-of-motion exercises, strengthening, and touch-down weight bearing. Patients progress to partial and full weight bearing as motion and strength return.

Because soft tissue impingement is the most often the result of ankle sprain, a physical therapy program designed to strengthen and restore proprioception is continued until full strength and mobility are achieved.

CONCLUSIONS

Anterior soft tissue impingement is a frequent cause of chronic ankle pain after ankle sprain. Presenting symptoms include vague and persistent pain in the area of the anterolateral gutter and occasionally the sinus tarsi. Pain is typically absent at rest and is exacerbated with activity. Physical examination reveals pain with forced dorsiflexion of the ankle, and ligamentous instability is not found with anterior drawer testing. Fullness and swelling may be found in the area of the anterolateral gutter. Causes of the impingement include synovial hypertrophy, the distal fascicle of the AITFL, and an impinging AITFL.

Conservative treatment consisting of nonsteroidal anti-inflammatory drugs, bracing, steroid injections, physical therapy, and orthotics is usually enough to treat soft tissue impingement. If conservative treatment fails for longer than 3 months, arthroscopic débridement is a highly effective means of treatment. Care should be taken to thoroughly examine the entire ankle joint to avoid overlooking associated injuries and pathologic anatomy.

REFERENCES

1. Coughlin MJ, Mann RA, Saltzman CL. *Surgery of the Foot and Ankle.* 8th ed. St. Louis, MO: Mosby; 2006.
2. Ekstrand J, Tropp H. The incidence of ankle sprains in soccer. *Foot Ankle.* 1990; 11:41-44.
3. Sandelin J. *Acute Sports Injuries: A Clinical and Epidemiological Study* [dissertation]. Helsinki, Finland: University of Helsinki; 1988.
4. Morris LH. News notes. *J Bone Joint Surg.* 1943; 25:220.
5. McMurray TP. Footballer's ankle. *J Bone Joint Surg Br.* 1950;32B:68-69.
6. Wolin I, Glassman F, Sideman S, Levinthal DH. Internal derangement of the talofibular component of the ankle. *Surg Gynecol Obstet.* 1950; 91:193-200.
7. Waller JF. Hindfoot and midfoot problems of the runner. In Mack RP, ed. *Symposium on the Foot and Leg in Running Sports.* St. Louis, MO: Mosby–Year Book; 1982:64-71.
8. Guhl JF. Soft tissue synovial pathology. In: *Ankle Arthroscopy; Pathology and Surgical Techniques.* Thorofare, NJ: Slack; 1988:93-135.
9. Andrews JR, Drez DJ, McGinty JB. Symposium: arthroscopy of joints other than the knee. *Contemp Orthop.* 1984; 9:71-100.
10. Ferkel RD, Karzel RP, Del Pizzo W, et al. Arthroscopic treatment of anterolateral impingement of the ankle. *Am J Sports Med.* 1991; 19: 440-446.
11. Basset FH 3rd, Gates HS 3rd, Billys BJ, et al. Talar impingement by the anteroinferior tibiofibular ligament: a cause of chronic pain in the ankle after inversion sprain. *J Bone Joint Surg Am.* 1990;72A:55-59.
12. Lassiter TE Jr, Malone TR, Garrett WE Jr. Injury to the lateral ligaments of the ankle. *Orthop Clin North Am.* 1989; 20:629-640.
13. Jacobson KE, Liu SH. Anterolateral impingement of the ankle. *J Med Assoc Ga.* 1992; 81:297-299.
14. Liu SH, Raskin A, Osti L, et al. Arthroscopic treatment of anterolateral ankle impingement. *Arthroscopy.* 1994; 10:215-218.
15. Hauger O, Moinard M, Lasalarie JC, et al. Anterolateral compartment of the ankle in the lateral impingement syndrome: appearance on CT arthroscopy. *AJR Am J Roentgenol.* 1999; 173:685-690.
16. Rubin D, Tishkoff N, Britton C, et al. Anterolateral soft-tissue impingement in the ankle: diagnosis using MR imaging. *AJR Am J Roentgenol.* 1997; 169:829-835.
17. Huh Y-M, Suh J-S, Lee J-W, Song H-T. Synovitis and soft tissue impingement of the ankle: assessment with enhanced three-dimensional FSPGR MR imaging. *J Magn Reson Imaging.* 2004; 19:108-116.

SUGGESTED READINGS

van Dijk CN. Anterior and posterior ankle impingement. *Foot Ankle Clin.* 2006:11:663-683.

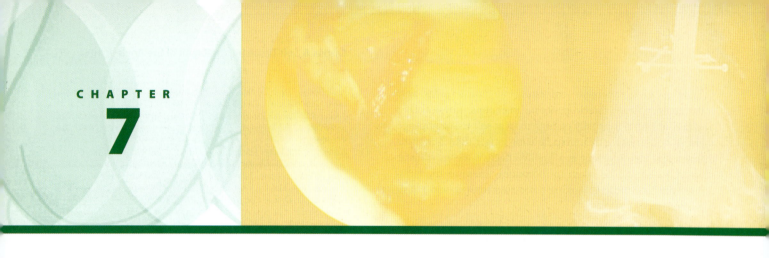

Anatomy, Evaluation, and Operative Setup for Posterior Ankle Arthroscopy

David Sitler

Arthroscopy of the posterior ankle was originally described as a diagnostic tool. As surgeons became more proficient with the technique, therapeutic procedures were incorporated.[1-5] The posterior portion of the ankle is often poorly visualized from traditional arthroscopic portals, and certain lesions are more easily dealt with by performing a dedicated posterior arthroscopy. Although the prone position and the proximity of the tibial neurovascular bundle have led some away from the technique, recent articles demonstrate that the procedure can be undertaken safely.[6]

To undertake a posterior arthroscopy, small joint arthroscopy skills, anatomic knowledge, and understanding the limitations of the procedure are necessary. This chapter outlines the pertinent anatomy, clinical entities that are treatable, indications, techniques, and postoperative care regimens.

ANATOMY

The anatomy of the posterior ankle can be divided into pertinent surface anatomy, relationships of deep structures and abnormal, congenital, or acquired deformities of the typical anatomy.

The posterior view of the ankle's surface anatomy includes the posterior edges of the malleoli, the Achilles tendon, and its insertion. Delineating these structures can guide marking of other structures in the superficial layers.

The sural nerve lies lateral to the Achilles tendon at a distance of approximately 1 cm form the lateral edge of the Achilles tendon at the level of the posterolateral portal. It courses obliquely away from the Achilles as it heads toward the lateral portion of the foot. Medially, the flexor hallucis longus (FHL) tendon is encountered first when moving from the margin of the Achilles tendon. Immediately adjacent to that is the tibial nerve. Further medially and anteriorly lie the posterior tibial artery and vein (Fig. 7-1).

Deep to the distal portion of the Achilles tendon lies the retrocalcaneal bursa. The posterior joint capsule is the next layer encountered. Deep to the capsule, the tibiotalar and subtalar

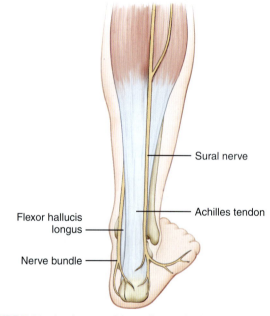

Sural nerve

Achilles tendon

Flexor hallucis longus

Nerve bundle

FIGURE 7-1 In the drawing of the surface and subcutaneous anatomy, notice the course of the sural nerve.

joints are apparent, as is the posterior process of the talus with a medial and more often prominent lateral tuberosity.

In dealing with surgical conditions in the posterior hindfoot, certain pathologic anatomic variations can be encountered. Retrocalcaneal bursitis, refractory os trigonum syndrome, hindfoot impingement, FHL tenosynovitis and stenosing tenosynovitis, and posterior osteochondral lesions of the talus are pathologic entities that can be identified and treated with posterior ankle arthroscopy. Loose bodies that are unreachable from anterior portals can be removed posteriorly.

Retrocalcaneal bursitis is primarily treated nonoperatively, but refractory symptoms can be treated with bursa excision through the arthroscope. The normal bursa is encountered routinely in posterior arthroscopy, because it is often the first potential space developed.

Os trigonum syndrome is marked by pain in the posterior ankle, especially with plantar flexion weight bearing. The os trigonum is an accessory ossicle that represents an unfused lateral tuberosity of the posterior process of the talus. A painful os trigonum can be the result of acute fracture of a large tuberosity of the same structure.

Tenosynovitis of the FHL can develop as an overuse injury, often with plantar flexion weight bearing and particularly in the en point toe position in ballet dancing. This reactive synovitis from overuse can lead to pain and triggering in the posteromedial ankle.

CLINICAL EVALUATION

The diagnostic clinical encounter begins with a thorough history of the chief complaint. Important personal information from the patient includes a history of operations or injuries to the feet or ankles. A history of all symptoms and previous treatments is elicited. The relative successes of nonoperative treatments are documented. Activities at the time symptoms began are recorded, as are activities that aggravate the symptoms.

Examination of the affected and unaffected leg begins with appropriate exposure of the patient. The legs from the knees down are bare and without socks and shoes. The examination progresses from standing alignment to observation of gate to seated examination. Range of motion, strength, and sensory and vascular status are assessed before provocative maneuvers are used. Gaits are described with a focus on pain-mediated gaits (i.e., antalgic or foot flat), those indicative of joint stiffness (i.e., vaulting), and those indicative of neurologic disorders (i.e., foot-drop, steppage, or circumduction).

The weight-bearing and non–weight-bearing alignment of the hindfoot are assessed. The alignment of the forefoot is recorded with the hindfoot stabilized in neutral. The range of motion of the tibiotalar and subtalar joints is examined. Strength testing of the ankle plantar flexors and dorsiflexors are compared with the unaffected side. Testing of the peroneal and posterior tibial tendons is carried out with the foot in a dorsiflexed position. Isolated strength testing of the FHL is indicated if pathology is suspected.

Some resistive strength testing maneuvers are provocative examinations. Further provocative examinations include direct palpation the posterior talus, palpation of the FHL in the tarsal tunnel, palpation of the Achilles tendon insertion, and a posterior ankle impingement test, which is performed by forcing plantar flexion in a slightly inverted foot.

Retrocalcaneal Bursitis

Retrocalcaneal bursitis is a disease of the tissue adjacent to the insertion of the Achilles tendon on the calcaneus. Some authorities think that it part of a spectrum of disease that includes calcific insertional Achilles tendinitis and that it is not as much an inflammatory phenomenon as it is a fibroproliferative disease of the Achilles insertion, akin to lateral epicondylitits.[5] A prominent

posterosuperior part of the calcaneus (i.e., Haglund's deformity) contributes to the symptoms is some patients.[2,3,7,8]

Symptoms typically manifest as overuse injuries with a bimodal pattern. There is pain and sometimes swelling or bony deformity at the insertion of the Achilles tendon. Pain often occurs with resisted strength testing and with forced dorsiflexion.

Radiographs can reveal a calcaneal spur or intrasubstance calcific tendinosis. The posterosuperior process of the calcaneus is evaluated by measuring the superior calcaneal angle and observing the parallel pitch lines.

Treatment mainstays are anti-inflammatory medications and immobilization. A stretching program is often used after the initial discomfort has diminished. Night splinting can be recommended during periods of provocative activity.

Surgical treatment is reserved for failure of maximal nonoperative treatment. Treatment is often directed at adjacent, secondarily inflamed structures if no obvious insertional disease is present. The retrocalcaneal bursa and fat pad are completely excised. Calcaneal exostectomy is often combined with the excision. The postoperative course is further immobilization.

Watson and colleagues[8] described a series of patients with retrocalcaneal bursitis with or without calcific insertional tendinitis. They found that patients without obvious insertional disease fared better than those with a spur. There was a 93% satisfaction rating, with an average time to maximal improvement of 5 months.[8]

Os Trigonum Syndrome

The os trigonum syndrome is the primary cause for the posterior ankle impingement syndrome. Typically, patients have a history of a hyper-plantar flexion or inversion injury, or they have a slow, insidious onset of symptoms in the setting of increased activities, indicating an overuse injury. The overuse injury often occurs in runners and dancers. Physical examination reveals pain with direct posterior palpation and in response to the posterior ankle impingement test.

Nonoperative treatment consists primarily of immobilization and nonsteroidal anti-inflammatory medications. Casting for a period of 4 to 6 weeks with regimented anti-inflammatory medications can relieve symptoms in most patients. For those with recurrent or recalcitrant symptoms, excision of the os trigonum can alleviate pain. Open excision has long been used successfully, but there have been complications related to infection and hematoma.[9]

Great success with arthroscopic excision has been reported.[2-4] Scholten and colleagues thought they were better able to address soft tissue impingement syndromes with posterior arthroscopy. They followed 55 patients for a minimum of 2 years, with none lost to follow-up. They found a significant increase in the American Orthopaedic Foot and Ankle Society (AOFAS) hindfoot score (75 to 90) and no degenerative changes on repeat radiographs.[2]

Flexor Hallucis Longus Tenosynovitis

FHL tenosynovitis has long been described in ballet dancers and in athletes with rapid start and stop (toe-off) running, such as soccer players. The repeated stress causes as tenosynovitis, which becomes painful with repetitive use. Rest and omission of painful activities typically alleviate symptoms.

Symptoms can develop in the midfoot at the knot of Henry, in the tarsal tunnel, and more proximally. Differentiating pain in these three areas is necessary to predict the potential surgical avenues available for treatment.

Long-standing symptoms may lead to the formation of a nodular thickening of the FHL in the area of the tarsal tunnel. If the thickening becomes ensnared on the flexor retinaculum, a triggering or catching sensation may be reported by the patient. The patient may report long periods of the great toe being stuck in a flexed position.

Nonoperative treatment is curative in most patients. The mainstay of therapy, as with os trigonum syndrome, is immobilization and anti-inflammatory medications. Some physicians advocate the use of corticosteroid injections into the triggering nodule, as is commonly used in the hand. For recurrent or recalcitrant symptoms, tenosynovectomy with surgical release of the FHL slip or posterior edge of the FHL sheath can be curative.

From the posterior arthroscopic portals, the FHL and the stout edge of the FHL sheath can easily be identified and released. Débridement of the stenosing tenosynovitis can be carried out on the tendon.

Michelson and coworkers reported a 67% success rate with nonoperative treatment. All of their patients who failed nonoperative treatments had successful outcomes after an open approach to the FHL at the proximal portion of the fibro-osseus tunnel.[10]

DIAGNOSTIC IMAGING

Plain Radiographs

Weight-bearing radiographs of the affected foot and ankle are mandatory. Other helpful images include the contralateral foot and ankle views, axial and lateral heel views, long leg alignment films, and specialized views of the subtalar joint. The radiographs are evaluated for alignment, stress reaction, acute bony pathology, and chronic disease.

Views of the ankle are evaluated for obvious fractures, including an osteochondral fracture of the talus. The tibiotalar joint is assessed for symmetry of the joint space and for degenerative changes, including anterior and posterior osteophytic disease. An os trigonum or fracture of a prominent lateral tubercle of the posterior process of the talus can be seen on the lateral view. Axial and lateral heel views are used to evaluate the calcaneus posterosuperior process, and they typically provide a good view of the posterior facet of the subtalar joint (Fig. 7-2).

Computed Tomography

Computed tomography (CT) provides valuable information for evaluating subchondral bone in the setting of an osteochondral lesion of the talus (OLT). Subchondral cysts in the talus are seen on CT. The size and surrounding bone structure of these lesions is evaluated better than with magnetic resonance imaging (MRI).

CT can show the bony detail of the os trigonum. The os can be an unfused ossification center with a fibrous connection, or it

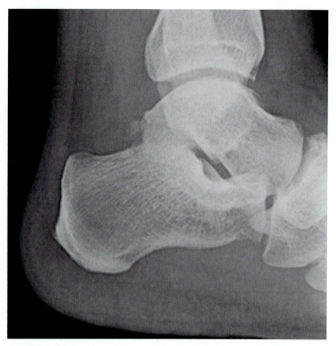

FIGURE 7-2 The lateral radiograph shows an os trigonum and a prominent posterosuperior process of the calcaneus.

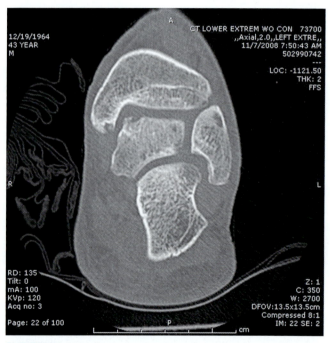

FIGURE 7-3 Coronal computed tomography shows a posteromedial osteochondral lesion of the talus.

can be a symptomatic, fully fused, large tubercle of the posterior process of the talus. A fracture of the os shows obvious cortical discontinuity on CT (Fig. 7-3).

Magnetic Resonance Imaging

MRI provides the greatest amount of information about involved soft tissues. The tendon can be evaluated on standard sequences, but the fluid-sensitive, fat-suppressed images delineate most pathologies better. In these sequences, tendons are typically very

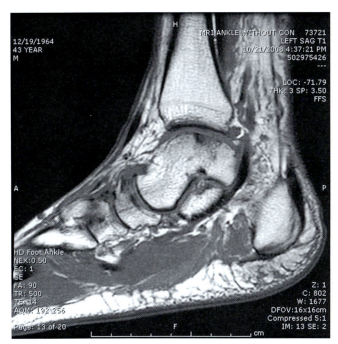

FIGURE 7-4 A sagittal magnetic resonance imaging shows the same osteochondral lesion of the talus (seen in Figure 7-3. Notice the large area of signal change.

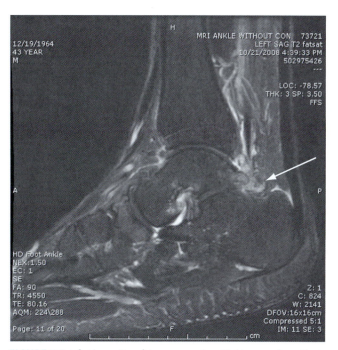

FIGURE 7-5 A fluid-sensitive, fat-suppressed sagittal image of a patient shows a symptomatic os trigonum *(arrow)* and posterior ankle impingement.

dark and homogeneous. Tendons may be torn, split, or surrounded by fluid, which is indicative of tenosynovitis. Attention is focused on the FHL tendon and the anatomy of the posterior neurovascular bundle for operative planning.

The fat-saturated and fluid-sensitive, fat-suppressed MR images are useful for evaluation of bone. In the fat-saturated images, the bone marrow has high signal intensity, and subchondral and cortical bone tissues are dark.

In the region of the OLT, the fat-sensitive sequence can show decreased signal intensity in subchondral bone, indicative of edema. Decreased signal intensity can be seen in the cartilage overlying the defect, possibly indicating calcified fibrocartilage in the defect. On the fluid-sensitive sequence, undermining of an unstable cartilage flap can be seen. Fluid-filled cysts are identified. High intensity signal in the bone marrow beneath the OLT indicates inflammation and continued injury (Fig. 7-4).

The same signal characteristics hold true for the MRI evaluation of the os trigonum. Edema in the ossicle or in the adjacent posterior talus indicates ongoing injury, supporting its role as the pain generator (Fig. 7-5).

Fluid about the FHL tendon can be seen clearly on fluid-sensitive sequences, and it is an indicator of ongoing inflammation and edema in the tendon. Tendon nodules, hypertrophy, and tears are also identified (Fig. 7-6).

An inflamed retrocalcaneal bursa is bright on fluid-sensitive images, and Achilles tendon pathology is identified as fusiform swelling of the tendon, intrasubstance fluid near the insertion, or the low-intensity signal of calcified material in the tendon substance.

Bone Scan

A three-phase bone scan can be useful in the diagnosis of overuse injuries, particularly a stress fracture that may be causing symp-

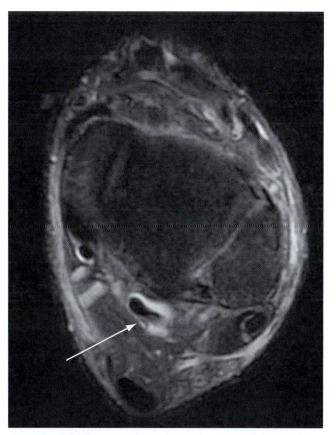

FIGURE 7-6 In a fluid-sensitive, fat-suppressed image of a patient with flexor hallucis longus tendonitis, notice the fluid signal around the tendon *(arrow)*.

toms similar to those of the discussed pathology. Active OLT and symptomatic os trigonum syndrome should have increased uptake on the bone scan.

TREATMENT

Surgical Technique

The patient is placed in the prone position. All bony prominences are well padded, and the operative leg is supported on a pad to allow the foot to lie in a neutral position and to provide space to manipulate the foot during the procedure. A thigh tourniquet is placed, and the lower extremity is prepared to the knee (Fig. 7-7).

The Achilles tendon, medial malleolus, and lateral malleolus are palpated and marked. The approximate course of the sural nerve and the posteromedial neurovascular bundle are drawn on the skin. The level of the tibiotalar joint is estimated by palpating the tips of the malleoli and the anterior and posterior joint while moving the foot (Fig. 7-8).

The posterolateral portal is established 5 mm distal to the estimated level of the tibiotalar joint and adjacent to the Achilles tendon. Using an 18-guage needle, 20 mL of arthroscopy fluid is injected into the joint to expand the capsule (see Fig. 7-7). A nick is created in the skin only, and a small hemostat is used to bluntly dissect toward the lateral aspect of the joint. A small joint arthroscopy canula for a 2.7- or 3.0-mm, 30-degree arthroscope with two stopcock valves is placed in this portal. Inflow fluid is placed on one valve, and suction or gravity drainage is attached to the other. By alternating opening the valves, blood can be cleared from the joint and visibility obtained.

The medial portal is established with direct arthroscopic guidance. The entry location in the skin is at the same level as the lateral portal and is adjacent to the Achilles tendon. An 18-guage spinal needle is used to ensure the pathway of the medial portal enters lateral to the FHL. By staying lateral to the FHL the medial neurovascular structures are protected from damage by the arthroscopic instruments (Fig. 7-9).

Instruments are inserted into the joint through the medial portal. A 4-mm, short, plastic cannula may be used to facilitate safe passage of instruments through this portal (Fig. 7-10).

A small amount of the posterior capsule is excised to facilitate visibility of the joint. Because the subtalar joint is close the tibiotalar joint, care must be taken to enter the proper joint. A system-

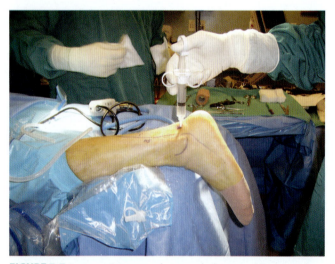

FIGURE 7-7 An operating room photograph shows positioning and setup. Notice that the foot is free to allow manipulation. Arthroscopy fluid is being injected where the lateral portal will be established.

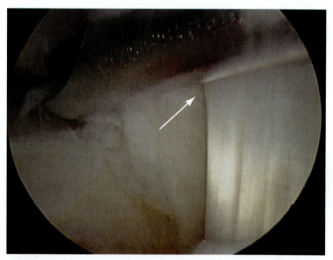

FIGURE 7-9 Arthroscopic view of a shaver being passed lateral to the flexor hallucis longus tendon *(arrow)* in the left ankle.

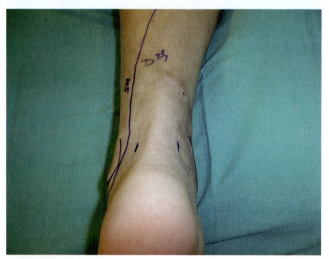

FIGURE 7-8 A clinical photograph of the posterior ankle shows the surface anatomy and portal sites drawn with a skin marker.

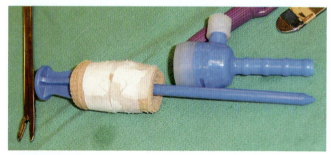

FIGURE 7-10 Modification of the plastic cannulas allow shorter instruments to be used.

atic diagnostic examination of the joint starts at the posteromedial talus (Fig. 7-11).

The talar dome and tibial articular surfaces should be inspected. Access to the posterior portion of the dome is obtained by dorsal flexing the ankle to deliver the articular portion posteriorly (Fig. 7-12). An OLT can be addressed. Loose cartilage and bone fragments are mobilized with a blunt spatula and removed with small joint graspers. Microfracturing or drilling of these lesions can be performed as indicated (Fig. 7-13).

The posterior portion of the talus and tibia is viewed. This is the area of the os trigonum. For patients with os trigonum syndrome, the process is excised. Sharp and dull spatulas are used to mobilize the bone. The fragment is removed through the medial portal (Fig. 7-14). If the piece is large, a pituitary rongeur is used to remove the process in small pieces (Figs. 7-15 and 7-16).

The FHL is inspected in the posteromedial joint. Tendonoscopy can be performed to inspect the integrity of the tendon.

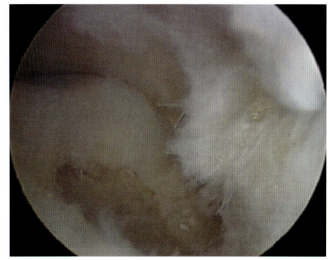

FIGURE 7-13 Arthroscopic view after excision of cartilage and bone from the osteochondral lesion of the talus seen in Figure 7-12.

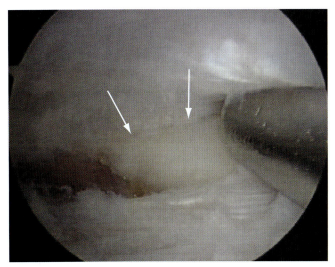

FIGURE 7-11 Minimal posterior capsule is excised to visualize the joint. The posterior articular surface of the talus is seen *(arrows)*.

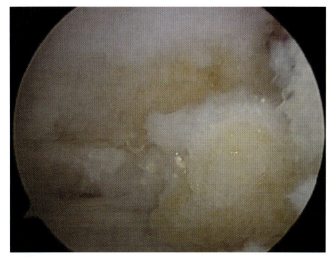

FIGURE 7-14 Arthroscopic view of removal of the bone and fibrous tissue of an os trigonum through the medial portal.

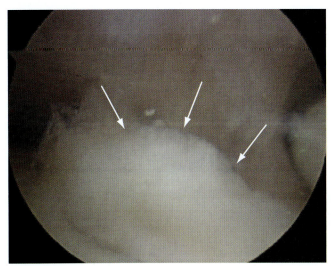

FIGURE 7-12 Arthroscopic view of loose cartilage over a posteromedial osteochondral lesion of the talus *(arrows)*.

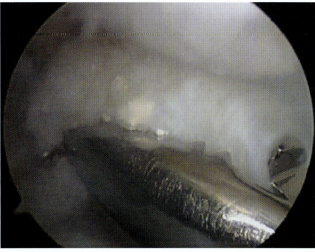

FIGURE 7-15 Arthroscopic view after a large os trigonum was partially removed by fragmentation.

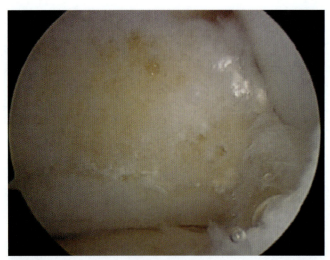

FIGURE 7-16 Arthroscopic view after complete removal of an os trigonum. The subtalar joint can be seen.

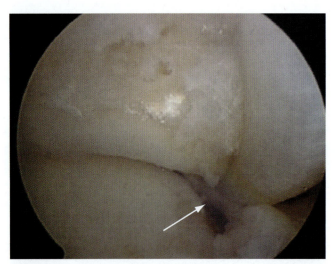

FIGURE 7-17 Arthroscopic view after the flexor hallucis longus tendon sheath has been released *(arrow)*. The subtalar joint and medial calcaneus can be seen.

Tenosynovitis is débrided with a small joint shaver. If there is triggering or constriction of the tendon, the FHL sheath can be released with arthroscopic scissors. The sheath can usually be released to the level of the sustentaculum talus of the calcaneus under direct arthroscopic visualization (Fig. 7-17).

The arthroscope is transferred to the medial portal. It can be placed through the plastic cannulas. If the plastic cannulas are replaced with the cannulas for the arthroscope, a switching stick should be used to ensure the instruments remain lateral to the FHL. The lateral gutter and the posterolateral joint are visualized. Loose bodies, often found in this portion of the ankle, are removed.

Retrocalcaneal endoscopy is performed if indicated. The arthroscope can be transferred between the portals, depending on the area of the retrocalcaneal space that needs to be visualized and instrumented. The bursa is removed with a motorized shaver. A Haglund deformity is removed with a burr. Intraoperative fluoroscopy is used to ensure an adequate amount of the posterosuperior process is removed.

The instruments are removed from the joint. The portals are sutured with nonabsorbable suture. Dressing sponges and a figure-eight compressive wrap are applied.

PEARLS & PITFALLS

- Placing the lateral portal distal to the joint and adjacent to the Achilles tendon avoids injury to the sural nerve.
- Passing instruments lateral to the FHL is important to avoid the medial neurovascular structures.
- Most small joint instruments and shavers are too short to be used through the plastic cannulas. The cannulas can be modified by cutting it short. Sterile padding is wrapped around the blunt trocar so that it can be used safely.
- A microfracture awl with a narrow shaft should be used to allow insertion and manipulation in the small joint space.

Postoperative Protocol

Arthroscopic procedures produce less soft tissue trauma, which allows early motion. Active range of motion is started on postoperative day 1. The dressing is removed on postoperative day 3 and replaced with small adhesive dressings. The compressive wrap is usually worn until postoperative day 7.

All patients are issued crutches after the procedure. Weight bearing is advanced as tolerated after postoperative day 3. However, if a microfracture procedure was performed, weight bearing is delayed for 6 weeks. Formal physical therapy is used for patients who have trouble regaining motion and strength.

CONCLUSIONS

Posterior ankle arthroscopy has evolved well beyond a simple diagnostic procedure. A better understanding of the anatomy in relation to portal placement has led to techniques to protect the structures at risk. Advancement of arthroscopic equipment allows us to treat more pathologic conditions in the posterior ankle.

REFERENCES

1. Ferkel RD, Scranton PE Jr. Arthroscopy of the ankle and foot. *J Bone Joint Surg Am.* 1993; 75:1233-1242.
2. Scholten PE, Sierevelt LN, van Dijk CN, Hindfoot endoscopy for posterior ankle impingement. *J Bone Joint Surg Am.* 2008;90:2665-2672.
3. van Dijk CN, van Dyk GE, Sholten PE, Kort NP. Endoscopic calcaneoplasty. *Am J Sports Med.* 2001; 29:185-189.
4. McGillion S, Cann LB. Posterior ankle arthroscopy: indications, limitations and outcomes [abstract]. *J Bone Joint Surg Br.* 2009;91B:211.
5. Willits K, Sonneveld H, Amendola A, et al. Outcome of posterior ankle arthroscopy for hindfoot impingement. *Arthroscopy.* 2008; 24:196-202.
6. Sitler DF, Amendola A, Bailey CS, et al., Posterior ankle arthroscopy: an anatomic study. *J Bone Joint Surg Am.* 2002;84A:763-769.
7. Yodlowski ML, Scheller AD Jr, Minos L. Surgical treatment of Achilles tendinitis by decompression of the retrocalcaneal bursa and the superior calcaneal tuberosity. *Am J Sports Med.* 2002; 30:318-321.
8. Watson AD, Anderson RB, Davis WH. Comparison of results of retrocalcaneal decompression for retrocalcaneal bursitis and insertional Achilles tendinosis with calcific spur. *Foot Ankle Int.* 2000; 21:638-642.
9. Abramowitz Y, Wollstein R, Barzilay Y, et al. Outcome of resection of a symptomatic os trigonum. *J Bone Joint Surg Am.* 2003;85A:1051-1057.
10. Michelson J, Dunn L. Tenosynovitis of the flexor hallucis longus: a clinical study of the spectrum of presentation and treatment. *Foot Ankle Int.* 2005; 26:291-303.

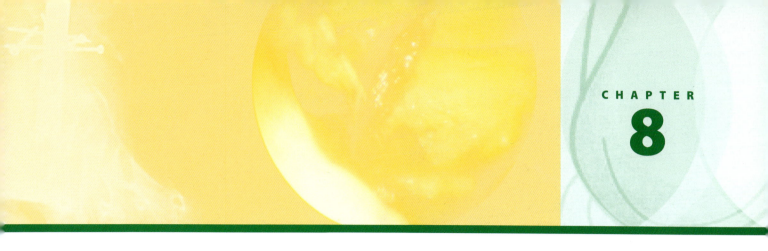

Posterior Ankle Arthroscopy for Conditions Causing Ankle Pain:
Os Trigonum, Posterior Ankle Soft Tissue Impingement, Flexor Hallucis Longus Stenosis, Haglund's Deformity, and Other Considerations

John E. Femino

Posterior ankle arthroscopy is an increasingly used technique that allows the orthopedic surgeon to address a number of causes of posterior ankle pain.[1-4] This minimally invasive technique has several advantages over traditional open surgical approaches to the posterior ankle, which can involve extensive dissection because of the depth of the ankle from the posterior skin. Concerns for wound healing problems in this high-tensile area of skin are minimized by the use of small arthroscopy portals, which often eliminates the need for postoperative immobilization and speeding recovery. One concern with using arthroscopic techniques in the posterior ankle region is the potential for neurovascular injuries.[5] However, with application of good anatomic knowledge of the posterior ankle region and the use of proper technique, this approach has proved to be safe and effective.[3-6] The magnification provided by the arthroscope allows the surgeon to work with greater precision and enhances the safety of the procedure. Several common causes of posterior ankle pain that are readily treated with posterior ankle arthroscopy are described in this chapter.

OS TRIGONUM

Os trigonum syndrome has been described in association with posterior ankle impingement in activities involving extreme plantar flexion, such as classical ballet and soccer. Also, a symptomatic os trigonum can be associated with tenosynovitis of the flexor hallucis longus (FHL) tendon.[7-10]

Normal and Pathologic Anatomy

Symptomatic os trigonum syndrome can be caused by repetitive forced plantar flexion, as seen in ballet dancers and soccer players, although symptoms can arise in other athletes and in nonathletes after acute ankle injuries. The normal talus has a posteromedial and a posterolateral tubercle. The posterolateral tubercle provides attachment for the fibrous component of the beginning of the tunnel for the FHL tendon. An enlarged posterolateral tubercle is called a trigonal process, and one that is separated from the body of the talus is called an os trigonum. Sarrafian summarized four large series totaling 2142 talus specimens, and the incidence of os trigonum ranged from 2.2% to 7.7%.[11] In some cases, an apparent os trigonum may represent nonunion of a fractured trigonal process after forced plantar flexion, but this has no bearing on clinical decision making or treatment.

History and Physical Examination

Athletes with posterior ankle pain due to an os trigonum have complaints similar to those of any patient with posterior ankle impingement; pain is worsened with plantar flexion. Posterior ankle pain can be vague by patient history, and the presence of FHL tenosynovitis can further diffuse the pain sensation. The physical examination finding of tenderness anterior to the Achilles tendon and retrocalcaneal bursa is strongly suggestive of posterior ankle impingement and can be elicited from both the posterolateral and the posteromedial sides of the ankle. This

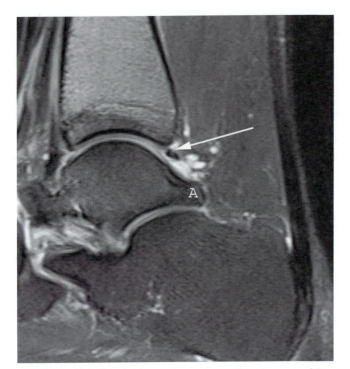

FIGURE 8-1 T2 MRI sagital image shows a large trigonal process of the talus (A), which can also cause posterior impingement like an os trigonum. The posterior soft tissue impingement lesion *(arrow)* is the torn deep component of the posterior tibial-fibular ligament which is shown detached from the posterior tibial plafond. This transverse ligament an displace into the ankle joint.

is particularly true when an unstable os trigonum is present. FHL tenosynovitis adds to the posteromedial tenderness in some cases. Extreme passive plantar flexion can exacerbate the pain, but this increase in pain is not specific for os trigonum, because it can also be found in cases of posterior soft tissue impingement.

Diagnostic Imaging

Radiographs are helpful for demonstrating the presence of an os trigonum or large trigonal process. Magnetic resonance imaging (MRI) is the preferred test for assessing the pathoanatomy of the os trigonum, which is best demonstrated by bone marrow edema of the os trigonum and adjacent talus. MRI is also helpful in differentiating other causes of posterior ankle pain and impingement, such as FHL tenosynovitis, loose bodies, posterior soft tissue impingement, and occult osteochondral lesions (Fig. 8-1).[12] Fluoroscopy can be used to guide injection of the os trigonum for diagnostic purposes.[13] Ultrasound can also be used to assess the pathoanatomy of the posterior ankle.[14]

Indications and Contraindications

Posterior ankle arthroscopy is indicated for patients with unresolved pain from os trigonum impingement. There are no notable contraindications to posterior ankle arthroscopy. The absence of a posterior tibial pulse behind the medial malleolus is an indication to review an MRI to assess the vascular anatomy.

Treatment Options

Conservative Management

Nonoperative treatments may include activity modification, nonsteroidal anti-inflammatory medications, and immobilization for 4 to 8 weeks.

Arthroscopic Technique

The patient is placed in the prone position, and a thigh tourniquet is typically used to avoid tethering of the muscles of the posterior leg. The knees are padded, and a bump is placed anterior to the distal tibia, with the ankle and foot allowed to hang over the end of the table so that the ankle and hallux can be passively dorsiflexed during the procedure. Distraction is not needed, and the arthroscopist can lean against the sole of the foot to increase dorsiflexion, minimizing the need for assistance.

The ankle joint is marked anteriorly by placing a skin marker across the joint line of the dorsiflexed ankle. Two portals are made on either side of the Achilles tendon, 1 to 2 cm inferior to the anterior ankle joint line at approximately the level of the tip of the fibula (Fig. 8-2). This position allows adequate access to the ankle and subtalar joints. Alternatively, fluoroscopy can be used to confirm portal position. After the skin incisions are made, it is essential to use a fine, straight hemostat to spread tissues anterior to the Achilles tendon and make a puncture directly in the midline through the fascia separating the superficial and deep posterior compartments (Figs. 8-3 and 8-4). After this ventral fascia is penetrated, the hemostat is directed laterally and then advanced anteriorly in a posterolateral position behind the ankle. The hemostat can then be spread during removal to open the fascial opening. This is performed from both portals. It is important to maintain this method of placing instruments into the deep posterior compartment. Introducing instruments through this midline fascial opening from the superficial posterior compartment and initially directing instruments laterally protects the posteromedial neurovascular structures (Fig. 8-5).

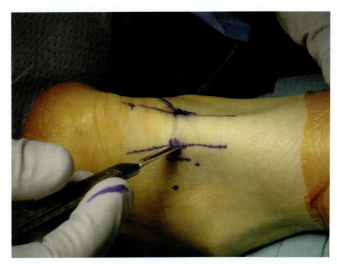

FIGURE 8-2 The incision for posterior ankle arthroscopy portal is made directly next to the Achilles tendon and angled anteriorly toward the midline.

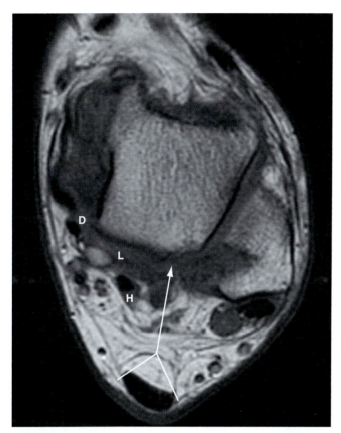

FIGURE 8-3 Axial magnetic resonance imaging the direction of the posterior ankle arthroscopy portals *(white lines and arrow)*. D, flexor digitorum tendon; H, flexor hallucis longus tendon; L, loose body.

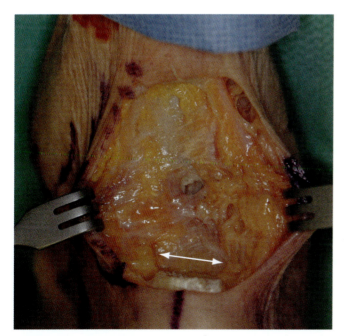

FIGURE 8-4 Cadaver shows a midline fascial opening from the superficial posterior compartment into the deep posterior compartment. The Achilles tendon has been removed *(arrow)*.

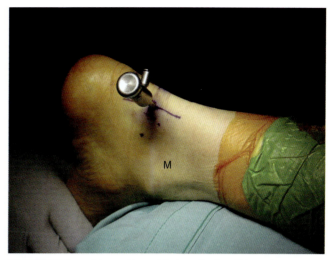

FIGURE 8-5 A medial portal is used for introduction of the arthroscope. Notice that the trocar is directed toward the posterolateral ankle after it has been passed through the midline fascial opening (M) medial malleolus.

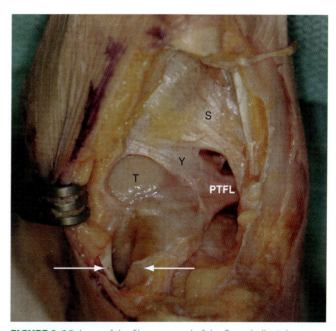

FIGURE 8-6 Release of the fibrous tunnel of the flexor hallucis longus tendon *(arrows)*. PTFL, posterior tibiofibular ligament; S, superficial posterior tibiofibular ligament; T, posterior talar body; Y, tibial slip or intermalleolar ligament.

Initially, the arthroscope is placed through the medial portal and a soft tissue débrider through the lateral portal. Loose connective tissues behind the ankle joint are removed to demonstrate the superficial posterior tibiofibular ligament (PTFL) (Fig. 8-6). The ankle is dorsi and plantar flexed to identify the articular margin, and the os trigonum posterior to this point can then be cleared of lateral soft tissues. Some fibers of the posterior talofibular ligament are attached to the os trigonum, but the remainder of the PTFL attachment onto the talus should be preserved (Fig. 8-7). The subtalar joint is identified, and the clearing of soft tissues around the os trigonum continues, using the joint line of the ankle and subtalar joint as boundaries. Medially, the

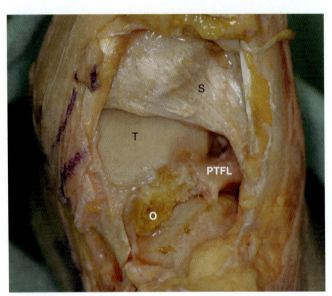

FIGURE 8-7 Surface of the removed trigonal process. Notice the remaining attachment of the posterior tibiofibular ligament (PTFL). S, superficial posterior tibiofibular ligament; T, posterior talar body.

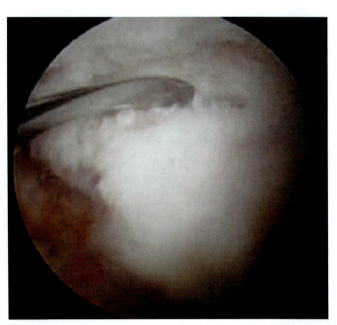

FIGURE 8-9 Freer elevator is used to mobilize the fibrous junction of os trigonum.

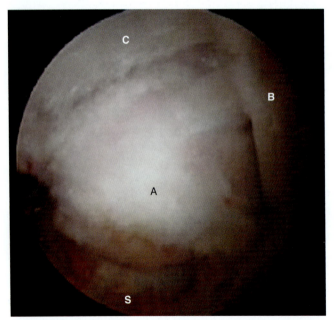

FIGURE 8-8 The arthroscopic view shows the os trigonum (A), flexor hallucis longus tendon (B), torn deep posterior tibiofibular ligament (C), and subtalar joint line (S).

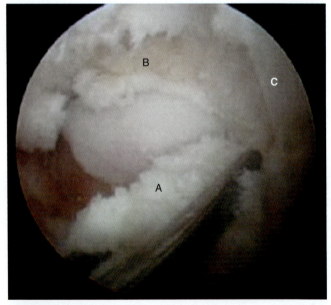

FIGURE 8-10 The arthroscopic view shows a hemostat removing the os trigonum (A), the posterior talus exposed after removal of the os trigonum (B), and the flexor hallucis longus tendon (C).

FHL tendon can be identified by moving the great toe into dorsiflexion. The FHL is used to mark the most medial boundary of the dissection (Fig. 8-8). The proximal attachment of the FHL tunnel is released from the os trigonum, which also serves to release the FHL, relieving any stenosis of the muscle or tendon simultaneously. At this point, the scope should be able to visualize the os trigonum well, and a freer elevator or similar blunt elevator can be used to probe the os and the fibrous junction between the os and the posterior talus (Fig. 8-9). In many cases, this junction can be loosened with a combination of the freer

elevator and the shaver. Alternatively, a bipolar or unipolar cautery device may be used to strip the soft tissues, including the posterior talofibular ligament and the attachment of the FHL tendon sheath, from the os trigonum. After it is free, the os trigonum can be removed with a hemostat through either portal, although the posterolateral portal often works better (Fig. 8-10). It may be necessary to extend the portal enough to allow for the removal of a large os in some cases. Final inspection and débridement of the edges of the excision site can be performed. It is not uncommon for the calcaneal articular surface of the subtalar joint

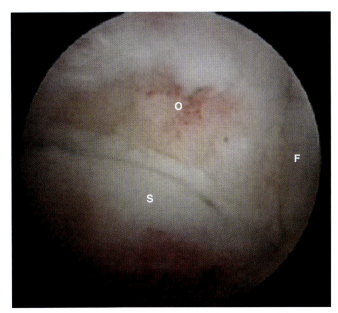

FIGURE 8-11 The posterior talus is exposed after removal of the os trigonum (O). F, flexor hallucis longus tendon; S, calcaneal side of subtalar joint.

to be exposed posteriorly, because the os trigonum often has an articular surface that corresponds to the calcaneal side of the joint (Fig. 8-11).

A word of caution is warranted about the use of an osteotome in cases of partially fused os trigonum or large trigonal processes. The angle achieved with an osteotome is often not steep enough to avoid penetration of the posterior talar body and can extend too far anteriorly, even with extreme dorsiflexion of the ankle joint. A curved osteotome may give a false sense of avoiding this problem. In some cases, it is best to use an arthroscopic burr to remove bony prominences rather than to perform an unintended osteotomy into the talar body. The portals can be closed with 3-0 nonabsorbable suture, and a bulky, soft dressing can be placed.

PEARLS & PITFALLS

- Patient positioning is critical to allow for adequate motion of the ankle and hallux during the procedure. This is accomplished by placing a bump beneath the anterior leg and having the patient's ankle and foot slightly overhanging the end of the table.
- Ankle and calf tourniquets are avoided so that the posterior leg musculature is not tethered by the tourniquet.
- Because of the required precision of the procedure, it is preferable to use general anesthesia so that patient movement will not interfere with the surgery. The prone position makes it impossible to convert to a general anesthetic without repositioning.
- Portal placement and instrument passage, as described earlier, are critical to the success and safety of the procedure. Portals are made on the medial and lateral margins of the Achilles tendon. Blunt spreading though the superficial posterior compartment fascia directly anterior to the Achilles tendon allows access to the deep posterior compartment. Instruments are directed to the posterolateral ankle first, and then work can proceed toward the medial side at the level of the ankle joint.

- The FHL tendon is the medial boundary of all dissection, and motion of the hallux is helpful to locate the FHL.
- The ankle should be dorsiflexed fully if an osteotome is being used to remove an os trigonum. Even with care, it is easy to cut into the talar body. The use of fluoroscopy can help to determine whether the appropriate angle can be achieved. An arthroscopic burr is a good alternative in such cases.
- Large bone fragments may require extension of the lateral portal for removal. If further arthroscopy is needed, the incision can be sutured to maintain fluid pressure.

Postoperative Rehabilitation Protocol

The ankle is dressed with a bulky soft dressing, and weight bearing is allowed as tolerated, usually with crutches for the first week. Active and passive motion of the hallux is encouraged as tolerated. In some cases, a removable cast boot is helpful for early mobilization during the first few weeks. Sutures are usually removed 10 to 14 days after surgery, and rehabilitation is advanced with low-impact aerobic exercises and ankle and hallux dorsiflexion stretches as tolerated. Regaining full active strength of the hallux can sometimes be difficult, and formal physical therapy may be warranted for retraining.

Summary

Posterior ankle arthroscopy is an effective and minimally invasive technique for removal of an os trigonum. The magnification of the arthroscope allows for very precise surgical technique with minimal dissection. The excellent visualization of all of the posterior ankle structures also allows for related pathologies to be evaluated and treated simultaneously. As with all posterior ankle arthroscopic procedures, adhering to the basic rules of portal placement and instrument passage are key to the safety of the technique.

POSTERIOR ANKLE SOFT TISSUE IMPINGEMENT

"Posterior ankle impingement syndrome" was long used as a general phrase to describe posterior ankle pain that is worsened with plantar flexion of the ankle.[15,16] Over time, a more anatomic approach to diagnosing the cause of posterior ankle pain has evolved, and posterior ankle soft tissue impingement is now recognized as a separate, although often associated, condition resulting from posterior bony impingement. Posterior ankle soft tissue impingement results from either a tear of the deep portion of the PTFL from the posterior rim of the tibial plafond or a tear of the posterior portion of the deep deltoid ligament (DDL).[17-19]

Normal and Pathologic Anatomy

The ligaments of the posterior ankle have been well described and are pictured in Figure 8-6.[20] The PTFL is composed of a deep and a superficial component. The superficial fibers are visible from the posterior view and fan out in a superior and medial direction from the fibular attachment to attach broadly on the tibia. The deep portion is a thick band that lies anterior to the superficial ligament and extends across the back of the ankle joint to the medial malleolus. It is not easily seen from the posterior view in an intact

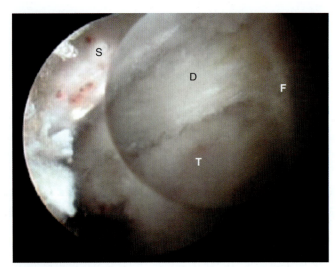

FIGURE 8-12 Posterior soft tissue impingement from torn deep posterior tibiofibular ligament (D). Figure 8-1 is a magnetic resonance image of the same patient. F, flexor hallucis longus tendon; S, superficial posterior tibiofibular ligament; T, talus.

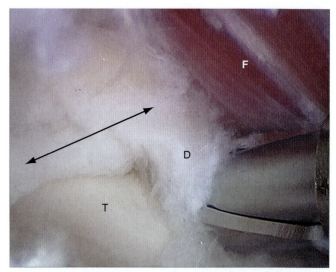

FIGURE 8-14 Débridement of posteromedial soft tissue impingement (D) anterior to the flexor hallucis longus tendon (F). The *arrow* indicates the torn medial side of the deep portion of the posterior tibiofibular ligament. T, talus.

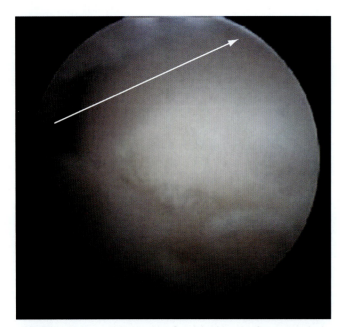

FIGURE 8-13 Posterolateral ankle after débridement of posterior tibial-fibular ligament. The *arrow* indicates the previous location of the unstable ligament.

specimen. The deep band forms a labral rim of the posterior tibial plafond and increases the coverage of the posterior talus.

When the deep band is torn from the attachment on the tibial plafond, it becomes hypermobile and can displace into or out of the ankle joint, creating painful impingement symptoms. If the torn ligament is unstable, it usually lies in an inferior and more posterior position and can then be readily visualized from the posterior arthroscopic view (Fig. 8-12). If posterior impingement is suspected and the ligament is not visualized in this manner, a probe can be passed into the ankle joint and stability can be tested by pulling posteriorly on the ligament to determine whether it is displaced out of the joint. From the anterior ar-

throscopic view, posterior impingement is often not easily visualized with joint distention, but the ligament can be displaced into the ankle joint with posterior pressure, giving clear evidence of the instability and impingement.

After débridement of the unstable deep PTFL is completed, the posterolateral talar dome is well visualized (Fig. 8-13). Posteromedial impingement due to a torn DDL occurs when torn fibers of the ligament remain flipped up into the posteromedial tibiotalar articulation, where the scar tissue mass creates impingement with ankle motion, particularly in plantar flexion. This configuration is not easily visualized on the initial posterior arthroscopic approach, because it lies anterior to the FHL tendon (Fig. 8-14). Often, there is surrounding scar tissue in the area, which can include the PTFL, and this lesion may be visualized only after initial débridement in this area.

History and Physical Examination

Posterior ankle pain that is worsened by plantar flexion is the typical complaint with any posterior impingement problem. An ankle injury involving twisting or hyper-plantar flexion can often precede the onset of pain. The physical examination is consistent with posterior soft tissue impingement when gentle pressure over the back of the ankle recreates the pain experienced with passive plantar flexion. Crepitus or a palpable or audible snap may be appreciated. Posteromedial soft tissue impingement can be difficult to discern from posterior tibial tendonitis, tarsal tunnel syndrome, and FHL tendonitis, but the focal nature of the tenderness and the exacerbation with passive plantar flexion strongly suggest the diagnosis.

Diagnostic Imaging

A lateral radiograph may show an os trigonum or a large trigonal process, which can cause posterior impingement, but the presence of one of these findings does not rule out the possibility of associated soft tissue impingement. MRI has become a very helpful tool in assessing the anatomy of the posterior soft tissues of the an-

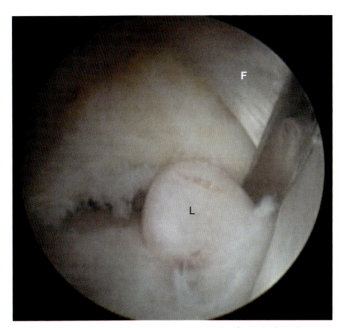

FIGURE 8-15 Loose body (L) seen anterior to the flexor hallucis longus (F). Figure 8-3 shows a magnetic resonance image of the same patient.

kle.[18,21-24] The finding of detachment of the deep PTFL from the plafond on the sagittal MRI views is diagnostic for injury to the ligament and can suggest the degree of displacement possible (see Fig. 8-1). The normal DDL is well visualized on MRI, and injury to it can be clearly detected.[18] A mass of soft tissue resulting from a ligament tear that is displaced can be visualized. Magnetic resonance arthrography may help in some cases to better delineate the anatomy of an impingement lesion and to assess for other pathologies such as loose bodies (Fig. 8-15). Ultrasound has also been described as a useful method of studying the posteromedial ankle and evaluating for impingement. Although it is a growing area of diagnostic radiology, this powerful diagnostic tool remains a specialized skill that requires expert knowledge of foot and ankle anatomy and pathology.[14,18]

Indications and Contraindications

Posterior ankle arthroscopy is indicated for patients with unresolved pain from posterior soft tissue impingement. There are no notable contraindications to posterior ankle arthroscopy. The absence of a posterior tibial pulse behind the medial malleolus is an indication to assess the vascular anatomy on MRI.

Treatment Options

Conservative Management

Rest, ice, anti-inflammatory medications, steroid injections (preferably image guided), and activity modification avoiding forced plantar flexion have been recommended. Casting for 3 to 4 weeks after an acute injury can be considered as for any severe ankle sprain. Taping of the ankle to prevent full plantar flexion can help an athlete return to sport immediately but may not aid the long-term healing.

Arthroscopic Technique

Positioning, portal placement, tourniquet placement, and anesthesia are performed in standard fashion as for a prone ankle arthroscopy. On the initial inspection of the posterolateral ankle, the talus is often obscured by the deep portion of the torn PTFL. When the ligament ruptures from its attachment on the rim of the posterior tibial plafond, it often falls into a more inferior position and lies below the superficial portion of the ligament (see Fig. 8-12). Alternatively, the ligament may be displaced into the ankle joint and can be mobilized with the use of an arthroscopic probe to pull it posteriorly, revealing the instability. The residual attachment to the posterior tibial plafond can be variable, and in some cases the ligament may be attached only at the origin and insertion points. A combination of arthroscopic débriders and cutters is effective to extract the unstable ligament, which usually entails removing the majority of it. Débridement of the tibial slip (intermalleolar ligament) may be necessary in some cases as a part of this débridement (see Figs. 8-6 and 8-7).

Excision of a posteromedial soft tissue impingement lesion is performed by gaining access to the area just anterior to the FHL tendon. If concomitant débridement of the PTFL is required, the medial portion must be débrided simultaneously. An arthroscopic probe can be used to retract the FHL tendon, allowing inspection of the posterior aspect of the medial gutter of the ankle. Normally, the posterior fibers of the DDL can be visualized in their anatomic location and the gutter is clearly visible. If the gutter is obscured by a displaced portion of a torn DDL, a small débrider can be advanced lateral and anterior to the FHL tendon (see Fig. 8-14). I prefer a small end-cutting shaver (2.9 to 3.5 mm) to débride this lesion, because the shaver will be pointing directly at the lesion. One great advantage of the posterior arthroscopic approach for this lesion is that, under the magnification of the arthroscope, a very precise débridement can be performed quite safely, without the morbidity of open dissection in this location. Figure 8-15 shows a small loose body anterior to the FHL tendon that was contributing to posteromedial impingement in this the patient, a football lineman, along with concomitant posterior soft tissue impingement and painful os trigonum (see Figs. 8-8 and 8-12).

PEARLS&PITFALLS

- Initial inspection should determine whether the deep portion of the PTFL is low lying; if not, an arthroscopic probe should be used to determine whether the ligament is unstable and can be displaced posteriorly.
- Posteromedial soft tissue impingement cannot be visualized until the area anterior to the FHL can be visualized.
- An arthroscopic probe or blunt elevator can be used to retract the FHL from the medial portal, and the scope can be used to visualize the lesion from the lateral portal.
- After it is in position, the débrider acts to retract the FHL
- An end-cutting débrider (2.9 to 3.5 mm) allows for efficient removal of the impingement lesion, because the instrument will be pointing straight at the lesion.

Postoperative Rehabilitation Protocol

The ankle is dressed with a bulky soft dressing, and weight bearing is allowed as tolerated, usually with crutches for the first week. In some cases, a removable cast boot is helpful for early mobilization during the first few weeks. Sutures are usually removed 10 to 14 days after surgery, and rehabilitation is advanced with low-impact aerobic exercises and ankle and hallux dorsiflexion stretches are encouraged as tolerated. A night splint is used for the first 4 to 6 weeks to avoid posterior scarring in a plantar-flexed position.

Summary

Posterior ankle soft tissue impingement is readily addressed by posterior arthroscopic treatment. Compared with open surgical débridement, greater precision is possible because of the magnification afforded by the arthroscope, and soft tissue dissection is minimized by avoiding surgical dissection through the medial neurovascular and tendon structures.

FLEXOR HALLUCIS LONGUS STENOSIS

FHL stenosis has been described in relationship to os trigonum impingement.[8,10,24-26] However, understanding of the spectrum of FHL pathology is growing, and recent reports have even suggested a relationship to the genesis of hallux rigidus.[27,28]

Normal and Pathologic Anatomy

The FHL tendon enters a fibro-osseous tunnel that begins behind the talus in a groove formed by the posterolateral and posteromedial tubercles of the talus (see Fig. 8-6).[29] Many symptomatic patients seem to have a primary stenosis of the entrance to the tunnel, caused by a low-lying muscle belly of the flexor hallucis, which creates a tethering of the muscle and chronic irritation of the muscle and surrounding tenosynovium (Fig. 8-16).[8,10,24,26,28] This can be seen in some cases to result in

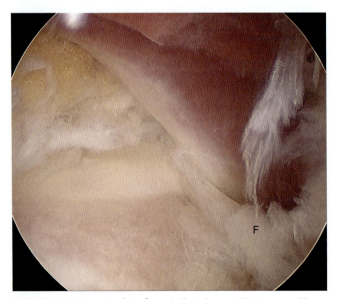

FIGURE 8-16 Stenosis of the flexor hallucis longus (FHL) is caused by a low-lying muscle belly. F, impingement at the fibrous tunnel of the FHL.

atrophy of the chronically compressed distal end of the muscle.[14] The fact that FHL stenosis and os trigonum impingement occur more frequently in ballet dancers and soccer players may have as much to do with the dynamic function of the FHL for the specialized demands of these activities as with the frequent plantar flexion that they require.[30]

History and Physical Examination

The history of FHL stenosis is often closely related to one of the posterior ankle pathologies; however, when found in isolation, it can have a more diffuse presentation. As with other tendinopathies, the symptoms of FHL stenosis can radiate up and down from the location of mechanical irritation. Patients may present with medial rather than posterior ankle pain, and the pain may radiate up the medial calf or behind the ankle or be manifested in the first metatarsophalangeal joint.[8,24,26,28] Physical examination often reveals focal tenderness over the entrance to the FHL tunnel. This tenderness is increased with passive dorsiflexion of the ankle and hallux, which puts the tendon on stretch and delivers the muscle belly more distally, recreating the stenosis. This area can be specifically palpated by placing direct pressure from posterior to anterior, medial to the Achilles tendon and posterior to the tarsal tunnel. The tendon can be confirmed to be directly palpated in most patients, and, with motion of the hallux, the muscle encroachment can be felt and seen as the muscle bulges beneath the skin. Direct palpation from the medial side of the ankle is not sufficient to determine whether the pain results from the posterior tibial nerve or from the FHL. Another finding that suggests FHL stenosis is pseudohallux rigidus, which is loss of passive dorsiflexion of the hallux with ankle dorsiflexion, with support under the first metatarsal head simulating weight bearing.[28]

Diagnostic Imaging

Diagnostic studies for defining FHL stenosis and tenosynovitis include MRI, ultrasonography, and tenography.[14,23,31-33] The value of imaging studies is in their ability to rule out other causes of posteromedial ankle pain and to define causes of posterior ankle pain that may be associated, such as os trigonum or posterior soft tissue impingement. FHL stenosis can be associated with increased fluid around the entrance to the FHL tunnel and surrounding edema, as seen on a T2-weighted sequence in the sagittal or axial views. Although there can be a natural communication with the ankle joint, a discordant amount of fluid on MRI or ultrasonography suggests FHL tendonitis. Dynamic ultrasound studies can reveal the impingement: the normal linear striations of the tapered distal muscle belly become bunched up as it encroaches on the FHL tunnel.[14,31] In some cases, the increased fluid may be seen as far distal as the midfoot, which on MRI is best seen on a coronal image.

Indications and Contraindications

Arthroscopic FHL release is indicated if pain is not relieved after conservative treatment. It is indicated for both isolated cases of FHL stenosis and those cases with other associated pathology of the posterior ankle. If indications for other procedures, such as tarsal tunnel release, are found along with FHL stenosis, an open approach should be chosen. Release of the tarsal tunnel from an endoscopic approach cannot be recommended at this time. The absence of a posterior tibial pulse behind the medial malleolus is an indication to assess the vascular anatomy through MRI review.

Treatment Options

Conservative Management

Nonoperative treatment of FHL tenosynovitis can include specific stretching exercises, a night splint, anti-inflammatory medications, ice, and activity modification or short-term immobilization.[28] If these measures fail to provide satisfactory improvement or relief of pain within 6 to 8 weeks, release of the FHL sheath, with or without distal muscle débridement, can be considered. Ultrasound-guided injections of the tendon sheath have been described,[31] but I do not advocate local steroid injection for this problem.

Arthroscopic Technique

Positioning and portal placement are the same as for any prone ankle arthroscopy procedure, as described previously. The FHL tendon is identified by movement of the hallux, and the amount of stenosis in full passive ankle and hallux dorsiflexion is observed. The degree of muscle débridement required can be considered based on this observation (see Fig. 8-16). The attachment of the fibrous tunnel on the posterolateral tubercle is released with an end-cutting arthroscopic débrider until the subtalar joint is visualized, indicating complete release of the tunnel from the talus (Fig. 8-17). At that point, the FHL is again examined through full passive dorsiflexion, and débridement of any low-lying muscle fibers is carefully performed. The suction on the débrider should be limited so as not to draw the adjacent peri-neural fat into the débrider tip. At the conclusion of the release and débridement, the FHL tendon should move freely through full passive motion, without any muscle impingement on the posterior talus (Fig. 8-18).

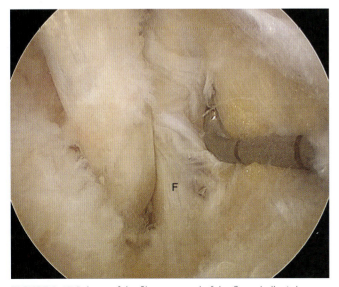

FIGURE 8-17 Release of the fibrous tunnel of the flexor hallucis longus from the posteromedial talus. Notice the transverse orientation of the fibers of the fibrous tunnel (F).

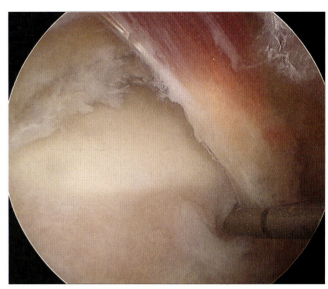

FIGURE 8-18 After release of the fibrous tunnel and débridement of the low-lying flexor hallucis longus (FHL) muscle belly, there is no further stenosis.

PEARLS & PITFALLS

- Positioning is critical to allow for full motion of the ankle and hallux into dorsiflexion.
- The FHL should be approached in typical fashion, by starting with the arthroscopic approach on the posterolateral side of the ankle and working toward the medial side.
- The FHL is identified by moving the hallux into and out of dorsiflexion with the ankle dorsiflexed.
- Initial evaluation of the amount of muscle encroachment is helpful to determine how much muscle needs to be débrided.
- The release of the fibrous tunnel attachment onto the postero-lateral tubercle of the talus begins superiorly and continues inferiorly until the subtalar joint is released.
- Final dynamic examination in full dorsiflexion should be performed to ensure that enough of the distal muscle belly has been resected.
- A small end-cutting débrider (2.9 to 3.5 mm) is helpful, because it will be pointing directly at the FHL tunnel and muscle.
- Care must be taken to not apply too much suction, to avoid taking perineural fat into the débrider.

Postoperative Rehabilitation Protocol

Postoperative treatment consists of a soft compressive dressing and splinting of the ankle in neutral position in a removable cast boot. Full weight bearing is allowed and encouraged. Early active and passive motion is important for regaining FHL function. It is not uncommon for the patient to experience FHL weakness and a sense of loss of active control in the early postoperative period. Formal physical therapy can be helpful to retrain and strengthen the joint. A night splint may be used for several months or until full function returns and is helpful to avoid postoperative scarring in equinus during sleep.

Summary

Posterior ankle arthroscopy is a safe and effective method for releasing the FHL tunnel and relieving FHL stenosis.[4,34,35] Minimal dissection allows for early return to function and less risk of wound problems. Associated pathology of the posterior ankle can be effectively treated simultaneously.

HAGLUND'S DEFORMITY

Posterior heel pain is related to a number of pathologies involving the Achilles tendon and its insertion.[36] Insertional problems of the Achilles tendon include painful impingement of the tendon and associated bursitis over a prominence of the posterior-superior calcaneal tuberosity (Fig. 8-19). Haglund described a case of excision of this prominent bone and proposed impingement of the bone on the Achilles tendon as the etiology of retrocalcaneal bursitis. He recommended removal of the bony prominence in addition to excision of the bursa, which was advocated as sole treatment of the problem at that time.[37] Essentially the same treatment was performed by various open approaches for the remainder of the 20th century. Several investigators have reported uniformly good results and few complications for the endoscopic excision of this bony impingement and bursa.[38-44]

Normal and Pathologic Anatomy

The upper third of the posterior surface of the calcaneus is composed of a pre-Achilles fibrocartilaginous bursal surface; the lower

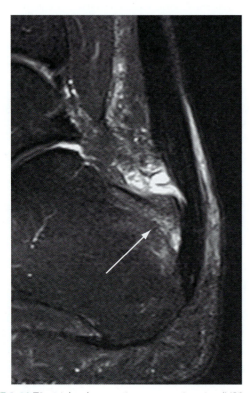

FIGURE 8-19 T2-weighted magnetic resonance imaging (MRI) shows bone marrow edema within the Haglund deformity *(arrow)*. High signal intensity superior and posterior to the bony prominence demonstrates the MRI finding of bursitis. Some degenerative changes with intermediate signal intensity changes in the Achilles tendon are seen in the area of impingement.

two thirds of the posterior calcaneal surface provides insertion for the Achilles tendon.[45] Prominence of the bony surface of the upper third of this surface creates an impingement syndrome of the Achilles tendon which has been associated with tight shoes and hard heel counters. Associated bursal inflammation and Achilles tendon degeneration are the result of the chronic mechanical impingement.

History and Physical Examination

A history of posterior heel pain is nonspecific, but the association of pain with tight closed-heel shoes is an indication of insertional Achilles tendon problems. Patients often state that only open-heel sandals or clogs are comfortable. A visible prominence is typically seen, although thickening of the Achilles insertion and intratendinous calcification can also account for posterior prominence in cases of more advanced tendon degeneration at the insertion. Physical examination reveals tenderness over the Achilles tendon above the insertion and over a more superior prominence. Tenderness just anterior to the Achilles tendon indicates bursitis, which is commonly associated.

Diagnostic Imaging

A lateral radiograph of the calcaneus may reveal a large bony prominence and intratendinous calcifications and may be helpful for surgical planning, especially if intraoperative fluoroscopy is used to judge resection of bone. MRI and ultrasonography can be helpful to determine the degree of tendon degeneration and bursal inflammation (see Fig. 8-19).

Indications and Contraindications

Endoscopic débridement of a Haglund deformity is indicated if nonoperative treatment has failed to relieve pain (reported in 10% to 50% of cases).[39,42,46,47] Endoscopic treatment of posterior Achilles pathology is not indicated in cases where extensive tendinosis requires direct surgical débridement of the Achilles insertion with detachment and reattachment. However, Achilles tendinosis can be treated by percutaneous longitudinal tenotomy, which may extend the use of minimally invasive surgery in some cases.

Treatment Options

Conservative Management

Conservative treatment has been reported to be successful in 50% to 90% of cases of posterior heel pain; it may be less effective in cases of significant bony impingement.[46,48] Achilles tendon stretching, night splints, gel pads, footwear modification, ice, anti-inflammatory medications, relative rest, immobilization, and injections have been reported to be of benefit. Steroid injections may help with pain caused by inflammation but are believed to carry a risk of weakening the Achilles tendon, potentially leading to rupture. If steroids are used, temporary immobilization for several weeks could help prevent tendon rupture. I do not recommend steroid injections around the Achilles tendon.

Endoscopic Technique

The technique of endoscopic Haglund resection has been described by several authors.[38,39,41-44] Both supine and prone positions have been suggested. I prefer the supine position, because the most pos-

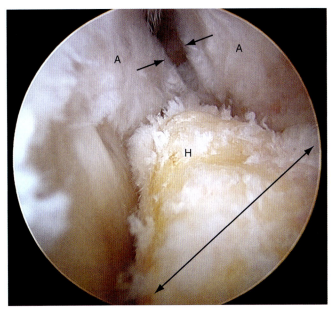

FIGURE 8-20 Endoscopic view of a Haglund deformity (H) of the same patient as in Figure 8-19. The line of resection is indicated by a *long arrow*. The *short arrows* demonstrate the location of the portal through the medial side of the U-shaped Achilles tendon insertion (A). This location allows for a direct line of action for the burr to débride down to the top of the central tendon insertion.

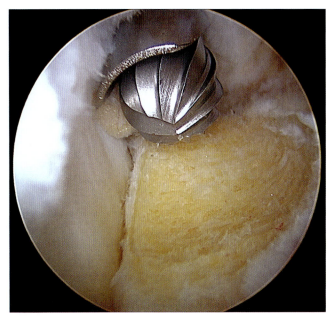

FIGURE 8-22 Arthroscopic view of the favorable working direction for the burr allowed by portal placement through the sides of the Achilles insertion.

terior portion of the resection is more ergonomically reached. Although it has been recommended to place the medial and lateral portals anterior to the tendon, I prefer to place them just anterior to the anterior surface of the central tendon, passing through the medial and lateral margins of the U-shaped insertion and directly into the pre-Achilles space (Figs. 8-20 and 8-21).[49] The advantage of this position is that it allows the arthroscopic burr to easily pass parallel to the tendon insertion, creating a flush surface across the entire posterior calcaneus (Fig. 8-22). The initial débridement of the bursa and fibrofatty tissue dorsal to the calcaneal tuberosity al-

lows for exposure of the Haglund deformity. After the soft tissues are cleared, the arthroscopic burr is used to remove all of the impinging bone. A fluoroscope can be used to confirm satisfactory resection of bone compared to the preoperative radiographs, and this can be compared with visual inspection (Fig. 8-23). Percutaneous longitudinal tenotomy can be used to treat associated degen-

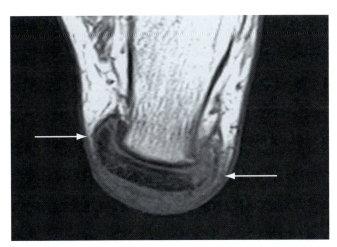

FIGURE 8-21 T1-weighted magnetic resonance image shows the U-shaped insertion of the Achilles insertion *(arrows)*. Portal placements through the sides of this insertion provide for direct access across the bony deformity. This enables precise débridement with an arthroscopic burr up to the margin of the central Achilles tendon insertion.

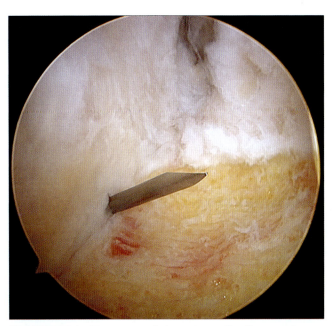

FIGURE 8-23 An 18-gauge needle is used to confirm fluoroscopic assessment of débridement with the arthroscopic appearance.

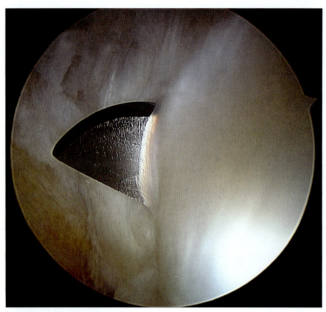

FIGURE 8-24 Longitudinal tenotomy through the area of tendinosis is performed under direct visualization. Several parallel incisions are made.

erative Achilles tendon with visualization through the arthroscope (Fig. 8-24).[50] Nonabsorbable sutures are used to close the portals, and a bulky soft dressing is used with a removable cast boot for immediate weight bearing. There should be no real risk of compromise to the tendon insertion, because the scope allows precise débridement up to the beginning of the tendon insertion. Elevation is encouraged for the first 48 hours to diminish the risk of significant bone bleeding postoperatively.

PEARLS&**PITFALLS**

- Supine position is more ergonomic for débridement of the most posterior portion of the bony impingement adjacent to the Achilles insertion.
- Adequate clearance of the foot from the bed facilitates use of instruments and the arthroscope.
- Posterior portal placement is advantageous for débridement adjacent to the tendon with the burr being parallel to the anterior tendon surface.
- Fluoroscopy may be helpful to judge the extent of bone excision.

Postoperative Rehabilitation Protocol

Because the insertion of the Achilles tendon is not compromised by an endoscopic approach for excision of the bony prominence, immediate partial weight bearing is allowed with crutches for comfort. In some cases, a short period in a removable cast boot facilitates mobilization. A night splint is used to avoid equinus. Physical therapy may begin 1 week after surgery, after the portals have become well sealed. A program of graduated strengthening and stretching is progressed over 4 to 6 weeks, and low-impact aerobic exercises, which can include pool therapy, are begun after the sutures are removed at about 2 weeks. Jogging on a treadmill is allowed as tolerated after 6 to 8 weeks, depending on whether

percutaneous tenotomy was performed. Unrestricted athletic activity is allowed after 10 to 12 weeks.[41,44] A maintenance program for stretching and focused strengthening of the soleus muscle is instituted for the next 6 months. A heel lift can be used during the first 6 weeks if the patient has a tight heel cord, but this does not obviate the need for a good preoperative and postoperative stretching program.[39]

Summary

Endoscopic excision of Haglund's deformity is a safe and minimally invasive alternative to traditional open Haglund excision techniques. The return to sporting activities is usually shorter, and the risk of complications, including wound complications, is lower.[38,39,41,44]

OTHER CONSIDERATIONS

The treatment of posterior talar osteochondral lesions is possible through posterior ankle arthroscopy, provided they are far enough posterior. This is not typical for most posteromedial osteochondral lesions and the available literature is limited. One concern is that drilling such a lesion can be done safely only through the posterolateral portal, and an alternative transosseous approach cannot be done at favorable angle because of the posterior slope of the talus. In the future, specialized instruments to allow protected drilling from a posteromedial approach may make this feasible without significant risk to the neurovascular and tendinous structures at the posteromedial ankle.

REFERENCES

1. Jerosch J. Subtalar arthroscopy—indications and surgical technique. *Knee Surg Sports Traumatol Arthrosc.* 1998;6:122-128.
2. Van Dijk CN, Van Bergen CJ. Advancements in ankle arthroscopy. *J Am Acad Orthop Surg.* 2008;16:635-646.
3. Scholten PE, Sierevelt IN, Van Dijk CN. Hindfoot endoscopy for posterior ankle impingement. *J Bone Joint Surg Am.* 2008;90:2665-2672.
4. Willits K, Sonneveld H, Amendola A, et al. Outcome of posterior ankle arthroscopy for hindfoot impingement. *Arthroscopy.* 2008;24:196-202.
5. Keeling JJ, Guyton GP. Endoscopic flexor hallucis longus decompression: a cadaver study. *Foot Ankle Int.* 2007;28:810-814.
6. Phisitkul P, Junko JT, Femino JE, et al. Technique of prone ankle and subtalar arthroscopy. *Tech Foot Ankle Surg.* 2007;6:30-37.
7. Bruns J, Eggers-Stroder G. [Os trigonum syndrome]. *Sportverletz Sportschaden.* 1991;5:155-158.
8. Hamilton WG, Geppert MJ, Thompson FM. Pain in the posterior aspect of the ankle in dancers: differential diagnosis and operative treatment. *J Bone Joint Surg Am.* 1996;78:1491-1500.
9. Iovane A, Midiri M, Finazzo M, et al. [Os trigonum tarsi syndrome: role of magnetic resonance]. *Radiol Med.* 2000;99:36-40.
10. Kolettis GJ, Micheli LJ, Klein JD. Release of the flexor hallucis longus tendon in ballet dancers. *J Bone Joint Surg Am.* 1996;78:1386-1390.
11. Sarrafian SK, ed. *Anatomy of the Foot and Ankle: Descriptive, Topographic, Functional.* 2nd ed. Philadelphia, PA: JB Lippincott; 1993:47-55.
12. Sanders TG, Rathur SK. Impingement syndromes of the ankle. *Magn Reson Imaging Clin North Am.* 2008;16:29-38, v.
13. Jones DM, Saltzman CL, El-Khoury G. The diagnosis of the os trigonum syndrome with a fluoroscopically controlled injection of local anesthetic. *Iowa Orthop J.* 1999;19:122-126.
14. Femino JE, Jacobson JA, Craig CL, Kuhns LR. Dynamic ultrasound of the foot and ankle: adult and pediatric applications. *Tech Foot Ankle Surg.* 2007;6:50-61.
15. Hedrick MR, McBryde AM. Posterior ankle impingement. *Foot Ankle Int.* 1994;15:2-8.
16. Henderson I, La Valette D. Ankle impingement: combined anterior and posterior impingement syndrome of the ankle. *Foot Ankle Int.* 2004; 25:632-638.

17. Jaivin JS, Ferkel RD. Arthroscopy of the foot and ankle. *Clin Sports Med.* 1994;13:761-783.

18. Koulouris G, Connell D, Schneider T, Edwards W. Posterior tibiotalar ligament injury resulting in posteromedial impingement. *Foot Ankle Int.* 2003;24:575-583.

19. Liu SH, Mirzayan R. Posteromedial ankle impingement. *Arthroscopy.* 1993;9:709-711.

20. Sarrafian SK, ed. *Anatomy of the Foot and Ankle: Descriptive, Topographic, Functional.* 2nd ed. Philadelphia, PA: JB Lippincott; 1993:159-165, 174-186.

21. Bureau NJ, Cardinal E, Hobden R, Aubin B. Posterior ankle impingement syndrome: MR imaging findings in seven patients. *Radiology.* 2000; 215:497-503.

22. Lee JC, Calder JD, Healy JC. Posterior impingement syndromes of the ankle. *Semin Musculoskelet Radiol.* 2008;12:154-169.

23. Robinson P. Impingement syndromes of the ankle. *Eur Radiol.* 2007; 17:3056-3065.

24. Hamilton WG. Stenosing tenosynovitis of the flexor hallucis longus tendon and posterior impingement upon the os trigonum in ballet dancers. *Foot Ankle.* 1982;3:74-80.

25. Marotta JJ, Micheli LJ. Os trigonum impingement in dancers. *Am J Sports Med.* 1992;20:533-536.

26. Sammarco GJ, Cooper PS. Flexor hallucis longus tendon injury in dancers and nondancers. *Foot Ankle Int.* 1998;19:356-362.

27. Kirane YM, Michelson JD, Sharkey NA. Contribution of the flexor hallucis longus to loading of the first metatarsal and first metatarsophalangeal joint. *Foot Ankle Int.* 2008;29:367-377.

28. Michelson J, Dunn L. Tenosynovitis of the flexor hallucis longus: a clinical study of the spectrum of presentation and treatment. *Foot Ankle Int.* 2005;26:291-303.

29. Sarrafian SK, ed. *Anatomy of the Foot and Ankle: Descriptive, Topographic, Functional.* 2nd ed. Philadelphia, PA: JB Lippincott; 1993:171, 174.

30. Femino JE, Trepman E, Chisholm K, Razzano L. The role of the flexor hallucis longus and peroneus longus in stabilization of the ballet foot. *J Dance Med Sci.* 2000;4:86-89.

31. Mehdizade A, Adler RS. Sonographically guided flexor hallucis longus tendon sheath injection. *J Ultrasound Med.* 2007;26:233-237.

32. Na JB, Bergman AG, Oloff LM, Beaulieu CF. The flexor hallucis longus: tenographic technique and correlation of imaging findings with surgery in 39 ankles. *Radiology.* 2005;236:974-982.

33. Peace KA, Hillier JC, Hulme A, Healy JC. MRI features of posterior ankle impingement syndrome in ballet dancers: a review of 25 cases. *Clin Radiol.* 2004;59:1025-1033.

34. Lui TH. Arthroscopy and endoscopy of the foot and ankle: indications for new techniques. *Arthroscopy.* 2007;23:889-902.

35. Van Dijk CN. Hindfoot endoscopy for posterior ankle pain. *Instruct Course Lect.* 2006;55:545-554.

36. Clain MR, Baxter DE. Achilles tendinitis. *Foot Ankle.* 1992;13:482-487.

37. Haglund P. Beitrag zur Klinik der Achillessehne. *Zeitschr Orthop Chir.* 1928;49:49-58.

38. Jerosch J, Schunck J, Sokkar SH. Endoscopic calcaneoplasty (ECP) as a surgical treatment of Haglund's syndrome. *Knee Surg Sports Traumatol Arthrosc.* 2007;15:927-934.

39. Leitze Z, Sella EJ, Aversa JM. Endoscopic decompression of the retrocalcaneal space. *J Bone Joint Surg Am.* 2003;85:1488-1496.

40. Lohrer H, Nauck T, Dorn NV, Konerding MA. Comparison of endoscopic and open resection for Haglund tuberosity in a cadaver study. *Foot Ankle Int.* 2006;27:445-450.

41. Morag G, Maman E, Arbel R. Endoscopic treatment of hindfoot pathology. *Arthroscopy.* 2003;19:E13-E13.

42. Van Dijk CN. Anterior and posterior ankle impingement. *Foot Ankle Clin.* 2006;11:663-683.

43. Van Dijk CN, Van Dyk GE, Scholten PE, Kort NP. Endoscopic calcaneoplasty. *Am J Sports Med.* 2001;29:185-189.

44. Ortmann FW, McBryde AM. Endoscopic bony and soft-tissue decompression of the retrocalcaneal space for the treatment of Haglund deformity and retrocalcaneal bursitis. *Foot Ankle Int.* 2007;28:149-153.

45. Sarrafian S, ed. *Anatomy of the Foot and Ankle: Descriptive, Topographic, Functional,* 2nd ed. JB Lippincott; 1993:60-65.

46. Davis PF, Severud E, Baxter DE. Painful heel syndrome: results of nonoperative treatment. *Foot Ankle Int.* 1994;15:531-535.

47. McGarvey WC, Palumbo RC, Baxter DE, Leibman BD. Insertional Achilles tendinosis: surgical treatment through a central tendon splitting approach. *Foot Ankle Int.* 2002;23:19-25.

48. Sammarco GJ, Taylor AL. Operative management of Haglund's deformity in the nonathlete: a retrospective study. *Foot Ankle Int.* 1998;19: 724-729.

49. Lohrer H, Arentz S, Nauck T, et al. The Achilles tendon insertion is crescent-shaped: an in vitro anatomic investigation. *Clin Orthop Relat Res.* 2008;466:2230-2237.

50. Maffulli N, Testa V, Capasso G, et al. Results of percutaneous longitudinal tenotomy for Achilles tendinopathy in middle- and long-distance runners. *Am J Sports Med.* 1997;25:835-840.

Instability of the Ankle and Subtalar Joints

Sameh A. Labib ● John Louis-Ugbo ● Jordan L. Goldstein

Ankle sprains are the most common sports-related injuries, and they account for almost 10% of emergency department visits. Most ankle sprains are inversion-type sprains that injure the lateral ankle ligaments. Chronic lateral ankle instability develops in 20% to 30% of patients after acute ankle sprains despite adequate nonoperative treatment.[1] The cause of chronic lateral ankle instability after ankle injury is not well understood and is probably multifactorial. Symptoms may result from inadequately healed torn ligaments or ligaments that have healed in a stretched manner.[2] Generalized hyperlaxity, strength and proprioception deficits are likely contributing factors.

ANKLE INSTABILITY

Anatomy and Physiology

Stability of the ankle joint depends on the contributions of bony architecture, ligamentous attachments, and the dynamic stability provided by muscles around the ankle.[3] The ankle is a composite joint that includes the distal tibiofibular syndesmosis and a diarthrodial mortise between the distal tibia and fibula and the talus. The subtalar joint provides sagittal rotation about a single oblique axis, from the neck of the talus to the lateral wall of the calcaneus. In the coronal plane, the axis of the ankle runs medial cephalad to lateral caudad, with a mean angulation of 82 ± 4 degrees in relation to the tibia (Fig. 9-1).

The ankle joint axis tends to change throughout the functional arc range of motion from dorsiflexion to plantar flexion. The distal fibula moves distally with weight bearing, deepening the mortise and increasing ankle stability. The talus is not as well contained by the mortise during plantar flexion compared with dorsiflexion, because the talus is wider anteriorly than posteriorly. The dorsal surface of the talus has a slight longitudinal groove that corresponds to a longitudinal ridge on the tibial plafond. The ridge and groove help to confer transverse plane stability to the tibiotalar joint. The distal fibula gives attachment to the

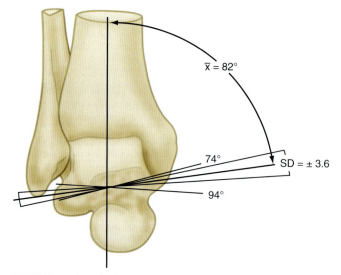

FIGURE 9-1 The subtalar joint provides sagittal rotation about a single oblique axis from the neck of the talus to the lateral wall of the calcaneus. In the coronal plane, the axis of the ankle runs medial cephalad to lateral caudad, with a mean angulation of 82 ± 4 degrees in relation to the tibia.

lateral ligaments of the ankle joint, and its posterior aspect is grooved to accept the tendons of the peroneus longus and peroneus brevis muscles.[4] Bony anatomic variations may contribute to increased ankle instability. For example, Scranton and colleagues showed that the fibula is located more posterior in patients with instability.[5] One study compared hindfoot varus measurements on computed tomography (CT) scans of patients with lateral ankle instability to those of patients without instability and found a statistically significant increased amount of varus in patients with instability.[6]

The ankle ligaments provide supplemental stability to the ankle and also contribute to hindfoot stability. Ligaments of the ankle joint include the syndesmotic ligaments, the deltoid ligament complex, and the lateral collateral ligaments. The syndesmotic ligaments include the anterior inferior and posterior inferior tibiofibular ligaments and the strong interosseous ligament.

The deltoid ligament is formed by four to six main ligaments on the medial side. Four of these are always constant; from anterior to posterior, they are the anterior tibiotalar ligament (ATTL), the tibionavicular ligament (TNL), the calcaneotibial ligament (CTL), and the posterior tibiotalar ligament (PTTL). Occasionally, calcaneonavicular and tibiospring ligaments can be part of the deltoid ligament. The deltoid ligament includes superficial and deep parts. The superficial ligaments cross two joints, namely the ankle and the subtalar joints. The deep ligaments cross only the ankle joint, though the demarcation is not always absolutely clear.[3,7] The deltoid ligament is the primary restraint against pronation and abduction of the talus, with the superficial and deep components equally effective.[7]

The lateral ankle joint ligamentous complex provides primary restraint to inversion and consists primarily of three structures: the anterior talofibular ligament (ATFL), the calcaneofibular ligament (CFL), and the posterior talofibular ligament (PTFL) (Fig. 9-2). Intimate knowledge of the anatomy is paramount to the success of surgical reconstruction. The ATFL, which is possibly a thickening of the joint capsule, is the most anterior structure. It averages about 24.8 mm in length and 7 mm in width and is the weakest and most easily injured of the ankle ligaments (Fig. 9-3). It originates about 10 mm proximal to the tip of the fibula and inserts on the lateral aspect of the talus, on average 18 mm superior to the subtalar joint.[3,7,8] The ATFL courses obliquely from posterolateral to anteromedial with respect to the tibiotalar joint. It resists internal rotation of the talus as well as anterior translation. The CFL is a round,

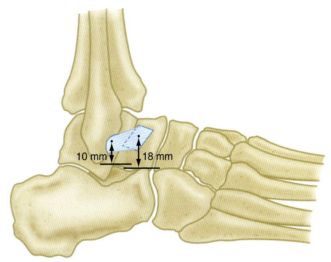

FIGURE 9-3 The anterior talofibular ligament (ATFL), which is possibly a thickening of the joint capsule, is the most anterior structure. It has an average length of about 24.8 mm and width of 7 mm, and it is the weakest and most easily injured of the ankle ligaments.

cordlike, extracapsular structure that originates from the inferior medial surface of the distal fibula. It extends posteroinferiorly, deep to the peroneal tendons, and attaches on a small tubercle on the lateral calcaneal surface, on average 13 mm inferior to the subtalar joint and posterior to the long axis of the fibula.[3] It is about 35.8 mm long and 5.3 mm wide (Fig. 9-4). The CFL is vertical and coplanar with the fibula at 10 to 20 degrees of ankle dorsiflexion. In that position, it resists inversion and becomes the primary ankle stabilizer and a secondary subtalar joint stabilizer.[8,9]

Isolated rupture of the PTFL is rare because it is the strongest and least vulnerable of the lateral ankle ligaments. The PTFL originates from the posterior portion of the distal fibula and in-

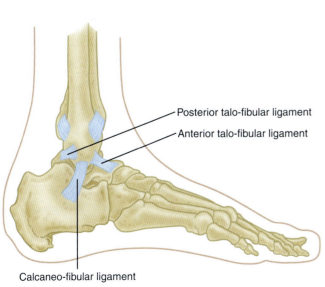

FIGURE 9-2 The lateral ankle joint ligamentous complex provides primary restraint to inversion and consists primarily of three structures: the anterior talofibular ligament (ATFL), the calcaneofibular ligament (CFL), and the posterior talofibular ligament (PTFL).

Posterior talo-fibular ligament
Anterior talo-fibular ligament
Calcaneo-fibular ligament

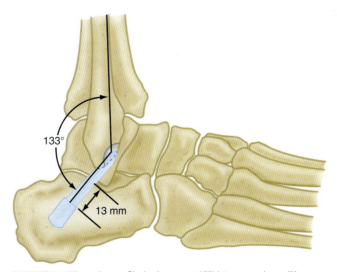

FIGURE 9-4 The calcaneofibular ligament (CFL) is a round, cordlike, extracapsular structure that originates from the inferior medial surface of the distal fibula. It extends posteroinferiorly, deep to the peroneal tendons, and attaches on a small tubercle on the lateral calcaneal surface, on average 13 mm inferior to the subtalar joint and posterior to the long axis of the fibula. It is about 35.8 mm long and 5.3 mm wide.

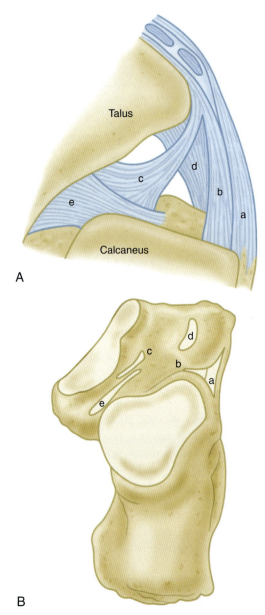

FIGURE 9-5 The lateral subtalar joint is further stabilized by the interosseous talocalcaneal ligament (ITCL), the cervical ligament, the inferior extensor retinaculum, and the lateral talocalcaneal ligament (LTCL).

serts onto the lateral tubercle of talus posteriorly. It may be injured in combination with rupture of the ATFL and CFL in severe ankle sprains and ankle dislocations.[7,10] The lateral subtalar joint is further stabilized by the interosseous talocalcaneal ligament (ITCL), the cervical ligament, the inferior extensor retinaculum, and the lateral talocalcaneal ligament (LTCL) (Fig. 9-5). In a biomechanical study, Tochigi and Amendola showed the ITCL to be the main stabilizer of the subtalar joint.[11]

The musculotendinous units that cross the ankle joint provide secondary or dynamic stability to the ankle and hindfoot. The most important of these are the laterally positioned peroneal tendons, which are the primary evertors of the ankle[12]; the tibialis posterior tendon; and the toe flexors medially. In a cadaveric study, Hatch and Labib demonstrated that the peroneal tendons, along with the superior peroneal retinaculum (SPR), provide static resistance to anterior talar displacement with the ankle in neutral position. In that study, sectioning of the retinaculum and removal of the tendons caused an average increase of 15% in anterior ankle displacement, indicating that the peroneal tendons may impart some static stability to the ankle joint.[13] This finding may explain the increased incidence of peroneal tendon problems in patients with chronic ankle instability.

Mechanisms of Chronic Lateral Ankle Instability

When the ankle is dorsiflexed, the talus fits snugly into the mortise and the ATFL is loose, but when the foot is plantar flexed, the ATFL becomes vertical and serves as the primary stabilizing structure of the ankle in inversion. Injury to the ATFL occurs with inversion of a plantar-flexed ankle with or without internal rotation. Commonly, the CFL is injured in combination with injury to the ATFL. Injures to the CFL occur with inversion of a dorsiflexed ankle. Subtalar ligament injury may be in continuum with a CFL injury. It has been shown that rupture of the ATFL occurs as an isolated injury in 50% to 75% of cases. With increasing force, the CFL also is ruptured. A rupture of the ATFL and the CFL occurs in 15% to 25% of cases. Isolated rupture of the CFL happens in approximately 1% of patients, and injury to the PTFL is extremely rare.[8-10,14] Isolated ligament injuries of the deltoid ligament are infrequent.

Chronic lateral ankle instability results when the injured ligaments do not regain the mechanical integrity necessary to stabilize the ankle against physiologic stress. Possible risk factors for ankle instability that have been implicated in the literature include (1) environmental factors, such as the condition of the playing field, the level of neuromuscular training, the position an athlete plays, and the available equipment[15] and (2) a patient's unique anatomy, including variations in ankle anatomy, multiligamentous laxity, limitation of ankle range of motion, a history of recurrent ankle sprain, diminished muscle strength, poor postural control and proprioception, and delayed muscle reaction time.[16] A varus tibial plafond alignment, a varus hindfoot alignment, and a posterior fibular position have also been proposed as possible predisposing factors in chronic ankle instability.[17]

Chronic lateral instability of the ankle usually manifests as a mechanical or a functional instability. Mechanical instability is objective abnormal motion of the talus relative to the ankle mortise, as measured on standardized stress radiographs or by clinical measurement of an anterior drawer sign or varus tilt.[7,15] Functional instability is manifested as a symptomatic feeling of the ankle's repeatedly giving way, combined with pain and difficulty walking on uneven terrain. Functional instability is most likely caused by increased laxity of the injured ligaments, inhibition of proprioceptive function, peroneal muscle weakness, or a combination of these factors.[7,15] Some patients manifest functional instability without the mechanical components or vice-versa.

PATIENT EVALUATION

History and Physical Examination

Patients with chronic lateral ankle instability usually present with a classic history of recurrent inversion sprain or giving way with lateral ankle pain and swelling that improves between episodes. Patients complain of difficulty on uneven terrain, most notably at night. Persistent ankle pain or mechanical locking usually indicates an intra-articular process such as chondral damage, synovitis, or loose body formation.

Physical examination should include an evaluation of gait, generalized laxity, and hindfoot varus malalignment (Fig. 9-6). Proprioception testing is done by asking the patient to balance on the affected foot (single leg balance) or to perform a single leg jump-landing test with comparison to the contralateral side.[18] Local ankle examination is often positive for tenderness to palpation over the affected ligaments with guarding, apprehension, and peroneal weakness.[19]

Clinical stress testing, including the talar tilt test and the anterior drawer test, may lead to the confirmation of a diagnosis of chronic ankle instability secondary to ligamentous insufficiency. The anterior drawer test is used to assess the ATFL. The talar tilt test evaluates the integrity of the CFL (Fig. 9-7). The talar tilt test also assesses subtalar instability in symptomatic patients. Thermann and colleagues described a provocative test for subtalar instability in which a varus stress to the calcaneus is applied with the ankle in 10 degrees of dorsiflexion and the talus locked in the ankle mortise. Subtalar pain or instability is considered a positive result.[20]

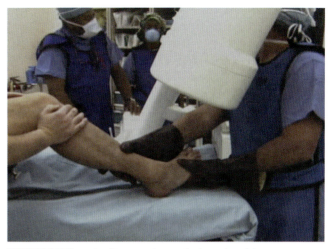

FIGURE 9-7 The talar tilt test evaluates the integrity of the calcaneofibular ligament (CFL).

Diagnostic Imaging

Radiographic evaluation of chronic ankle and subtalar instability is very important in ruling out the other differential diagnoses of chronic ankle pain. Plain radiographs in the standing position are used to evaluate hindfoot varus (Saltzman hindfoot view),[21] talus osteochondral lesions, or concomitant fractures. The Os subfibulare is nonunion of a distal fibula avulsion fracture of the ATFL insertion that may require repair (Fig. 9-8).

Radiographic tests of laxity demonstrating lateral instability (talar tilt test) and anterior instability (anterior talar translation tests) are pivotal in the objective assessment of ankle instability. These become even more pronounced and informative when performed with the patient under anesthesia (Fig. 9-9AR). How much talar translation or varus tilt is abnormal is a subject of much debate, with a wide range of values described in the literature.[4,22] However, a reasonable guideline is an absolute tibiotalar anterior translation of greater than 10 mm, or greater than 3 mm more than the opposite

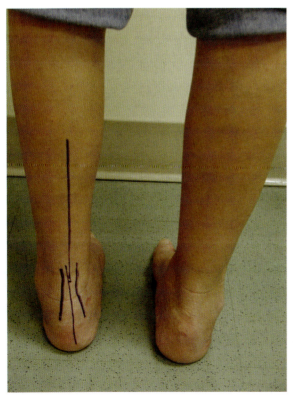

FIGURE 9-6 Physical examination should include an evaluation of gait, generalized laxity, and hindfoot varus malalignment (left foot).

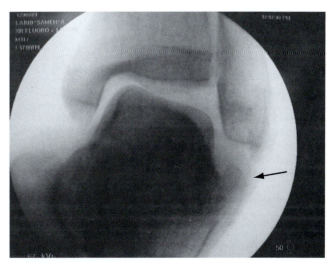

FIGURE 9-8 Os subfibulare is a nonunion of a distal fibula avulsion fracture of the anterior talofibular ligament (ATFL) insertion that may require repair.

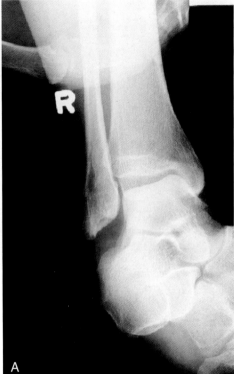

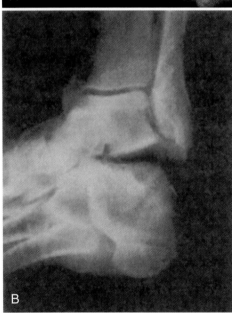

FIGURE 9-9 A, Radiographic tests of laxity demonstrating lateral instability (talar tilt test) and R, anterior instability (anterior talar translation tests) are pivotal in the objective assessment of ankle instability. These become even more pronounced and informative when performed with the patient under anesthesia. A 30-degree cephalad view of a talar tilt stress test (Broden's view) is used to assess subtalar instability.

normal ankle. A varus talar tilt angle greater than 15 degrees on the affected side, or 10 degrees more than the normal side, is considered positive for chronic ankle instability.[4] A 30-degree cephalad view of a talar tilt stress test or a Broden view is used to assess subtalar instability (see Fig. 9-9). MRI examination has proved essential in the preoperative evaluation of ankle instability and ligament visualization. Concomitant talus osteochondral lesions, intra-articular im-

pingement, or peroneal tendon injuries are common MRI findings that need to be addressed at the time of surgery.[23]

TREATMENT

Indications and Contraindications for Surgical Treatment

Not all patients with ligamentous laxity require surgery. The principal indication for surgical intervention is recurrent giving-way or instability despite proprioceptive training in patients who have mechanical laxity. Relative contraindications to surgery include instability caused by collagen disease, coalitions of the tarsal bones, and functional instability without mechanical instability.[4,15,17] Absolute contraindications include advanced ankle arthritis, Charcot's neuroarthropathy, and neurologic conditions leading to muscle imbalance or paralysis.

Management of Chronic Lateral Ankle Instability

Before surgical treatment of chronic lateral ligament insufficiency is considered, a supervised rehabilitation program that is based on peroneal muscle strengthening and proprioception training should be completed. Ankle bracing is also beneficial.[16]

Although an all-arthroscopic procedure for lateral ankle instability is possible,[24] open repair remains the standard of care for ankle and subtalar instability.[16] Concomitant arthroscopy of the ankle joint followed by reconstruction of the ligaments is now common practice. This is particularly important because of the association of ankle instability with concomitant intra-articular pathology.[25]

Several procedures have been described for the treatment of ankle instability, and the success rate varies from 50% to more than 90% in most series in the literature.[17] These surgeries can be divided into secondary "native" ligament repair and imbrications (*anatomic*) and ligament reconstructions with free tendon grafts or transfers (*nonanatomic*). Three classic nonanatomic repairs—the Evans, Watson-Jones, and Chrisman-Snook techniques—were widely used in the past, with variable short- and long-term results.[15,16] Major disadvantages of nonanatomic techniques are the sacrifice of normal, well-functioning anatomic structures around the ankle joint (e.g., peroneal tendons) and the limitation of ankle motion with alteration of normal kinematics of the ankle, which leads to joint degeneration and skin- and nerve-related complications. Late deterioration is common with these procedures and results in increasing laxity, reduction of ankle function, and increased pain.[7,15,16,26]

Because of the drawbacks associated with nonanatomic procedures, anatomic reconstruction of the lateral ankle ligaments is regarded as the surgical treatment of choice for patients with chronic ankle instability. However, nonanatomic repair does still play a role in certain situations, such as in cases of failed surgical stabilization, absence of adequate ligament tissue, and joint hyperlaxity.[7] Anatomic reconstruction of the ankle ligaments involves suturing of the remnants of the original ligaments (as described by Brostrom) or reconstruction of the original ligament ends with reinforcement using adjacent tissues, including the periosteum or inferior extensor retinaculum (Gould modification of the Brostrom procedure).[27-29] Satisfactory long-term functional results after anatomic reconstruction using the Gould modification have been published.[29,30] The damaged or elongated remnants of the ATFL and CFL are divided, shortened 3 to 5 mm, and imbricated or reinserted into bone.

Preferred Surgical Treatment

The Gould modification of the Brostrom procedure for reconstruction of chronic lateral ankle instability is preferred. We prefer to perform an initial diagnostic arthroscopy before undertaking the repair of the lateral ankle ligaments. Chronic lateral ankle instability is associated with intra-articular pathology in up to 93% of cases, as described by Ferkel and others.[25,31,32] These intra-articular abnormalities include loose bodies, osteochondral defects, synovitis, adhesions, chondromalacia, and osteophytes. Failure to recognize or appreciate these abnormalities could compromise results of ankle instability repair.

Surgical Procedure

The patient is positioned supine on the operating table, and intravenous antibiotics are administered. A bump is placed under the hip of the operative side. An examination under anesthesia (EUA) with specific use of fluoroscopy is performed, to further document positive findings on the anterior drawer and talar tilt tests (see Fig. 9-9). After a proximal thigh tourniquet is placed, a thigh holder is positioned under the operative side with hip flexion at 60 degrees. To avoid compression of the neurovascular structures, the holder should not impinge on the popliteal fossa when the leg is flexed at the knee (Fig. 9-10). Skin preparation is then performed in a standard fashion.

After the extremity is draped, the medial and lateral malleoli, anterior tibialis tendon, superficial peroneal nerve, and standard arthroscopic portals are marked out. An Esmarch bandage or ace wrap is used to exsanguinate the leg, and the tourniquet is inflated. The leg is then placed in a Guhl noninvasive ankle distractor set (Smith and Nephew), and the appropriate tension is dialed to distract the joint. A 21-point diagnostic arthroscopic examination of the ankle is performed to ensure a thorough evaluation of the joint.[25] The arthroscopic procedure is described in other chapters of this text. Appropriate treatment of incidental lesions can be undertaken before the ligamentous repair. Care is taken to minimize fluid extravasations during the procedure. This is best accomplished with the use of low-pressure arthroscopy done in an expeditious manner. In our hands, the average ankle arthroscopy takes between 15 and 20 minutes.

Brostrom-Gould Repair

After the diagnostic arthroscopy, the leg is removed from the Guhl distractor, and the thigh holder is removed before the Brostrom-Gould repair is commenced (video 1). With the patient still lying supine, attention turned to the lateral ankle. At this time, the appropriate landmarks are marked out, including the distal fibula and superficial peroneal nerve (SPN). The skin incision depends on the planned surgical procedure. For a classic Brostrom repair, a curvilinear incision just anterior to fibula is used (Fig. 9-11A). This incision should start at the ankle joint line, 1 cm anterior to the distal fibula, and extend in a curvilinear fashion just inferior and posterior to the tip of the fibula, almost like a **C** shape for the left

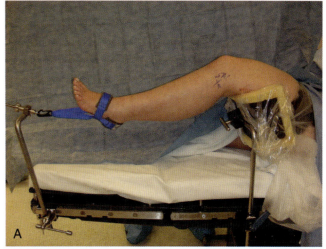
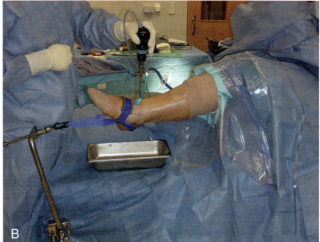

FIGURE 9-10 When the leg is flexed at the knee, the holder should not impinge on the popliteal fossa to avoid any compression of the neurovascular structures.

ankle and a backward **C** shape for the right ankle. If hindfoot varus correction with a valgus (Dwyer) calcaneal osteotomy will be necessary, a second incision is made posterior to the fibula and parallel to the peroneal tendons (see Fig. 9-11B). In the case of concomitant peroneal tendon involvement, the initial incision is changed to an extended, posteriorly based, lateral incision following the peroneal tendons. With this incision, an anterior flap is raised to expose the capsule and extensor retinaculum (see Fig. 9-11C). Care is taken to elevate full-thickness tissue flaps anteriorly, to expose the ATFL and the inferior extensor retinaculum, and inferiorly, to expose the peroneal tendons and the calcaneal tuberosity. It is important to identify and protect the intermediate dorsal cutaneous branch of the superficial peroneal nerve as it courses over the extensor retinaculum anterior to the fibula. We extend the skin incision and subcutaneous dissection posterior to the fibula to expose the calcaneus, because the CFL attachment is relatively posterior on the calcaneus. The lateral extent of the inferior extensor retinaculum is identified and mobilized for later reconstruction to the fibula (Fig. 9-12).

The peroneal sheath is incised, and the tendons are retracted from their sheath to expose the underlying CFL (Fig. 9-13). At

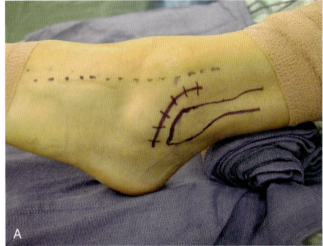

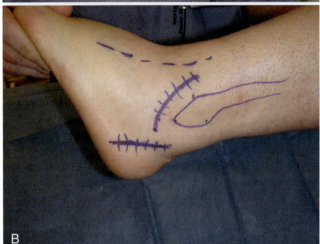

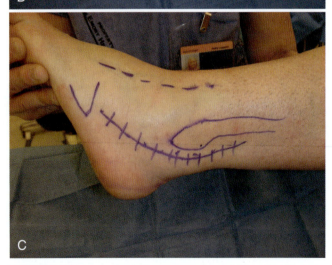

FIGURE 9-11 A, For a classic Brostrom repair, a curvilinear incision just anterior to fibula is marked out. **B,** If hindfoot varus correction with a valgus (Dwyer) calcaneal osteotomy will be necessary, a second incision is made posterior to the fibula and parallel to the peroneal tendons. **C,** In the case of concomitant peroneal tendon involvement, the initial incision is changed to an extended, posteriorly based, lateral incision following the peroneal tendons. With this incision, an anterior flap is raised to expose the capsule and extensor retinaculum.

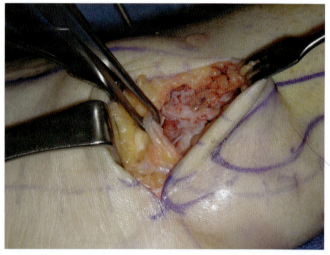

FIGURE 9-12 The lateral extent of the inferior extensor retinaculum is identified and mobilized for later reconstruction to the fibula.

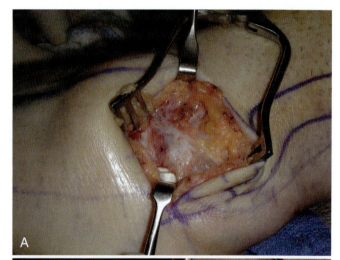

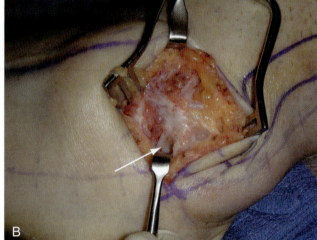

FIGURE 9-13 A and **B,** The peroneal sheath is incised, and the tendons are retracted from their sheath to expose the underlying calcaneofibular ligament (arrow).

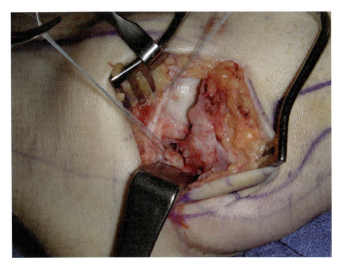

FIGURE 9-14 The anterior talofibular ligament is usually transected during the repair as the arthrotomy is made in line with the anterolateral capsule incision at the ankle joint.

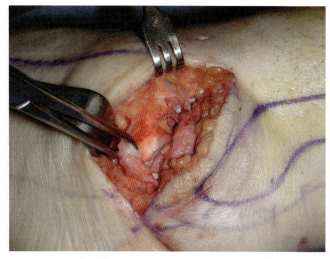

FIGURE 9-15 After all sutures are placed, the ankle is dorsiflexed and everted as for a posterior drawer test, and the ankle should be held in this position while all the sutures are tied.

this point, the torn edges of the ATFL and CFL or laxity within the ligaments can be identified. Often, the ATFL stump cannot be easily identified because it blends with the ankle joint capsule. The ATFL is usually transected during the repair as the arthrotomy is made in line with the anterolateral capsule incision at the ankle joint (Fig. 9-14). The talofibular joint space should now be visualized and inspected for any additional pathology, with care taken not to damage the underlying cartilage. The CFL is identified underneath the peroneals, and its laxity is assessed in dorsiflexion. If the remaining portions of either ligament appear too small to repair, the tissue is excised, and periosteum is elevated from the underlying fibula to create flaps for later repair to the residual ATFL and CFL.

A 2-0 fortified polyester suture (Fiberwire, Arthrex, Naples, FL) is used to imbricate the ATFL and capsule in a "pants over vest" fashion. This stitch starts on the distal side and then crosses over to the proximal side with a near-far–far-near sequence (see Fig. 9-14). The CFL is imbricated in a similar manner. All sutures should be placed before any knots are tied. After all sutures are placed, the ankle is held reduced in neutral and eversion while all sutures are tied (Fig. 9-15). If the ligaments have avulsed off of the bone rather than rupturing midsubstance, they can be repaired with suture anchors (minicorkscrew anchors) or tied over a bone bridge after a small trough is made for the ligaments. Sutures are then placed in the remaining capsular tissues and tied. We routinely perform the Gould modification in which the inferior extensor retinaculum is mobilized, advanced proximally over the area of reconstruction, and then repaired to the distal fibula periosteum with no. 0 nonabsorbable polyester suture (Fig. 9-16). To judge the adequacy of the repair, the foot is held up with the hip in full internal rotation and should maintain an everted position against gravity (i.e., negative gravity test) (Fig. 9-17). The tissues are then closed in layers with 2-0 Vicryl for the subcutaneous layer and 3-0 Monocryl for the skin. The extremity is placed in a well-padded splint after sterile dressings are applied, in a position of eversion and neutral ankle dorsiflexion.

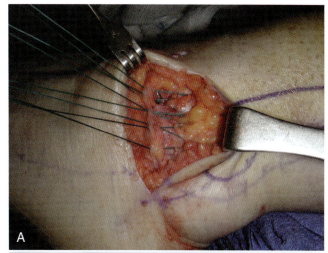

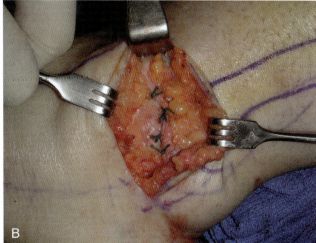

FIGURE 9-16 A and **B,** Sutures are placed in the remaining capsular tissues and tied. We routinely perform the Gould modification, in which the inferior extensor retinaculum is mobilized, advanced proximally over the area of reconstruction, and then repaired to the distal fibula periosteum with no. 0 nonabsorbable polyester suture.

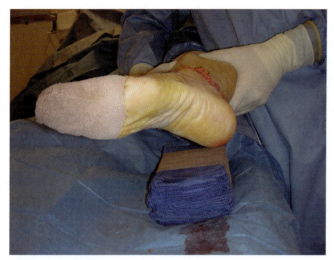

FIGURE 9-17 To judge the adequacy of the repair, the foot is held up with the hip in full internal rotation, and it should maintain an everted position against gravity (i.e., negative gravity test).

Special Considerations

A detailed preoperative examination is extremely helpful, because comorbid conditions can change the surgical plan. For example, if the patient displays peroneal pathology (peroneal instability, peroneal tear) on examination or on MRI, the operative plan should also address these issues. In such a case, the incision would be a posterior extensile incision around the fibula (to deal with both issues) rather than an anterior incision (see Fig. 9-11C).

Another important issue to evaluate is hindfoot varus (see Fig. 9-6). We agree with other authors that, in patients with chronic ankle instability and hindfoot varus, surgical reconstruction of the lateral ligamentous complex without addressing the hindfoot varus leads to higher failure rates. We believe that hindfoot varus is a predisposing factor to inversion ankle sprains, which, in turn, lead to injury of the lateral ligamentous complex. In such cases, one would plan on performing a concomitant calcaneal lateral closing wedge (Dwyer) osteotomy. There would be two laterally based incisions for this procedure: the standard anterior curvilinear incision for the Brostrom-Gould reconstruction and an oblique lateral incision over the posterior calcaneus for the osteotomy (see Fig. 9-11B).

It is also important to be mindful of the symptomatic os subfibulare, which is an avulsion fracture of the distal fibula that resulted in a nonunion. This fracture fragment usually contains the attachment site of the ATFL, with or without that of the CFL, and can result in lateral ligament instability. Sometimes this is not evident until stress radiographs are obtained (Fig. 9-18). The treatment for this condition is open reduction and internal fixation of the fracture fragment with a partially threaded cancellous screw (video 2). If the piece of bone is too small to be captured with a screw, suture anchors may be used for the repair.

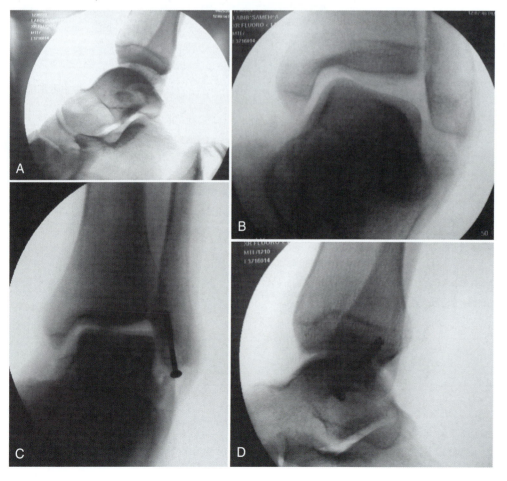

FIGURE 9-18 This fracture fragment usually contains the attachment site of the anterior talofibular ligament (ATFL), the calcaneofibular ligament (CFL), or both, and it can result in lateral ligament instability. Sometimes, this is not evident until stress radiographs are obtained.
A, Positive anterior drawer Xray;
B, Positive lateral tilt Xray with distal migration of OS subfibulare;
C, Screw fixation of OS subfibulare;
D, Negative anterior drawer Xrays SLP ORIF.

Postoperative Rehabilitation

The foot remains splinted with no weight bearing allowed for 3 weeks, after which the patient returns for a dressing change and further immobilization in a cast boot for 3 more weeks. Partial to full weight bearing is allowed from week 3 to week 6 postoperatively. At week 6, patient is referred to physical therapy for gait training, peroneal strengthening, and proprioceptive exercises. Daily flexion-extension range of motion exercise is allowed at week 3, but no inversion-eversion motion is permitted until week 12. The patients may return to activities as tolerated at 12 weeks. Patients undergoing a concomitant calcaneal osteotomy or open reduction and internal fixation of a distal fibula nonunion are placed in a non–weight-bearing cast for the initial 6 weeks.

REFERENCES

1. Garrick JG. The frequency of injury, mechanism of injury, and epidemiology of ankle sprains. *Am J Sports Med.* 1977;5:241-242.
2. Freeman M, Dean M, Hanham I. The etiology and prevention of functional instability of the foot. *J Bone Joint Surg Br.* 1965;47:678-685.
3. Burks RT, Morgans J. Anatomy of the lateral ankle ligaments. *Am J Sports Med.* 1994;22:72-77.
4. Clanton TO. Athletic injuries to the soft tissues of the foot and ankle. In: Coughlin MJ, Mann RA: *Surgery of the Foot and Ankle.* ed 7. St Louis, MO: Mosby, 1999:1090-1209.
5. Scranton PE Jr, McDermott JE, Rogers JV. The relationship between chronic ankle instability and variations in mortise anatomy and impingement spurs. *Foot Ankle Int.* 2000;21:657-664.
6. Van Bergeyk AB, et al. CT analysis of hindfoot alignment in chronic lateral ankle instability. *Foot Ankle Int.* 2002;23:37-42.
7. Ajis A, Younger A, Maffulli N. Anatomic repair for chronic lateral ankle instability. *Foot Ankle Clin.* 2006;11:539-545.
8. Rasmussen O. Stability of the ankle joint: analysis of the function and traumatology of the ankle ligaments. *Acta Orthop Scand Suppl.* 1985; 211:1-75.
9. Kjaersgaard-Andersen P, Wethelund J, Helmig P, et al. Effect of the calcaneofibular ligament on hindfoot rotation in amputation specimens. *Acta Orthop Scand.* 1987;58:135-138.
10. Lassiter TE Jr, Malone TR, Garret WE Jr. Injury to the lateral ligaments of the ankle. *Orthop Clin North Am.* 1989;20:629-640.
11. Tochigi Y, Amendola A, Rudert MJ, et al. The role of the interosseous talocalcaneal ligament in subtalar joint stability. *Foot Ankle Int.* 2004; 25:588-596.
12. Clarke HD, Kitaoka HB, Ehman RL. Peroneal tendon injuries. *Foot Ankle Int.* 1988;19:280-288.
13. Hatch GF, Labib SA, Hutton W. Role of the peroneal tendons and superior peroneal retinaculum as static stabilizers of the ankle. *J Surg Orthop Adv.* 2007;16:187-191.
14. Freeman M. Instability of the foot after injuries to the lateral ligament of the ankle. *J Bone Joint Surg Br.* 1965;47:669-676.
15. Watson AD. Ankle instability and impingement. *Foot Ankle Clin.* 2007; 12:177-195.
16. Maffulli N, Ferran NA. Management of acute and chronic ankle instability. *J Am Acad Orthop Surg.* 2008;16:608-615.
17. Coughlin MJ, Mann RA, Saltzman CL. *Surgery of the Foot and Ankle.* Philadelphia, PA: Mosby Elsevier; 2007:1467-1468.
18. Ross SE, Guskiewicz KM. Examination of static and dynamic postural stability in individuals with functionally stable and unstable ankles. *Clin J Sport Med.* 2004;14:332-338.
19. Renstrom AFH, Lynch SA. Acute ligament injuries of the ankle. *Foot Ankle Clin.* 1999;4:697-711.
20. Thermann H, Zwipp H, Tscherne H. Treatment algorithm of chronic ankle and subtalar instability. *Foot Ankle Int.* 1997;18:163-169.
21. Saltzman CL, El-Khoury GY. The hindfoot alignment view. *Foot Ankle Int.* 1995;16:572-576.
22. Scranton PE. Sprains and soft-tissue injuries. In: Pfeffer GB, ed. *Chronic Ankle Pain in the Athlete.* ed 1. Monograph series. Rosemont, IL: American Academy of Orthopedic Surgeons; 2000:3-20.
23. Griffith JF, Brockwell J. Diagnosis and imaging of ankle instability. *Foot Ankle Clin.* 2006;11:475-496.
24. Maiotti M, Massoni C, Tarantino U. The use of arthroscopic thermal shrinkage to treat chronic lateral ankle instability in young athletes. *Arthroscopy.* 2005;21:751-757.
25. Ferkel RD, Chams RN. Chronic lateral instability: arthroscopic findings and long term results. *Foot Ankle Int.* 2007;28:24-31.
26. Kaikkonen A, Kannus P, Jarvinen M. Surgery versus functional treatment in ankle ligament tears. *Clin Orthop Relat Res.* 1996;326:194-202.
27. Brostrom L. Sprained ankles. VI. Surgical treatment of "chronic" ligament ruptures. *Acta Chir Scand.* 1966;132:551-565.
28. Gould N, Seligson D, Gassman J. Early and late repair of lateral ligament of the ankle. *Foot Ankle.* 1980;1:84-89.
29. Hamilton WG, Thompson FM, Snow SW. Modified Brostrom procedure for lateral ankle instability. *Foot Ankle.* 1993;14:1-7.
30. Krips R, Van Dijk CN, Halasi PT, et al. Long-term outcome of anatomical reconstruction versus tenodesis for the treatment of chronic anterolateral instability of the ankle joint: a multi-center study. *Foot Ankle Int.* 2001;22:415-442.
31. Komenda G, Ferkel R. Arthroscopic findings associated with the unstable ankle. *Foot Ankle Int.* 1999;20:708.
32. Hintermann B, Boss A, Schäfer D. Arthroscopic findings in patients with chronic ankle instability. *Am J Sports Med.* 2002;30:402-409.

SELECTED READINGS

Berg EE. The symptomatic os subfibulare. *J Bone Joint Surg Am.* 1991; 73:1251-1254.

Lui TH. Arthroscopic-assisted lateral ligamentous reconstruction in combined ankle and subtalar instability. *Arthroscopy.* 2007;23:554.

Thordarson DB. *Foot and Ankle.* Philadelphia, PA: Lippincott Williams & Wilkins; 2004:242-246, 250-259.

Ankle Fractures

Beat Hintermann

Ankle fractures are common, and although joint stability can be regained by adequate reduction and internal fixation of the fracture, some patients have disabling, persistent pain even after joint congruity is completely restored.[1,2] Persistent pain may be associated with exercise or change in the weather, and there may be radiographic evidence of osteoarthritic changes. These features suggest that an articular cartilage lesion or another radiographically nondetectable lesion might have occurred at the time of injury and may be the cause of the pain.

Ankle injuries result from abnormal motion of the talus within the ankle mortise. Fractures of the malleoli can result from impact of the talus on the malleoli caused by rotational or translational forces. Fractures can also occur in tension, and the malleoli can be avulsed because of pull exerted by the intact collateral ligaments to the talus.[3,4]

Ankle fracture treatment is still based on classification criteria that were created in a time when the ankle was thought to be a simple hinge and only plain radiographs were available to assist diagnosis. This may explain why final results do not always correlate with the extent of bone damage and the reduction and stability achieved. It also suggests the need for specific studies to determine how and to what extent accompanying injuries are predictive factors for outcome in ankle fracture.

Hintermann and coworkers prospectively evaluated the arthroscopic findings in 288 consecutive patients with acute ankle fracture (148 male and 140 female patients; mean age, 45.6 years).[5] They found that, independent of fracture type, cartilage lesions were most frequently present on the talus and to a lesser extent on the tibia, fibula, and medial malleolus. The frequency and severity of cartilage lesions increased from type B to type C fractures, and there was an increase observed from subgroup 1 to subgroup 3 in both type B and type C

fractures. These findings support the belief that the severity of injury directly depends on the height of the fibula fracture. The fact that there was an unexpectedly high incidence of cartilage lesions in all fracture types may explain the observation from daily practice that the final results do not always correlate with the reduction and stability achieved. It seems that the fate of the fractured ankle (i.e., prognosis) may be determined to a significant extent during the accident itself, when the cartilage and other intra-articular and periarticular structures are injured.

Cartilage lesions apparently occur when the talus is rotated or translated in the loaded ankle mortise until the fracture occurs. This is especially true for type C fractures, and it is true to a lesser extent for type B fractures as long as the underlying mechanism is a pronation or rotation movement. Supination trauma, as typically seen in type A fractures, may critically stress the medial half of the joint, but the load forces may not be as high as in pronation or rotation trauma. Taga and colleaues[6] found cartilage lesions in the medial joint in 89% of 9 patients evaluated after an acute ankle sprain and in 95% of 22 patients with chronic ankle sprain. They found more cartilage lesions on the distal tibia than on the medial talus. They concluded that these injuries were mainly caused by local stress concentration. They found no correlation between the severity of the cartilage lesion and the degree of instability. This may support the belief that cartilage lesions occur to a significant extent at the time of the acute injury.

A higher incidence of cartilage lesions occurs in female patients than in male patients, and this can be explained by several factors. First, the cartilage may be less resistant to mechanical stress in females.[1] Second, the cartilage may have become more vulnerable with increasing age (because the age of the female patients was significantly higher).[5] Third, overall muscular and bony strength are lower in females, so that fracture probably occurs during an earlier phase of the injury, and with a higher incidence, exposing the articular surfaces to a higher risk of possible damage. This may be especially true for elderly patients.

Arthroscopy performed directly after ankle fracture can be used to visualize intra-articular lesions that cannot be detected on plain radiographs.[5,7] Cartilage lesions were found in 79.2% to 90.0% of patients examined arthroscopically.[5,8] The ligaments could not be identified by arthroscopy in all cases, and there were significant differences among the four ligaments; overall, more injuries to the ligaments were found than expected.[5] Although its role has not been established in the acute treatment of ankle fractures,[9] arthroscopy has proved to be valuable for providing detailed knowledge of the fractured ankle.[5,10] It has also been helpful in the treatment of symptomatic osteophytes after ankle fracture.[2]

The aim of this chapter is to give an overview of my own technique and experience in arthroscopic evaluation of the acutely fractured ankle. In particular, an attempt is made to define the role of arthroscopy when treating ankle fractures.

NORMAL AND PATHOLOGIC ANATOMY

The ankle joint consists of three bones that form the malleolar mortise. They are connected by a complex ligamentous apparatus to provide stability. However, a unique feature of the ankle joint is its high concentration of articular surfaces. Injuries can affect the ligaments alone or both ligamentous and bony structures. Typically, the result is an unstable ankle joint, particularly in cases involving bony structures (e.g., ankle fractures).

PATIENT EVALUATION

History and Physical Examination

Acute ankle fractures result from severe trauma, such as traumatic inversion, eversion, or rotation. In most instances, a combination of different movements leads to a typical injury pattern. The history sometimes is helpful to elucidate the exact mechanism of injury, but frequently the patient does not recall the exact combination of inversion, eversion, and rotational forces that occurred at the time of injury. Physical examination consistently reveals swelling and tenderness to palpation over the fractured bone. Ecchymosis usually occurs over the first 24 hours. It is important to remove any splinting material that may have been applied at the time of injury, in order to assess for deformity of the ankle that accompanies a fracture dislocation. The skin must be carefully assessed for compromise, and the presence of pulses in the foot should be documented, especially in cases of fracture dislocation. On rare occasions, open fractures may occur, even if the bony deformity is mild.

Diagnostic Imaging

Standard radiographs of the ankle are the main step in imaging for diagnosis of an acute ankle fracture. In more complex cases,

a computed tomography scan may be used to better visualize the injury pattern, in particular in regard to damage to the articular surfaces.

MANAGEMENT

Indications and Contraindications

Theoretically, every fractured ankle can be viewed by arthroscopy before open reduction and internal fixation (ORIF). However, arthroscopy may not be helpful in all fractured ankles. I recommend considering arthroscopic evaluation for cases in which the proposed fracture mechanism does not explain the extent of the lesion or the imaging findings do not explain the overall injury. For instance, if an intermediate fragment is suspected in the case of a posterior fracture, arthroscopy may be helpful in confirming the diagnosis and deciding whether an additional posteromedial approach should be performed to reposition and fix the posterior fragment properly. Likewise, if an injury to the deltoid ligament is present or suspected, arthroscopy can help determine whether reconstruction is advised. In some cases, arthroscopy may allow the surgeon to recognize an interposed deltoid ligament between talus and medial malleolus after closed reduction of the fracture.

Arthroscopy is generally contraindicated if there is significant damage to the skin or a poor soft tissue mantle is present, because it might provoke further injury to the soft tissues due to swelling caused by filling of the ankle joint.

Conservative or Operative Management

It is generally accepted that ORIF is the best treatment for unstable or dislocated ankle fractures.[11-15] Few investigators suggest that perfect reduction is required to achieve good long-term results. Bauer and associates studied 143 patients 30 years after they sustained an ankle fracture that was treated by closed methods and found that 82% were free of arthritis and 83% were free of symptoms.[11] In contrast, in a series by Beris and colleagues of 23 patients who had an ankle fracture with poor reduction, 78.3% developed osteoarthritis.[16] Accordingly, I limit nonoperative treatment to older or polymorbid patients with ankle fractures without dislocation.

Arthroscopic Technique

The patient is placed supine on the operating table. The knee is flexed to about 90 degrees using a knee holder; this allows the leg to assume a hanging position with the foot and ankle touching the table (Fig. 10-1). No ankle distraction device is used. To avoid iatrogenic lesions of the articular cartilage and soft tissue, the joint is first inflated with saline, and portals are created by blunt dissection. A 4.5-mm, 30-degree arthroscope is introduced into the ankle joint through a standard central anterior portal (Fig. 10-2). The liquid is evacuated, and the cavity is filled with saline. If necessary, accessory anteromedial or anterolateral portals, or both, are also used for insertion of instruments. Systematic arthroscopic examination, as described by Ferkel and Orwin,[1] is performed to visualize the internal structures.

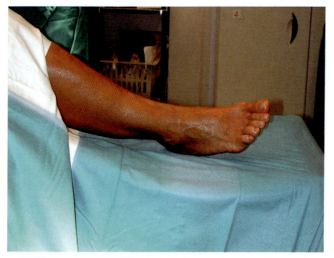

FIGURE 10-1 The knee is flexed over a knee holder so that the foot is in a hanging position. This allows free investigation of the ankle joint without the use of a distraction device.

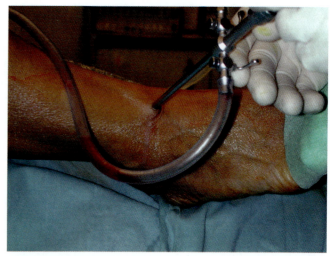

FIGURE 10-2 A central anterior portal is used. Landmarks are the lateral border of the anterior tibial tendon and the tibiotalar joint line.

Articular cartilage lesions are graded according to the depth of the lesion, as assessed by inspection and probing:

■ Grade 1: superficial lesion
■ Grade 2: fissuring or degeneration of less than one half of the thickness of the articular cartilage (Fig. 10-3)
■ Grade 3: fasciculation or degeneration of greater than one half of the thickness of the articular cartilage (Fig. 10-4)
■ Grade 4: erosion of the cartilage down to the subchondral bone (Fig. 10-5)

The anterior talofibular ligament (Fig. 10-6), calcaneofibular ligament, deltoid ligament (Fig. 10-7), and anterior (Fig. 10-8) and posterior (Fig. 10-9) tibiofibular ligaments (syndesmosis) are assessed by inspection and probing. Ligament injuries are graded according to the severity of the fiber tear and the degree of instability present: A partial lesion involves a tear of less than one half of the ligament without complete instability, whereas a complete lesion implies a tear of the complete ligament or bony avulsion of the ligament with instability.

Arthroscopy is also used to visualize the fracture pattern (Fig. 10-10) and to detect unexpected injuries to articular surfaces, such as impression (Fig. 10-11).

Figure 10-12 shows a case in which arthroscopy was beneficial for understanding of the injury pattern, removal of a loose fragment, and reduction of the deltoid ligament that was interposed between the medial malleolus and the talus.

Arthroscopy may be used for removal of free fragments (e.g., bone and cartilage fragments), for reduction of interposed soft tissues (e.g., capsular, ligaments), and to assist closed reduction and percutaneous fixation of a fracture (e.g., medial malleolus). It may also be used to check the obtained reduction, particularly in Maisoneuve-type fractures.

PEARLS & PITFALLS

1. Careful preoperative evaluation of the fractured ankle must be performed to detect the presence of an ankle fracture dislocation requiring immediate reduction or to detect an open ankle fracture.
2. Careful management of inflow for arthroscopy is critical. The minimum inflow pressure and flow rate that are required to achieve visualization should be used.
3. During arthroscopy of the fractured ankle, the soft tissues must be monitored at frequent intervals to be certain that the inflow fluid is not causing excessive swelling of the soft tissues of the calf, ankle, or foot.

Postoperative Rehabilitation Protocol

The postoperative rehabilitation is dictated by the type of fracture and the degree of stability achieved with ORIF. If the arthroscopic evaluation has detected damages to the articular cartilage, non–weight bearing may be advised up to 6 to 8 weeks after ORIF. In the case of detected injuries to the ligamentous structures, external stabilization may be advised.

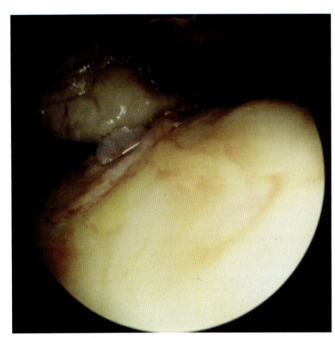

FIGURE 10-3 Grade 2 lesion of cartilage.

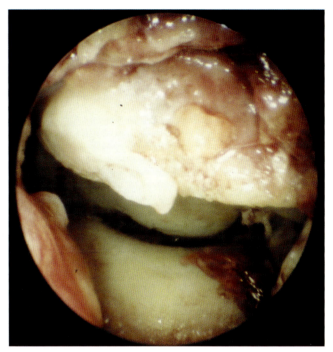

FIGURE 10-4 Grade 3 lesion of cartilage.

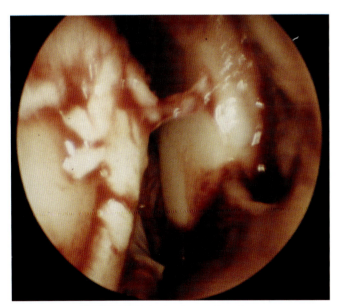

FIGURE 10-5 Grade 4 lesion of cartilage.

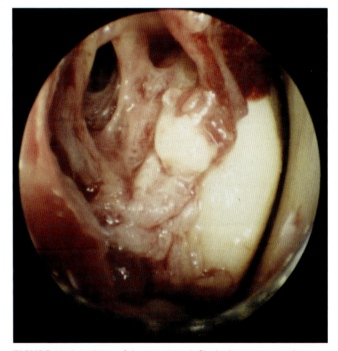

FIGURE 10-6 Avulsion of the anterior talofibular ligament together with the periosteum of external aspect of the fibula.

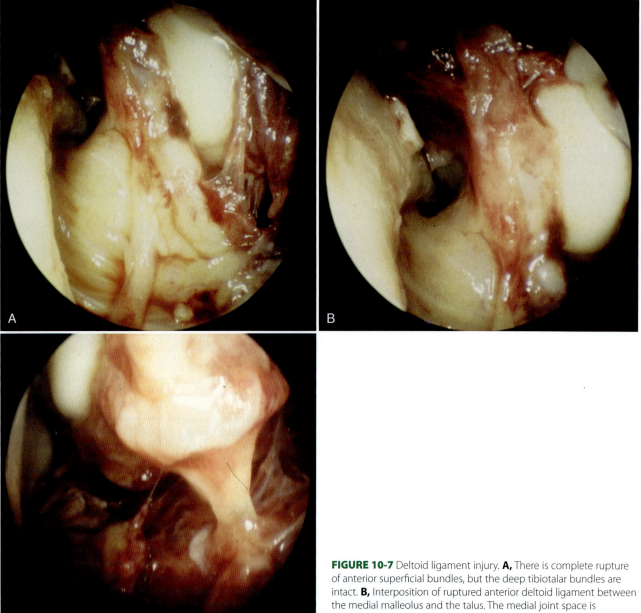

FIGURE 10-7 Deltoid ligament injury. **A,** There is complete rupture of anterior superficial bundles, but the deep tibiotalar bundles are intact. **B,** Interposition of ruptured anterior deltoid ligament between the medial malleolus and the talus. The medial joint space is markedly widened. **C,** Avulsion of the whole deltoid ligament from the medial malleolus.

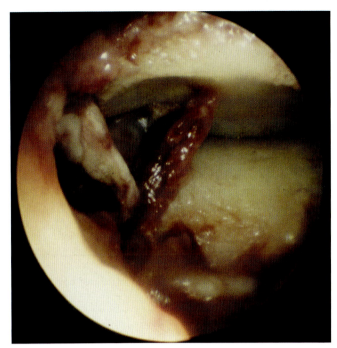

FIGURE 10-8 Distal avulsion of the anterior tibiotalar ligament (syndesmosis).

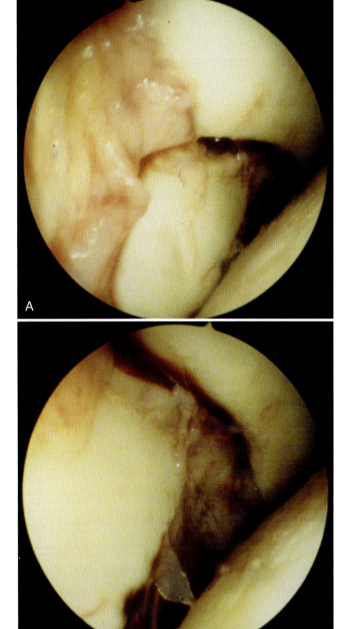

FIGURE 10-9 Rupture of the posterior tibiotalar ligament (syndesmosis). **A,** The fibula is subluxated in the anterior direction. **B,** Closer inspection shows the rupture of the posterior syndesmotic ligament.

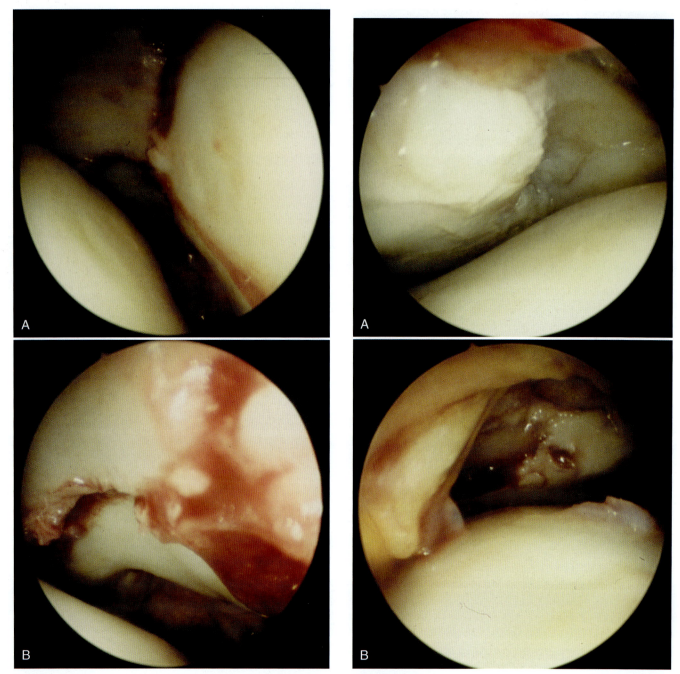

FIGURE 10-10 Fractures of tibial plafond. **A,** A third fragment is seen posteriorly between the fracture of medial malleolus and the tibial plafond. **B,** A posterior tibial fragment (i.e., Volkman fragment) is minimally displaced.

FIGURE 10-11 Impression fracture of the anteromedial tibial plafond. **A,** Impression fracture with preserved articular surface. **B,** Impression fracture with interrupted articular surface and extended cartilage lesion.

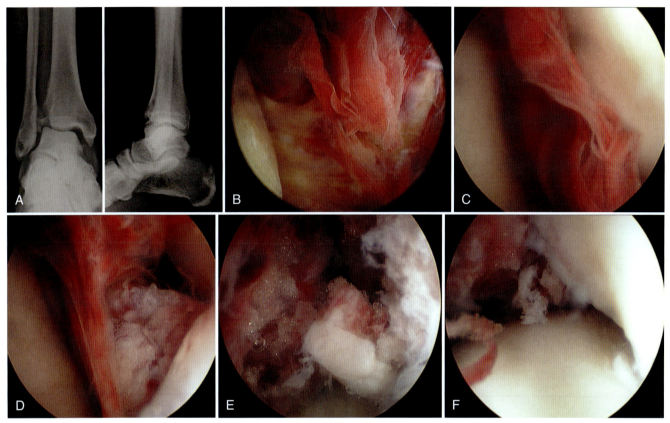

FIGURE 10-12 A 56-year-old man sustained an external rotation trauma of his right ankle when walking in the snow. **A,** Standard radiographs show a complex avulsion fracture of the syndesmosis and a marked widening of the distal tibiofibular space. An intermediate fragment is also suspected. **B,** The deltoid ligament shows an extended lesion. **C,** A part of the superficial deltoid ligament is interposed between medial malleolus and talus. **D,** Further inspection shows an extended rupture of the strong deep bundles of deltoid ligament, which are also interposed between the medial malleolus and the talus, resulting in marked widening of the medial gutter. **E,** Rupture of the anterior syndesmotic ligament with an intermediate osteocartilaginous fragment. **F,** After removal of the fragment, the lateral border of the tibial plafond and the ligamentous injury to the posterior syndesmotic ligament can be seen.

CONCLUSIONS

Arthroscopy may be beneficial for true understanding of the fractured ankle, especially in identifying associated intra-articular lesions and in recognizing the type and extent of instability. However, the significance of these findings is not yet clear, and it is uncertain whether addressing such issues in this setting will affect the outcome or treatment of these fractures. Further observation of patients is necessary to correlate final outcomes with intra-articular lesions and their treatment.

It appears that, even in ankle fractures that require conventional ORIF, arthroscopy may be useful to rule out occult intra-articular pathology. The added time and morbidity is minimal, and the procedure can be done with only manual distraction. Arthroscopy aids in the evaluation and treatment of chondral and osteochondral pathology as well as ligamentous injuries. It enables the surgeon to minimize the open approach and secondary damages to the surrounding tissues while performing ORIF. It is suspected, although not yet proved, that the postoperative range of motion improves more quickly after lavage and débridement of an acute ankle fracture.

REFERENCES

1. Ferkel RD, Orwin JF. Arthroscopic treatment of acute ankle fractures and postfracture defect. In: Ferkel RD, ed. *Arthroscopic Surgery*. New York, NY: Lippincott-Raven; 1996:185-200.
2. Van Dijk CN, Tol JL, Verheyen CC. A prospective study of prognostic factors concerning the outcome of arthroscopic surgery for anterior ankle impingement. *Am J Sports Med*. 1997;25:737-745.
3. Geissler WB, Tsao AK, Hughes JL. Fractures of the ankle. In: Rockwood C, Green DP, Bucholz RW, Heckman JD, eds. *Fractures in Adults*. New York, NY: Lippincott-Raven; 1996:2201-2266.
4. Tile M. Fractures of the ankle. In: Schatzker J, Tile M, eds. *The Rationale of Operative Fracture Care*. New York, NY: Springer; 1996:523-561.
5. Hintermann B, Regazzoni P, Lampert C, et al. Arthroscopic findings in acute fractures of the ankle. *J Bone Joint Surg Br*. 2000;82:345-351.
6. Taga I, Shino K, Inoue M, et al. Articular cartilage lesions in ankles with lateral ligament injury: an arthroscopic study. *Am J Sports Med*. 1993; 21:120-127.
7. Yoshimura I, Naito M, Kanazawa K, et al. Arthroscopic findings in Maisonneuve fractures. *J Orthop Sci*. 2008;13:3-6.
8. Thomas B, Yeo JM, Slater GL. Chronic pain after ankle fracture: an arthroscopic assessment case series. *Foot Ankle Int*. 2005;26:1012-1016.
9. Thordarson DB, Bains R, Shepherd LE. The role of ankle arthroscopy on the surgical management of ankle fractures. *Foot Ankle Int*. 2001; 22:123-125.
10. Loren GJ, Ferkel RD. Arthroscopic assessment of occult intra-articular injury in acute ankle fractures. *Arthroscopy*. 2002;18:412-421.

11. Bauer M, Bergstrom B, Hemborg A, et al. Malleolar fractures: nonoperative versus operative treatment: a controlled study. *Clin Orthop Relat Res.* 1985;199:17-27.

12. Yde J, Kristensen KD. Ankle fractures. Supination-eversion fractures stage II: primary and late results of operative and non-operative treatment. *Acta Orthop Scand.* 1980;51:695-702.

13. Phillips WA, Schwartz HS, Keller CS, et al. A prospective, randomized study of the management of severe ankle fractures. *J Bone Joint Surg Am.* 1985;67:67-78.

14. Makwana NK, Bhowal B, Harper WM, Hui AW. Conservative versus operative treatment for displaced ankle fractures in patients over 55 years of age: a prospective, randomised study. *J Bone Joint Surg Br.* 2001;83:525-529.

15. Rammelt S, Grass R, Zwipp H. Ankle fractures. *Unfallchirurg.* 2008;111:421-437.

16. Beris AE, Kabbani KT, Xenakis TA, et al. Surgical treatment of malleolar fractures: a review of 144 patients. *Clin Orthop Relat Res.* 1997;(341):90-98.

Osteochondral Lesions of the Talar Dome:
Anatomy, Etiology, and Evaluation

Steven Mussett ● W. Bryce Henderson ● Mark Glazebrook ● Johnny Tak-Choy Lau

TERMINOLOGY

Pathologic lesions involving the talar dome have been widely reported in the orthopedic literature, along with lesions of the cartilage and subchondral bone. *Osteochondritis dissecans* was historically described in 1887 as an inflammatory process of the bone cartilage interface that resulted in the loss of structural integrity.[1] This process has also been called *osteochondrosis dissecans*, and the pathogenesis was thought to be related to repeated trauma or spontaneous focal avascular osteonecrosis, resulting in the loss of structural support for the overlying articular cartilage.[2] Berndt and Harty[3] described the occurrence of talar articular injury in 1959 and attributed the primary cause of the traumatic lesions to these osteochondral fractures. The term *osteochondral defect* has been loosely used in the literature to refer to defects of the talus with traumatic or atraumatic causes. To encompass all previous terminology, these lesions are referred to as *osteochondral lesions* in this chapter.

NORMAL AND PATHOLOGIC ANATOMY

Ankle Anatomy and Cartilage Biology

The ankle represents a ginglymus joint, with the saddle-shaped trochlea articulating with the distal tibia. A congruent mortise is formed with the distal tibia and its malleolus and with the lateral malleolus of the fibula. The dome of the talus is trapezoidal, and on average the anterior aspect is 2.5 mm wider than the posterior aspect. Approximately 60% of the talus is covered with articular cartilage, and the thickness varies with location. The thickest area is the medial corner, and the thinnest area is in the lateral gutter.[4]

Topographic studies have shown significant differences in the mechanical properties of human ankle cartilage. Tibial cartilage is significantly stiffer than the corresponding talar articulating cartilage, and the softest tissue is found in the posteromedial and posterolateral talus.[5] Mean cartilage thickness is inversely related to the mean compressive modulus, with thicker cartilage found medially and thinner cartilage found laterally. These properties may explain the clinically observed findings of osteochondral lesions with repetitive overuse syndromes in medial lesions and acute traumatic events resulting in lateral lesions.

Pathology

Early reports on osteochondral lesions suggested a vascular insult as the primary cause. However, the current consensus supports a traumatic event or repeated insults as the inciting cause. In most cases, a history of trauma can be elicited from the patient. In their original work, Berndt and Harty[3] elicited a history of trauma in 90% of their patients studied. This finding has been reproduced by subsequent investigators.

There appears to be a discrepancy between lateral and medial lesions. Canale and Belding[6] retrospectively reviewed 31 osteochondral lesions and found that all of the lateral lesions were related to trauma, whereas only 64% of the medial lesions were related to a significant traumatic event. In a comprehensive review of the early literature, including more than 500 reported cases of osteochondral lesions, Flick and Gould[7] found that 98% of lateral lesions and only 70% of medial lesions were associated with a traumatic event. These findings support the theory that almost all lateral lesions occur as a result of trauma, whereas most medial lesions are traumatic in origin. The findings also suggest that there is an atraumatic cause for certain patients. In a series of 50 patients, Bauer and Ochsner[8] reported no history of trauma in 33 patients with deep medial lesions. They also demonstrated deep osteolysis close to the margin of the lesion, suggesting an atraumatic cause.[8] Reports of medial lesions occurring in identical twins and siblings with no history of trauma and the occurrence of bilateral talar dome lesions in up to 10% of cases further suggest an atraumatic cause in some patients.[9,10]

For osteochondral lesions with atraumatic causes, vascular ischemia is thought to be the precipitating factor, but other possible predisposing events may include vascular insufficiency, embolic phenomena, endocrine disorders, or genetic predisposition. It is unknown whether medial talar dome lesions due to acute or repetitive trauma have a natural history different from that of medial dome lesions of atraumatic origin.

INCIDENCE AND CLASSIFICATION

Epidemiology

The incidence of osteochondral lesions depends on the associated cause. Although early studies reported an incidence of osteochondral lesions of 6.5% with ankle sprains, improved imaging techniques and the use of arthroscopy have suggested that the incidence in cases of acute ankle injury is about 70%.[11-14] The prevalence is increased with associated trauma. Hinterman and colleagues[14] showed that 69.4% of 288 ankle fractures requiring open reduction and fixation had associated talar articular cartilage injury. Leontaritis and coworkers[13] reported a similar arthroscopic finding; the incidence of chondral injury was 74% in a series of 84 acute ankle fracture patients. The average age of occurrence is usually between 20 and 30 years, with a slight preponderance in men.[15]

Frequency of Lesion Location

Lesions of the talus are commonly located in two main areas: anterolateral and posteromedial. Central and posterolateral lesions have been reported, but they remain uncommon.

The biomechanical forces responsible for producing medial or lateral osteochondral lesions were investigated by Berndt and Harty[3] on a small number of cadavers. They were able to replicate these lesions in the laboratory using various combinations of ankle dorsiflexion and plantar flexion combined with inversion of the ankle joint. Lateral osteochondral lesions are caused by inversion with ankle dorsiflexion and subsequent internal rotation of the tibia on the talus, resulting in impaction with the face of the fibula. These lesions are usually shallow and wafer shaped, and they are thought to be caused by a tangential force vector that results in shearing forces.[16] Medial osteochondral lesions occur with inversion and plantar flexion of the foot. These lesions are deeper and cup shaped, factors that are related to impaction of the posteromedial talar dome on the tibial articular surface with a more perpendicular force vector. They tend to be more stable and have less of a tendency to displace compared with the shallower lateral osteochondral lesions.

Medial lesions occur more frequently than lateral lesions. It has been shown in cadaveric studies even without dissection of the lateral ligaments that peak pressures occur at the medial rim of the talus.[17] A biomechanical topographic study has shown that the softest cartilage of the talar dome is found at the most medial and lateral edge of the talus.[5] Lesions can involve the articular cartilage, underlying subchondral bone, and various depths of cancellous bone of the talus. Occasionally, a cystic component may develop beneath the articular cartilage, and this lesion may be overlooked by the inexperienced arthroscopist.

TABLE 11-1	Berndt and Harty Classification
Stage	**Description**
I	Small subchondral compression
II	Incomplete fragment avulsion
III	Complete fragment detachment undisplaced
IV	Complete fragment detachment displaced

Adapted from Berndt AL, Harty M. Transchondral fractures (osteochondritis dissecans) of the talus. J Bone Joint Surg Am. *1959;41A:988-1020.*

Classification

The most recognized classification system is that of Berndt and Harty.[3] It is unclear from their original paper whether it was based on radiographic imaging or intra-operative findings. However, it has traditionally been adopted as a radiographic staging system (Table 11-1).

With the advent of more advanced imaging, various investigators have introduced other classification systems. Ferkel and Scranton[18] developed a computed tomography (CT) classification system that corresponded with the original Berndt and Harty system and that included information on the amount of subchondral necrosis, cyst formation, and displacement of the fragment. A magnetic resonance imaging (MRI) classification has been introduced by Hepple and associates[19]. It includes information on the degree of bone and cartilage injury, amount of displacement, and subchondral cyst formation. The addition of more complicated imaging modalities has added to the description of the location of the lesion and degree of injury but has not changed operative management when the clinical course and chronicity of symptoms are included in the decision-making process. With remarkable foresight, Berndt and Harty[3] referred to their classification system as *arbitrary.* Although it is still the most recognized classification and is useful for research purposes and preoperative planning, the staging of patients has not changed operative management based on intra-operative findings.

PATIENT EVALUATION

History

Patients with an osteochondral lesion usually present with persistent pain in the ankle, which frequently is localized to the side of the lesion. In acute cases, the pain is accompanied by swelling, ecchymosis, and decreased range of motion. In a more chronic presentation, the pain is usually a dull ache in the ankle joint with associated stiffness. Crepitation, tenderness with weight baring and range of motion, mechanical clicking, and recurrent swelling should raise the suspicion of an osteochondral lesion. Uncommonly, the ankle joint may lock because of a loose bony fragment or cartilaginous flap. A thorough history of a traumatic event or instability should be elicited, and if absent, the factors predisposing to possible vascular insufficiency should be sought, including endocrine abnormalities; vascular, hematologic, and coagulation disorders; and any relevant family history. These patients should be questioned about symptoms in the contralateral ankle.

Physical Examination

Results of the physical examination vary, and there is no specific test to diagnose an osteochondral lesion. Inspection of the ankle may demonstrate acute injury with swelling and ecchymosis, or it may appear completely normal, as is often the case with delayed presentations. An attempt to elicit tenderness with palpation should be made by focusing on the common sites of osteochondral lesions. Posteromedial lesions may produce tenderness on palpation when the ankle is dorsiflexed and the region posterior to the medial malleolus is palpated. Anterolateral lesions demonstrate tenderness on palpation when the joint is palpated laterally with the ankle in plantar flexion. These findings are nonspecific because the tenderness is likely related to joint synovitis rather than the lesion itself. The joint should be taken through a range of motion to assess stiffness and to feel for crepitus and mechanical signs of clicking or locking. Ligamentous stability should be assessed to ascertain evidence of laxity, specifically of the lateral complex. The examination is completed with a thorough neurovascular assessment and examination of the contralateral ankle for comparison.

Diagnostic Imaging

Plain radiographs are the initial investigation of choice for a suspected lesion. Anteroposterior, lateral, and mortise views should be obtained on presentation. Radiographs obtained with the ankle in various degrees of plantar flexion and dorsiflexion may help demonstrate posteromedial and anterolateral lesions, respectively (Fig. 11-1).[20] Plain radiographs of the other ankle should be obtained to exclude bilateral lesions. Although useful as a primary investigation, radiographs are limited in their ability to demonstrate subtle subchondral cyst formation, and they provide no information on the status of the soft tissue.

CT provides valuable information on the involved bony architecture. Scans in the coronal and axial planes should be obtained for patients with persistent pain, even when initial radiographs appeared normal (Fig. 11-2). Baseline CT scans can accurately diagnose all lesions except for early (stage I) lesions. Information can be obtained on the size and location of bone fragments, the integrity of subchondral bone, and the presence or absence of cyst formation. Intra-articular injection of contrast can add to the diagnostic accuracy of cartilage lesions and provide information on the state of attachment of the osteochondral fragment to the talus.[21,22]

MRI affords an accurate assessment of the ankle's soft tissue structures, including the articular cartilage and supporting ligaments. Multiplanar evaluation is possible with no radiation exposure to the patient. Sequences can identify the size and location, and they provide information on the stability of the lesion (Figs. 11-3 and 11-4). DeSmet and colleagues[23] prospectively showed an excellent correlation between staging in MRI and arthroscopy and correctly predicted stable and unstable lesions in 92% of cases. MR arthrography (MRA) has become a useful adjunct to routine MRI and may provide more detail about the osteochondral lesion and afford improved preoperative planning (Fig. 11-5).

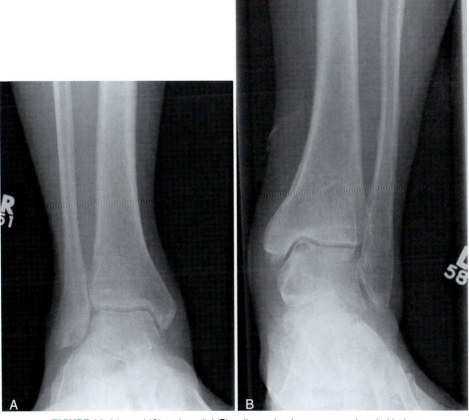

FIGURE 11-1 Lateral (**A**) and medial (**B**) radiographs show an osteochondral lesion.

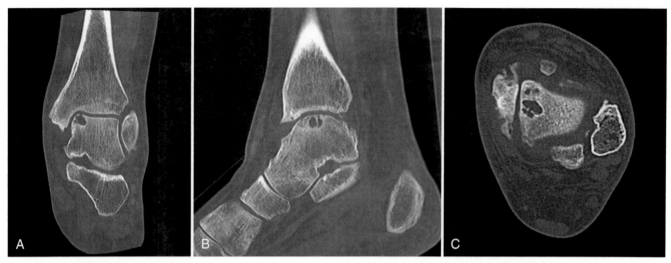

FIGURE 11-2 Coronal (**A**), sagittal (**B**), and axial (**C**) computed tomography views show a medial osteochondral lesion.

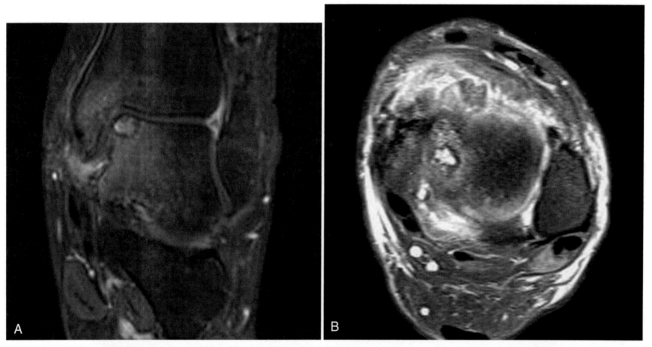

FIGURE 11-3 Coronal (**A**) and axial (**B**) T2-weighted MRI scans shows a medial osteochondral lesion.

Bone scintigraphic results correlate with osteochondral injury and can be used to discern which joint is causing clinical discomfort if other imaging modalities have not been helpful in locating the lesion.[24] It may also have a role in localizing CT to the specific area of uptake. More advanced imaging has largely replaced scintigraphy, but it still provides a valuable tool in the workup of persistent ankle pain for the surgeon without immediate access to CT or MRI.

Verhagen and coworkers[25] prospectively compared the patient's history and physical examination, plain radiographs, CT, MRI, and arthroscopy for diagnosing an osteochondral fracture of the talus or tibial plafond in 104 painful ankles with 35 lesions. Plain radiographs had a sensitivity of 70% and a specific-ity of 94%. CT had a sensitivity of 81% and a specificity of 99%. MRI showed a sensitivity of 96% and a specificity of 99%, whereas arthroscopy showed a sensitivity of 100% and a specificity of 97%. There was no statistically significant difference found between CT, MRI, and arthroscopy. CT had a better positive predictive value than other modalities, and MRI had a better negative predictive value.[25] Arthroscopy tended to miss the lesions on the tibial side, so the specificity of this diagnostic modality would like trend closer to 100% if only talar lesions were studied.

Stone[26] recommended an imaging protocol that may prove beneficial for the general orthopedist. On initial presentation, plain radiographs are obtained, and if acute pathology is

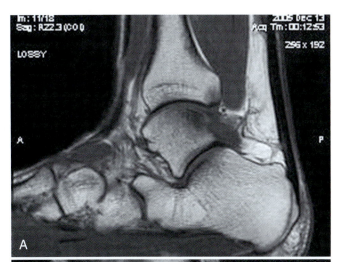

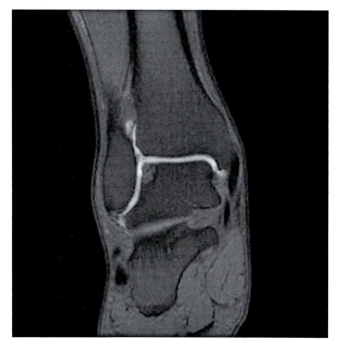

FIGURE 11-5 Coronal magnetic resonance arthrography shows a lateral osteochondral lesion.

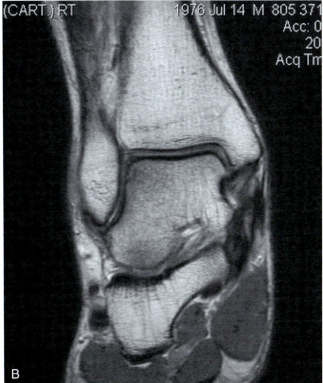

FIGURE 11-4 Coronal, T1-weighted (**A**) and sagittal, T2-weighted (**B**) MRI scans show a lateral osteochondral lesion.

recognized, a CT scan is obtained to delineate the size, location, and degree of displacement of the osteochondral fragment. If no pathology is seen, nonoperative management for a presumed soft tissue injury is initiated. If symptoms persist despite normal radiographs, MRI is recommended because of its ability to detect bony and soft tissue lesions that may be causing symptoms. CT and MRI are equivalent sources of information in the decision-making pathway for recognized lesions, but MRI can help to diagnose osteochondral lesion and other pathology without increased radiation exposure and should be the investigation of choice after plain film radiography for evaluation of persistent foot and ankle pain.

TREATMENT

Natural History and Recommended Treatment

The natural history of osteochondral lesions remains controversial because most patients receive some form of nonoperative or operative treatment. In a small series of 10 ankles with osteochondral lesions followed for more than 15 years, 4 of 6 ankles treated nonoperatively failed to heal, but the ankles remained asymptomatic. Osteoarthritis developed in only 2 of 10 ankles and was reported as an uncommon complication.[27] Further study by Bruns[28] showed that development of osteoarthritis was uncommon and that it occurred only to a mild degree in adult patients with osteochondral lesions.

Most published sources recommend nonoperative treatment for Berndt and Harty stage I and II lesions. Controversy exists for stage III lesions and lesions in the skeletally immature patient. In a systematic review of 210 patients, Tol and associates[29] found a success rate of 45% for nonoperative treatment of stage I and II lesions and medial stage III lesions. This nonoperative intervention included a period of immobilization and limited or no weight bearing.[29] Canale and Belding[6] showed that nonoperative and operative treatment of stage III lesions was equivalent, but the results of operatively treated lateral lesions were superior. This finding likely reflects the fact that medial lesions are deeper and inherently more stable than lateral lesions.

Results of operative treatment are varied and depend on the lesion's characteristics and the intervention provided. Tol and colleagues[29] found that excision, curettage, and drilling had an 85% success rate, whereas excision and curettage without drilling had a success rate of 78%, a difference that was not statistically significant. Operative intervention is recommended for

Berndt and Harty stage III and IV lesions and for smaller lesions with ongoing clinical symptoms. Stage V lesions (cystic) remain controversial, with evidence for and against operative intervention. Shearer and coworkers[30] showed that 71% of these lesions had good or excellent results at an average follow-up of 38 months. They suggested that these lesions usually run a benign course and remain stable with time, and unless progressive enlargement occurs, they do not warrant operative management. In contrast, Scranton and associates[41] suggested that type V cystic lesions have a poorer surgical prognosis, and they suggested that an aggressive surgical approach using osteochondral autografting was more appropriate for patients with large cystic lesions. Concern also exists about the urgency of intervening operatively if nonoperative management fails, but it is generally agreed that delaying operative intervention for a period of up to 12 months does not compromise the results of subsequent surgical treatment.[31]

For skeletally immature patients, most physicians have traditionally recommended a trial of nonoperative management for stage I, II, or III lesions because they retain the propensity to heal. This was disputed by Letts and colleagues[32], who reported a series of 26 lesions followed for a mean of 16 months. They reported good results for only 37.5% of all patients with stage I, II, or III lesions treated with immobilization and protected weight bearing.[32] The trend will likely be toward treating skeletally immature patients with the same principles as applied to the adult population, with a trial of nonoperative treatment for stable stage I or II lesions and operative intervention for stages III and IV.

The indications for operative and nonoperative treatment of osteochondral lesions remain controversial because most published series do not provide an accurate description of the size and site of the involved lesions.[26] When making treatment decisions, it is important to consider patient characteristics (e.g., age, activity) and lesion characteristics (e.g., size, site, stability, chronicity). Based on these characteristics, a decision can be made to treat with nonoperative regimens or with surgical intervention.

Nonoperative Management

Nonoperative management is aimed at reducing the associated synovitis, relieving pain, and maintaining range of motion. Nonsteroidal anti-inflammatory drugs and physiotherapy together with a period of restricted weight bearing are indicated. During the acute presentation, cast or brace immobilization may be beneficial. The duration of weight-bearing restriction required is not clearly defined because this factor has been poorly controlled in most published series. An injection of local corticosteroid into the joint may help to reduce inflammation, but this effect is temporary and is not routinely recommended. Chondroprotective agents may have some role, but no objective evidence exists to support their use in osteochondral lesions.

Operative Treatment

Operative management of osteochondral lesions is indicated for lesions that have failed nonoperative intervention and for larger, inherently unstable lesions. Many methods of operative management are available, and recommended guidelines continue to be published and presented on a regular basis, although no firm evidence-based guideline exists to aid in the operative decision-making process for osteochondral lesions.

The principles of operative intervention are to relieve pain and restore joint function by the removal of loose bodies, stabilization of the adjacent interface of bone and articular cartilage, and removal of any necrotic subchondral bone at the base of the lesion. The cause of pain in patients with an osteochondral lesion of the talar dome is unclear but probably is related to the presence of loose bodies or to unstable bone margins, because the articular cartilage itself has no nerve innervation. The primary goal of pain relief may be achieved in most patients by débridement procedures combined with some form of treatment of the base to stimulate the formation of fibrocartilage, such as curettage, abrasion, drilling, or microfracture. The secondary goal of prevention of development of degenerative arthritis is more difficult to define because there are no long-term studies to document the prevention of degenerative changes by other forms of articular cartilage replacement or regeneration.

Treatment can be accomplished by open or arthroscopic means, depending on the location of the lesion and the expertise of the surgeon. Operative management includes primary fixation or intervention using techniques of nontissue transplantation or tissue transplantation for the treatment of an irreparable or chronic osteochondral lesion (Table 11-2). Many techniques have been described, and they often are based on the patient's age and the stage and size of the osteochondral lesion. Am in-depth review of all techniques is beyond the scope of this chapter, but an overview of the available techniques follows.

We recommend arthroscopic débridement associated with any technique of subchondral bone penetration (i.e., curettage, drilling, or microfracture) for osteochondral lesion of the talus that is less than 15 mm in diameter (see Fig. 11-1). This approach aims at promoting revascularization of the lesion and creating stability with a healthy rim of attached cartilage and a

TABLE 11-2 Surgical Intervention Options

Nontissue transplantation
Primary internal fixation
Primary intervention
Excision or débridement
Curettage
Drilling
Microfracture
Tissue transplantation
Autologous bone graft
Osteochondral autograft transplantation
Single plug
Mosaicplasty
Osteochondral allograft transplantation
Autologous chondrocyte transplantation
Autologous stem cell transplantation

base of bleeding subchondral bone. Thorough débridement of the degenerative cartilage together with a secondary intervention (e.g., drilling) does make a significant difference in lesion grade over time and is recommended.[33] These techniques are simple, are cost effective, and have shown good results, as reported in the literature for primary and revision procedures. However, the base of the lesion is filled with fibrocartilage, and although this is usually sufficient for smaller lesions, the inferior mechanical properties compared with hyaline cartilage may lead to earlier failure in larger lesions. Other techniques are recommended for larger lesions, but the exact size is controversial. Some surgeons suggests that lesions should be no larger than 1.5 cm^2 and 7 mm deep and lesions that fail to respond to arthroscopic débridement and subchondral bone penetration.[34]

For larger lesions and lesions that fail to respond to arthroscopic débridement and subchondral bone penetration, management options include tissue transplantation with autograft tissue (i.e., osteochondral autologous transfer system [OATS] or mosaicplasty) or allograft tissue (i.e., fresh allograft or fresh-frozen allograft). Common guidelines suggest lesions with a diameter of more than 10 mm are best suited to tissue transplantation. OATS and mosaicplasty harvest full-thickness osteochondral plugs from a donor site and implant these plugs into the osteochondral lesion's site using an interference fit. Donor site cartilage appears to remain as type II collagen with normal articular proteoglycans and microarchitecture. However, the border area of most grafts is filled in with fibrocartilage.[35-37] These techniques have shown good or excellent results (mostly level IV evidence) during short-term to intermediate-term follow-up. Results are less promising in older patients with larger lesions, and concern still exists about donor site morbidity and the considerable mechanical differences between knee and ankle cartilage. The use of osteochondral allografts negates the risk of donor site morbidity but comes with a low risk of disease transmission. Short-term and intermediate-term results with fresh and fresh-frozen allograft transplantation are promising, with most grafts incorporating and functioning reasonably well at long-term follow-up.[38]

Autologous chondrocyte implantation has gained popularity based on its reported success in treating lesions of the knee Koulalis and colleagues[39] have reported good or excellent results with no complications for their small series of patients, and Whittaker and coworkers[40] reported a 90% rate of good or excellent results in their series; the defect was filled in all cases. This method can treat larger lesions and, with careful technique, can address shoulder lesions. However, it is costly, requires staged procedures, and is associated with a longer recovery period. Despite these factors, autologous chondrocyte implantation remains a favorable approach for certain osteochondral lesions involving the talus, such as large, noncystic lesions in younger patients. Autologous stem cells have also been implanted on acellular scaffolds or mixed within the implanted matrix. These pluripotential cells are thought to have the ability to organize and recreate structural tissue, including chondral and subchondral anatomy.

PEARLS & PITFALLS

- The primary cause of osteochondral lesions is trauma, and the incidence is high when associated with an ankle fracture.
- Patients with atraumatic osteochondral lesions warrant workup for secondary predisposing causes.
- Further imaging is recommended for patients with ongoing symptoms after adequate initial management of an ankle sprain.
- CT is recommended for lesions visible on plain radiographs, but MRI proves more useful for patients with chronic pain with an undetermined cause.
- Definitive management is based on patient characteristics (e.g., age, activity) and characteristics of the osteochondral lesion (e.g., site, size, stability, chronicity).
- The natural history of these lesions is controversial, but it appears that late development of osteoarthritis is uncommon and, if present, remains mild.
- The incidental finding of an osteochondral lesion in an asymptomatic patient does not require surgical intervention.
- For patients requiring intervention, a thorough assessment of the lesion's characteristics is required to determine the optimal technique to minimize complications and afford the best possible outcome.

Postoperative Rehabilitation

Postoperative management is based on each patient's individual intervention. For simple arthroscopic débridement and subchondral bone penetration there is no consensus on whether immediate weight bearing or protected weight bearing is best. For patients undergoing initial primary fixation or intervention other than simple débridement a period of limited or non-weight bearing for six weeks is recommended. The guidelines for transplantation have not been established with the literature suggesting limited weight bearing from two up to twelve weeks. There appears to be more consensuses on range of motion with active and passive range initiated as soon as can be tolerated by the patient. For intervention requiring bone healing, rehabilitation begins after healing is demonstrated with the goal of restoring ankle range of motion with active and passive exercises progressed to strength and proprioception training tailored to the patients need.

REFERENCES

1. Barrie HJ. Osteochondritis dissecans 1887-1987. A centennial look at Konig's memorable phrase. *J Bone Joint Surg Br.* 1987;69:693-695.
2. Pappas AM. Osteochondrosis dissecans. *Clin Orthop Relat Res.* 1981; (158):59-69.
3. Berndt AL, Harty M. Transchondral fractures (osteochondritis dissecans) of the talus. *J Bone Joint Surg Am.* 1959;41A:988-1020.
4. Sugimoto K, Takakura Y, Tohno Y, et al. Cartilage thickness of the talar dome. *Arthroscopy.* 2005;21:401-404.
5. Athanasiou KA, Niederauer GG, Schenck RC Jr. Biomechanical topography of human ankle cartilage. Ann Biomed Eng 1995;23:697-704.
6. Canale ST, Belding RH. Osteochondral lesions of the talus. *J Bone Joint Surg Am.* 1980;62:97-102.
7. Flick AB, Gould N. Osteochondritis dissecans of the talus (transchondral fractures of the talus): review of the literature and new surgical approach for medial dome lesions. *Foot Ankle.* 1985;5:165-185.
8. Bauer RS, Ochsner PE. [Nosology of osteochondrosis dissecans of the trochlea of the talus.] *Z Orthop Ihre Grenzgeb.* 1987;125:194-200.
9. Anderson DV, Lyne ED. Osteochondritis dissecans of the talus: case report on two family members. *J Pediatr Orthop.* 1984;4:356-357.

10. Woods K, Harris I. Osteochondritis dissecans of the talus in identical twins. *J Bone Joint Surg Br.* 1995;77:331.

11. Coltart WD. Aviator's astragalus. *J Bone Joint Surg Br.* 1952;34B:545-566.

12. Bosien WR, Staples OS, Russell SW. Residual disability following acute ankle sprains. *J Bone Joint Surg Am.* 1955;37A:1237-1243.

13. Leontaritis N, Hinojosa L, Panchbhavi VK. Arthroscopically detected intra-articular lesions associated with acute ankle fractures. *J Bone Joint Surg Am.* 2009;91:333-339.

14. Hintermann B, Regazzoni P, Lampert C, et al. Arthroscopic findings in acute fractures of the ankle. *J Bone Joint Surg Br.* 2000;82:345-351.

15. Chew KT, Tay E, Wong YS. Osteochondral lesions of the talus. *Ann Acad Med Singapore.* 2008;37:63-68.

16. Anderson I.F, Chrichton KJ, Grattan-Smith T, et al. Osteochondral fractures of the dome of the talus. *J Bone Joint Surg Am.* 1989;71:1143-1152.

17. Bruns J, Rosenbach B, Kahrs J. [Etiopathogenetic aspects of medial osteochondrosis dissecans tali.] *Sportverletz Sportschaden.* 1992;6:43-49.

18. Ferkel RD, Scranton PE Jr. Arthroscopy of the ankle and foot. *J Bone Joint Surg Am.* 1993;75:1233-1242.

19. Hepple S, Winson LG, Glew D. Osteochondral lesions of the talus: a revised classification. *Foot Ankle Int.* 1999;20:789-793.

20. Stroud CC, Marks RM. Imaging of osteochondral lesions of the talus. *Foot Ankle Clin.* 2000;5:119-133.

21. Ragozzino A, Rossi G, Esposito S, et al. [Computerized tomography of osteochondral diseases of the talus dome.] *Radiol Med.* 1996;92:682-686.

22. Heare MM, Gillespy T 3rd, Bittar ES. Direct coronal computed tomography arthrography of osteochondritis dissecans of the talus. *Skeletal Radiol.* 1988;17:187-189.

23. De Smet AA, Fisher DR, Burnstein MI, et al. Value of MR imaging in staging osteochondral lesions of the talus (osteochondritis dissecans): results in 14 patients. *AJR Am J Roentgenol.* 1990;154:555-558.

24. Schimmer RC, Dick W, Hintermann B. The role of ankle arthroscopy in the treatment strategies of osteochondritis dissecans lesions of the talus. *Foot Ankle Int.* 2001;22:895-900.

25. Verhagen RA, Maas M, Dijkgraaf MG, et al. Prospective study on diagnostic strategies in osteochondral lesions of the talus. Is MRI superior to helical CT? *J Bone Joint Surg Br.* 2005;87:41-46.

26. Stone JW. Osteochondral lesions of the talar dome. *J Am Acad Orthop Surg.* 1996;4:63-73.

27. McCullough CJ, Venugopal V. Osteochondritis dissecans of the talus: the natural history. *Clin Orthop Relat Res.* 1979;(144):264-268.

28. Bruns J. [Osteochondrosis dissecans tali. Results of surgical therapy.] *Unfallchirurg.* 1993;96:75-81.

29. Tol JL, Struijs PAA, Bossuyt PMM, et al. Treatment strategies in osteochondral defects of the talar dome: a systematic review. *Foot Ankle Int.* 2000;21:119-126.

30. Shearer C, Loomer R, Clement D. Nonoperatively managed stage 5 osteochondral talar lesions. *Foot Ankle Int.* 2002;23:651-654.

31. O'Farrell TA, Costello BG. Osteochondritis dissecans of the talus. The late results of surgical treatment. *J Bone Joint Surg Br.* 1982;64:494-497.

32. Letts M, Davidson D, Ahmer A. Osteochondritis dissecans of the talus in children. *J Pediatr Orthop.* 2003;23:617-625.

33. Takao M, Uchio Y, Kakimaru H, et al. Arthroscopic drilling with débridement of remaining cartilage for osteochondral lesions of the talar dome in unstable ankles. *Am J Sports Med.* 2004;32:332-336.

34. Giannini S, Vannini F. Operative treatment of osteochondral lesions of the talar dome: current concepts review. *Foot Ankle Int.* 2004;25:168-175.

35. Lee CH, Chao KH, Huang GS, Wu SS. Osteochondral autografts for osteochondritis dissecans of the talus. *Foot Ankle Int.* 2003;24:815-822.

36. Baltzer AW, Arnold JP. Bone-cartilage transplantation from the ipsilateral knee for chondral lesions of the talus. *Arthroscopy.* 2005;21:159-166.

37. Hangody L, Kish G, Módis L, et al. Mosaicplasty for the treatment of osteochondritis dissecans of the talus: two to seven year results in 36 patients. *Foot Ankle Int.* 2001;22:552-558.

38. Gross AE, Agnidis Z, Hutchison CR. Osteochondral defects of the talus treated with fresh osteochondral allograft transplantation. *Foot Ankle Int.* 2001;22:385-391.

39. Koulalis D, Schultz W, Heyden M. Autologous chondrocyte transplantation for osteochondritis dissecans of the talus. *Clin Orthop Relat Res.* 2002;(395):186-192.

40. Whittaker JP, Smith G, Makwana N, et al. Early results of autologous chondrocyte implantation in the talus. *J Bone Joint Surg Br.* 2005;87:179-183.

41. Scranton PE, Frey CC, Feder KS. Outcome of osteochondral autograft transplantation for type-V cystic osteochondral lesions of the talus. *J Bone Joint Surg Br.* 2006;88:614-619.

Osteochondral Lesions of the Talar Dome:
Débridement, Abrasion, Drilling, and Microfracture

Thomas O. Clanton ● Brian Weatherby

Osteochondral lesions of the talus (OLTs) have various names and presentations. After the diagnosis is clear from the history, physical examination, and appropriate imaging studies, the treatment plan can be outlined for the patient. Nonoperative treatment with immobilization and no weight bearing remains a valid alternative, particularly for the patient without evidence of separation of the lesion.

The recommendations in this chapter pertain primarily to the patient who has presented with pain or mechanical symptoms that necessitate intervention or to the patient who has failed prior nonoperative management. In such cases, surgery is indicated, and the most thought-provoking decision for the surgeon and the patient becomes the exact procedure that will produce the best overall outcome for correcting the problem.

Since the introduction of arthroscopy, the most common operative treatments rendered for OLT have been a continuation of what had been performed previously through standard incisions, such as excision of a loose fragment, débridement of the lesion, drilling, or abrasion and curettage. With the addition of the microfracture technique, as originally described for the knee by Steadman[1] and later modified to the ankle, these forms of treatment for OLTs are collectively known as *conventional surgical treatment.*

INDICATIONS AND CONTRAINDICATIONS

Several factors must be taken into consideration to select the most appropriate surgical procedure for a symptomatic OLT, including the location, size or depth, and grade or stage of the lesion. Patient-specific characteristics, such as age, body mass index (BMI), degree of ankle instability, ankle alignment, duration of symptoms, and previous surgery, also influence outcomes.[2-6]

The lesion's location does not technically limit the ability to perform the conventional surgical treatments discussed in this chapter as it does other restorative procedures, such as osteochondral autograft or allograft transplantation (i.e., osteoarticular transfer system [OATS]) or autologous chondrocyte implantation (ACI), which require greater access to the talar dome.[7] Schimmer and colleagues[8] found a trend toward a better prognosis for medial lesions, and Choi and associates[9] found that anterior lesions had better results than posterior lesions, although this was disputed in a large case series that showed no correlation between outcome and lesion location.[2,10] The location of the osteochondral lesion should not preclude treatment or greatly affect the outcome of lesions treated with conventional surgical treatment. It does however, have an impact on the use of specific surgical techniques (discussed later).

In contrast to the location of the lesion, size has proved to be an important prognostic indicator of the success of conventional surgical treatment. Good or excellent outcomes have been demonstrated in several studies in which the OLT was intraoperatively measured at less than 1.5 to 2.0 cm^2, with later studies advocating a cut-off size of 1.5 cm^2.[2,6,11,12] For lesions larger than 1.5 cm^2, OATS or ACI have been recommended by several surgeons.[13-15] These transplantation techniques have yielded good or excellent results.[16-18] Size may also be a determinant for internal fixation of acute, displaced osteochondral fragments in young patients. DeLee[19] advocated internal fixation for a fragment that is larger than one third of the size of the dome. Alternatively, Stone and coworkers[20] recommended that the lesion be at least 7.5 mm in diameter to warrant internal fixation.

Various grading and staging systems exist for the classification of OLTs, and each is driven by its own descriptors. Unfortunately, this has made the interpretation of results difficult for correlation of outcomes with stage or grade.[12] It is widely accepted that a higher stage has a worse prognosis, as seen in a case series that established a relationship between the arthroscopic stage of Ferkel and clinical outcome.[10]

The literature on this topic reflects the importance of separating lesions into two distinct categories: those that have a cystic component, reflecting an underlying bony defect, and those that do not.[3,4,6,21] Cystic lesions should then be further subdivided into two groups based on the presence or absence of an intact dome of overlying articular cartilage. Cystic lesions usually have poorer outcomes than noncystic lesions when treated with excision and curettage or with excision and drilling.[3,4,6] However, successful treatment outcomes for cystic lesions with an intact cartilage cap have been demonstrated with the technique of retrograde drilling from the lateral talar process or sinus tarsi and bone grafting.[21,22] This technique avoids violation of the intact talar dome cartilage while stimulating restoration of the underlying void. If a defect in the overlying cartilage is associated with a cystic lesion, it should be débrided and drilled or microfractured, and bone should be grafted to provide structural support for the replacement layer of fibrocartilage and any existing stable cartilage flap.

Accumulated experience in treating OLTs has taught us that factors associated with the individual patient can have a tremendous impact on the result of conventional surgical treatment.[2-6] Several case series with relatively long-term follow-up have suggested that acute lesions have significantly better clinical outcome scores than chronic lesions.[2-6] The threshold offered in most studies that delineates the two categories is a 12-month duration of symptoms. More controversy surrounds the influence of patient age on the outcome of OLT treatment. Three separate case series with a total of 386 patients revealed no significant correlation between patient age and outcome.[3,6,9] In contrast, two case series with a total of 122 patients revealed a significant association between patient age and outcome, with success more often seen in patients younger than 30 to 35 years and failure seen in patients 45 to 50 years old.[2,4]

With regard to patient weight (i.e., BMI), two small case series addressing OLTs failed to establish any relationship with outcomes.[3,23] The opposite viewpoint is supported by a large case series evaluating OLTs[2] and another large, prospective cohort study analyzing osteochondral lesions of the knee,[24] which showed a BMI grater than 28 to 30 to be a significant variable in predicting successful conventional surgical treatment.

Ankle instability has been an accepted cause of OLT, and surgically correcting ankle instability in the setting of a talar OLT should correlate with outcome. This has been clearly demonstrated by two independent studies,[2,8] and it is recommended that any patient with mechanical ankle instability undergo some type of anatomic ligament reconstruction at the time OLT is surgically addressed. Although it seems that the immobilization required after ligament reconstruction may impair the healing process stimulated by conventional surgical treatment and promoted by early passive motion and no weight bearing, this approach has not been confirmed.

Another patient-specific factor to take into consideration is prior conventional surgical treatment. Existing literature on this topic has exhibited inconsistent findings and led to controversy on the topic. Schuman and colleagues[25] showed that revision curettage and drilling had a poorer outcome (75% good or excellent results) compared with that of primary curettage and drilling (86%), and a case series[2] of 105 patients found that 17 patients who underwent repeat débridement and microfracture did not meet the criteria for a successful result, although they did improve their American Orthopaedic Foot and Ankle Society (AOFAS) scores by a mean of 17.2 points postoperatively. A different case series of 12 patients treated with repeat arthroscopic débridement and curettage reported overwhelmingly successful results.[26] Based on these findings, it is reasonable to recommend repeat conventional surgical treatment to address persistently symptomatic OLTs after a primary procedure, with the exception of cystic lesions.[3]

After processing all of the aforementioned factors, operative intervention using conventional options can be chosen as a valid treatment for an OLT. It is therefore helpful to compartmentalize the information presented into more concrete categories: indications, contraindications, and relative contraindications (Table 12-1). Conventional surgical treatment encompasses

TABLE 12-1

Indications	Contraindications	Relative Contraindications
Failure of nonoperative treatment	Size > 15 mm^2	One prior CST
Displaced fragments	Two prior CSTs	Age > 50
Small cystic and noncystic lesions	Large cystic lesion	BMI > 30
Size < 15 mm^2	Inadequate nonoperative treatment if indicated	Kissing lesion on the tibia
Age < 50 years	Acute lesion with attached subchondral bone > 7.5 mm diameter	
BMI < 30		
Presence of ankle instability		

BMI, body mass index; CST, conventional surgical treatment.

several different surgical techniques. In the treatment of non-cystic lesions, arthroscopic excision of loose fragments and débridement of the lesion are consistent approaches. Variability is introduced in the selection of drilling, abrasion and curettage, or microfracture as the additional maneuver. The medical literature shows no significant differences in outcome for these approaches. This has been demonstrated in studies directly comparing these surgical options[11,27] and by numerous other studies that show successful outcomes with each individual technique.[2,5,9,10,12,23] In the treatment of a lesion with a cystic component, the surgical technique directly impacts the outcome, and retrograde drilling with bone grafting should be performed when possible.[21,22]

TREATMENT
Conservative Management

In the evolution of treatment for osteochondral lesions, the nonoperative approach with protection from weight-bearing stresses began with the adolescent knee.[28-31] This approach was extended to the ankle until the classic study by Berndt and Harty, which included a careful analysis of 24 cases of OLT and a systematic review of the literature that included 191 lesions in 183 patients.[32] Their study found a 75% rate of poor results for the conservatively treated patients, and it confirmed that the results in children were no better than in adults. Over the ensuing 50 years, the nonoperative treatment of limited weight bearing and cast immobilization has continued to be the recommended treatment for Berndt and Harty stage 1 and 2 lesions, which are nondisplaced fragments that remain at least partially attached.[33-35] Because there are no adverse affects on the final outcome if surgery is delayed for up to 12 months, a trial of nonoperative treatment of these lesions is warranted.[35-37]

Another consideration in the nonoperative management of OLT, viscosupplementation, has gained attention. Viscosupplementation has been used as an approved treatment for arthritis of the knee for some time, and although it remains controversial, several studies have shown its effectiveness for use in the treatment of ankle arthritis.[38-40] This experience has been extrapolated to sporadic use for OLTs, and a prospective study has shown promising results. Mei-Dan and colleagues[41] demonstrated statistically significant decreases in pain and stiffness, with increases in functional scores over a 26-week follow-up period. In a patient who is adamantly averse to surgical intervention, viscosupplementation can be introduced as a potentially viable treatment option.

Unfortunately, the correlation between the radiographic grade and the actual condition of the articular cartilage is not very accurate, making it difficult to recommend treatment guidelines based solely on radiographic or CT images.[42] Magnetic resonance imaging (MRI) has become the standard for evaluation of the articular cartilage in osteochondral lesions, and findings correlate well with arthroscopic findings.[43] MRI studies should be obtained for all symptomatic lesions requiring treatment. The articular cartilage can then be analyzed to determine whether it remains contiguous at some point, allowing creation of a flap, or there is complete disruption of continuity, signaling an unstable pattern and warranting surgical intervention.

Arthroscopic Technique

The arthroscopic approach is the gold standard for treatment of OLTs. This technique facilitates visualization of the entire joint and avoids the morbidity associated with an open procedure. Advances in arthroscopic technology have provided small, fiberoptic, 2.7-mm arthroscopes with options of 30-degree and 70-degree viewing angles; more effective constructs to adequately distract the joint; and smaller versions of arthroscopic instruments. Not every OLT is directly accessible, and even the seasoned arthroscopic surgeon may have significant technical difficulty in addressing certain posterior lesions.

After standard visualization and working portals have been established, the joint is thoroughly visualized and photographed. Loose bodies within the joint should be identified and removed. In most circumstances, this means the arthroscope is in the anteromedial portal to begin the case. A probe can then be introduced through the anterolateral portal to locate and outline the lesion and to determine the integrity of the articular cartilage and underlying subchondral bone. Depending on the medial or lateral location and extent of the lesion, the arthroscope may be moved to the opposite portal to facilitate visualization and access. If at this point the lesion is seen to be too posterior to allow adequate evaluation, the posterolateral portal should be established without hesitation. The posteromedial portal is an option for posterior lesions, but extreme caution must be used in this area because of the potential for injury to the neurovascular bundle.

After the OLT is evaluated and proper access is obtained, the specific treatment is based on the type of lesion. At this stage, it is essential to have the necessary instrumentation and any special equipment potentially required to address unexpected situations (Box 12-1). This is best confirmed in the preoperative setting to ensure an unhindered operation.

The technique for most osteochondral lesions (i.e., those without underlying cystic lesions) is straightforward. Any loose,

---

Box 12-1 Special Instrumentation for Arthroscopic Treatment of an Osteochondral Lesion of the Talus

- Standard angled curettes (large variety)
- Small joint graspers
- Drill guide
- Small joint microfracture awls
- Power drill
- Long, 0.062-inch Kirschner wires
- 3.4- and 4.5-mm ring curettes
- Small, right-angle chisel

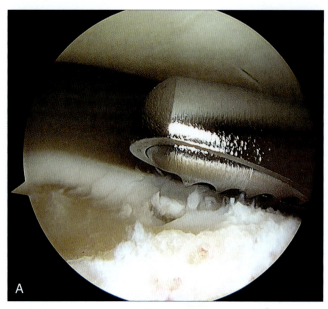

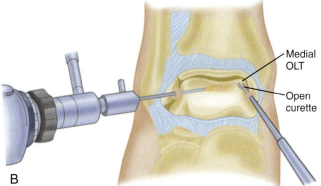

FIGURE 12-1 **A,** The arthroscopic image of an unstable osteochondral lesion on talar dome that is being débrided with a shaver. **B,** Drawing of arthroscopic débridement shows the scope in the anterolateral portal and the shaver in the anteromedial portal.

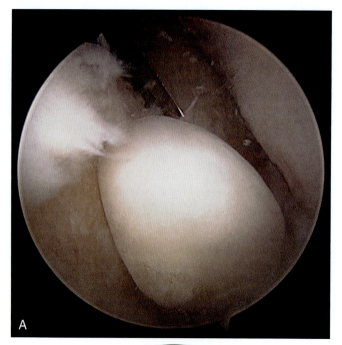

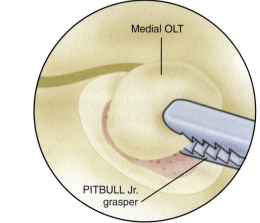

FIGURE 12-2 **A,** The arthroscopic image shows a loose osteochondral fragment being removed with a grasper. **B,** The drawing shows removal of an osteochondral fragment with a grasper.

unstable articular cartilage or osteochondral fragments must be débrided by shaving or curettage (Fig. 12-1) or by extracting the loose fragments from the joint with a grasper (Fig. 12-2). This leaves a defect in the articular surface with irregular margins that can be reformed into trephined edges with a small ring or regular curette (Fig. 12-3). Debris is removed from the joint with the shaver or a grasper, or both. If the basal layer of articular cartilage remains atop the defect, it is abraded or "scratched up" with a curette (Fig. 12-4). The surgeon can stop

at this point or proceed with drilling or microfracture of the lesion to further expose marrow elements to create a "super clot" (Fig. 12-5).

We use a 0.0625-inch Kirschner wire when drilling and standard or small microfracture awls for the microfracture technique. An assortment of angled awls is useful for penetrating the subchondral bone in a vertical orientation to the degree possible. The punctures are made to a depth of 2 mm and begin at the junction of normal cartilage with the osteochondral de-

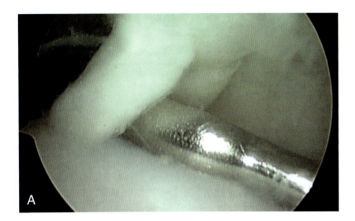

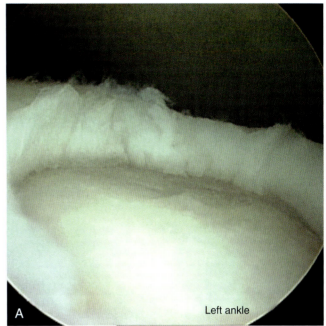

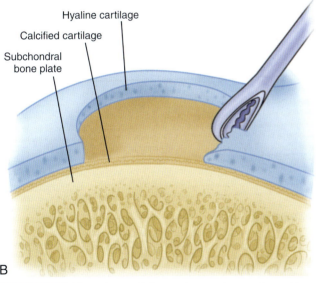

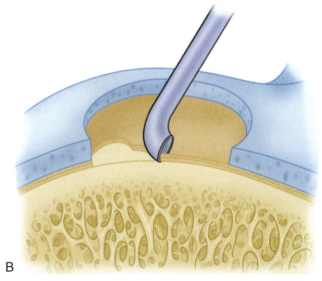

FIGURE 12-3 A, The arthroscopic image shows a ring curette pushing up a loose osteochondral fragment in preparation for trephining the edges. **B,** The drawing shows curettage of the osteochondral lesion to calcified cartilage layer with trephination of edge.

FIGURE 12-4 A, The arthroscopic image shows an osteochondral lesion at completion of curettage with removal of the calcified cartilage. **B,** The drawing shows curettage of the osteochondral lesion to remove the layer of calcified cartilage.

fect. After the perimeter of the lesion is microfractured, the pattern continues into the center of the lesion while keeping the holes 3 to 4 mm apart (Fig. 12-6). The shaver is again introduced to clean up the joint, and if used, the tourniquet is then released and the pump pressure reduced to confirm bleeding in the lesion (Fig. 12-7).

Technical aspects of antegrade drilling of OLTs depend on the location of the lesion. Anterolateral lesions are amenable to drilling through the anterolateral portal or through a separate anterior puncture in the capsule. The Kirschner wire can be introduced directly through the portal or placed through a guide, such as one of the meniscal repair cannulas used for inside-out repairs (Fig. 12-8). Plantar flexion of the ankle improves access to more posterior lesions. As in the microfracture technique described, drill holes should be placed at 3- to 4-mm intervals, beginning at the periphery of the lesion and working toward the center. Care is taken when drilling vertical walls not to perforate viable bone close to the overlying, intact subchon-

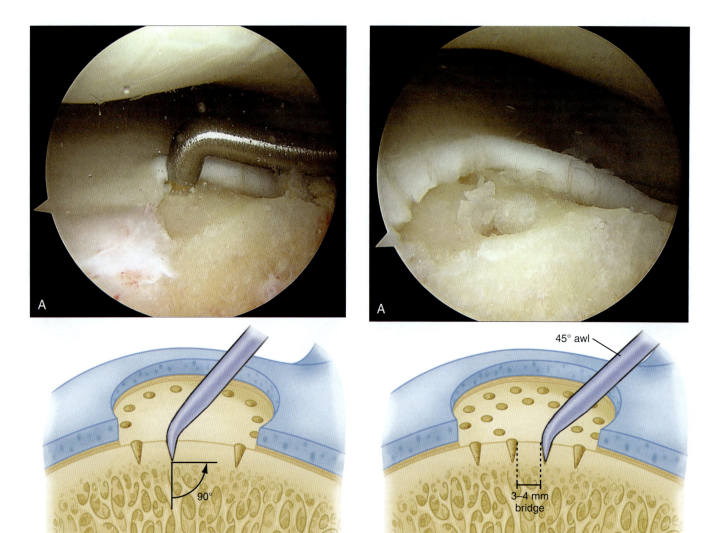

FIGURE 12-5 A, The arthroscopic image of microfracture being performed with a 90-degree awl. **B,** The drawing shows microfracture technique 1.

FIGURE 12-6 A, The arthroscopic image shows the osteochondral lesion after microfracture. **B,** The drawing shows of microfracture technique 2.

dral plate and therefore create a stress riser that may lead to further collapse. Drilling of posteromedial lesions may be facilitated by using a commercially available drill guide with a transmalleolar approach. The aiming guide arm is introduced into the joint with the tip placed into the center of the lesion under direct arthroscopic visualization. A percutaneous incision is made over the area of the medial malleolus as indicated by the location of the external trocar, and the trocar is then advanced down to bone. A 0.062-inch Kirschner wire is drilled through the trocar in a transmalleolar fashion and visualized entering the joint (Fig. 12-9). The ankle can be dorsiflexed and plantar flexed to drill multiple holes in the lesion through the same medial malleolar drill hole.

Any lesion encountered that maintains an intact cartilage roof with a cystic component and stable subchondral bone, although uncommon, is best treated with retrograde drilling and bone grafting[21,22] (Fig. 12-10). This technique involves the use of a transtalar approach accessed through a more distal anterolateral incision in the area of the sinus tarsi. After the additional incision is made and blunt dissection is carried out down to the talus, the arm of a commercially available drill guide is introduced into the ankle joint through the anteromedial or posterolateral portal with the arthroscope in the anterolateral or posterolateral portal. The tip of the aiming guide is directed to rest on top of the lesion's intact cartilage roof (Fig. 12-11). This can be assisted by the use of intraoperative C-arm fluoroscopy or, in some institutions, by

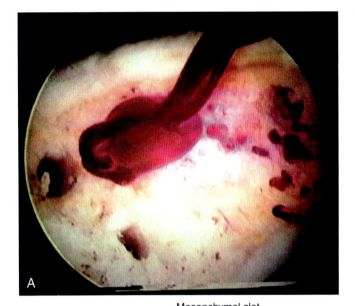

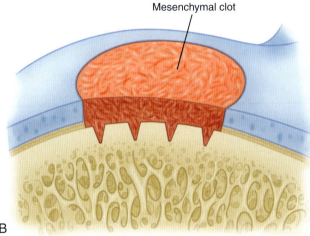

Mesenchymal clot

FIGURE 12-7 A, The arthroscopic image shows bleeding in the osteochondral lesion after microfracture. **B,** The drawing shows a mesenchymal clot formed in the osteochondral lesion after microfracture. (**A,** *From Ferkel RD, Zanotti RM, Komenda GA, et al. Arthroscopic treatment of chronic osteochondral lesions of the talus: long-term results. Am J Sports Med. 2008;36:7150-1761.*)

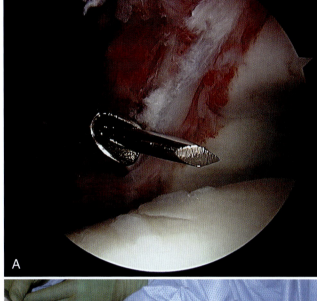

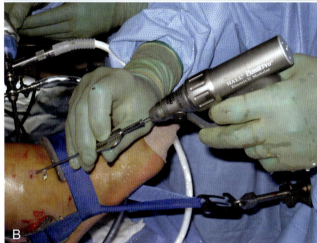

FIGURE 12-8 A, The arthroscopic image shows a 0.062-inch Kirschner wire placed through a meniscal guide to drill an osteochondral lesion. **B,** The arthroscope is placed in the anteromedial portal with a meniscal guide, and a Kirschner wire is placed through the anterolateral portal.

computer-assisted, three-dimensional guidance systems.[44] When the aiming guide is in place, a trocar is placed through the exterior arm of the drill guide into the sinus tarsi incision and down to talar bone. Using fluoroscopic guidance, a long Kirschner wire is then placed through the trocar and advanced up into the void of the cystic lesion but not through the stable subchondral bone. This position should be confirmed arthroscopically. The appropriate size of cannulated trephine drill is advanced over the Kirschner wire up to the tip, with care taken not to violate the roof. With an established tunnel leading to the lesion, the sub-chondral cyst can be curetted and bone grafted using autograft from the calcaneus or distal tibia (Fig. 12-12).

For a cystic lesion with unstable cartilage, standard or ring curettes are used to remove any loose articular cartilage flaps back to stable cartilage. The base of the lesion is inspected, and any unstable osteochondral fragment; soft, necrotic bone; or fibrous material is removed by curettage or shaving until viable bone is encountered (Fig. 12-13). The lesion must be thoroughly defined and débrided, including any portion that extends onto the vertical surfaces of the talus in the gutter.

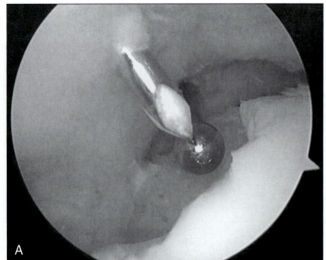

FIGURE 12-9 A, The arthroscopic image shows drilling through the medial malleolus, with the drill guide entering anteromedially for a posteromedial osteochondral lesion. **B,** The drawing shows a drill guide being used for transmalleolar drilling of an osteochondral lesion of a left ankle shoulder lesion. (**A**, *From Ferkel RD, Zanotti RM, Komenda GA, et al. Arthroscopic treatment of chronic osteochondral lesions of the talus: long-term results. Am J Sports Med. 2008;36:7150-1761).*

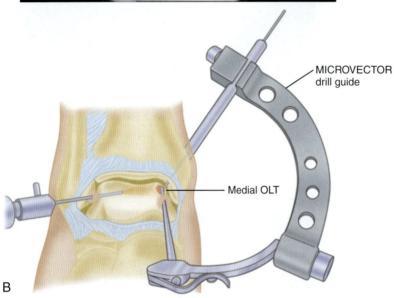

MICROVECTOR
drill guide

Medial OLT

B

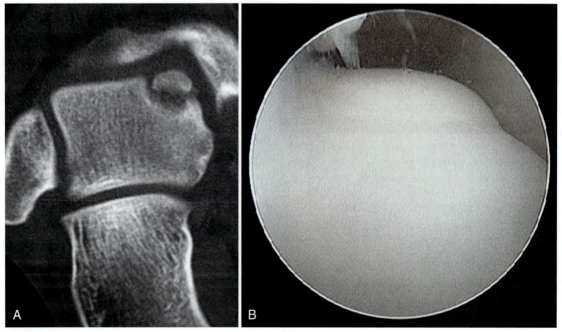

FIGURE 12-10 A, Coronal CT shows an osteochondral lesion of the medial talar dome with intact articular cartilage and an underlying cyst. **B,** Arthroscopic image of same osteochondral lesion shows intact articular cartilage.

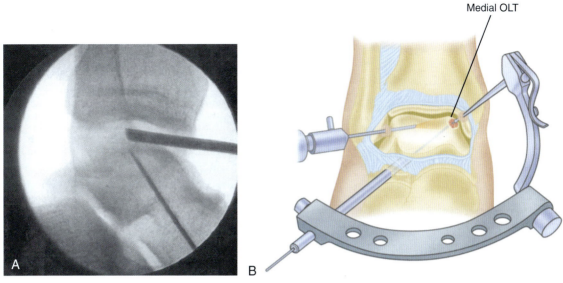

FIGURE 12-11 A, Fluoroscopy shows retrograde drilling of a medial osteochondral lesion of the talus (OLT). **B,** The drawing shows retrograde drilling of a medial OLT with a drill guide.

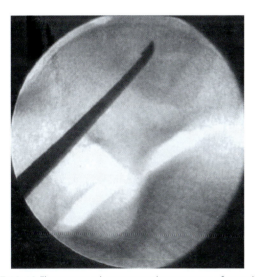

FIGURE 12-12 Fluoroscopy shows transtalar curettage of a medial osteochondral lesion of the talus.

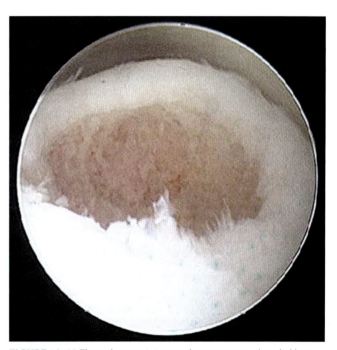

FIGURE 12-13 The arthroscopic image shows an osteochondral lesion of the talus after curettage to viable bone.

The remaining defect should be thoroughly inspected. If a hard sclerotic bony base is present that was not easily penetrated with the curettage performed, additional perforation with a microfracture awl or antegrade drilling is recommended to expose marrow elements to the defect (Fig. 12-14). Additional stimulation should be done if there is no punctate bleeding demonstrated after curettage when the inflow pressure is reduced or the tourniquet is released.

The cystic lesion may warrant open bone grafting after curettage and débridement have been done. There is no consensus regarding this issue, and no specific lesion size or depth to guide the indication of bone grafting has been established in the literature. Saxena and colleagues[45] performed autogenous bone grafting by open arthrotomy on all Hepple stage 5 lesions (i.e., subchondral cyst formation seen on MRI) found in athletes with 90% good or excellent outcomes and a mean time for return to activity of 20 weeks. We prefer to obtain autogenous bone graft from the calcaneus or distal tibia by using 6- or 8-mm bone graft harvester reamers, which are commercially available. The lesion must then be approached in an open fashion by an arthrotomy or osteotomy, depending on the location of the lesion, as described in detail by Muir and associates.[7]

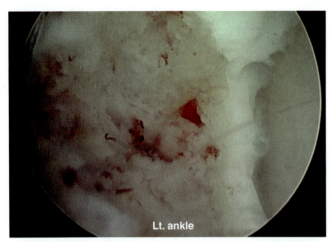

FIGURE 12-14 The arthroscopic image shows an osteochondral lesion of the talus after curettage and microfracture with early bleeding.

After the lesion is accessed, the bone graft should be tamped into place so that the void is tightly packed and no graft remnants are left prominent.

PEARLS&PITFALLS

PEARLS

- Nonoperative treatment is the recommended option for nondisplaced lesions that remain at least partially attached. Cast immobilization and limited weight bearing do not endanger surgical outcomes, even when surgery delayed up to 12 months.
- Preoperative planning with CT or MRI can guide the optimal portal placement and ensure adequate visualization and access for the working instruments.
- All conventional surgical methods (i.e., curettage, drilling, abrasion, and microfracture) have statistically similar results. The choice should depend on the surgeon's preference and access to the lesion.
- The surgeon should preplan the approach to the lesion through the sinus tarsi by use of a foot and ankle model and avoid injury to the lateral branch of the superficial peroneal nerve.
- Familiarity with the article by Muir and colleagues[7] can guide the surgeon's approach, particularly in the event that an open approach becomes necessary. It also can help the operator avoid an ill-conceived approach that will not allow access to the lesion.

PITFALLS

- The small, tight ankle (no ligamentous laxity) and posterior lesions warrant caution. They may be best addressed with an open approach from behind the malleoli.
- Avoid getting into the middle of the case and realizing that some of the instrumentation needed to address the lesion is missing.
- Transmalleolar drilling can be more difficult than other methods due to positioning of the guide and orientation of the malleolar hole to the lesion. Start with more direct methods when possible.
- Retrograde drilling is an advanced technique. Be prepared to abort and use a conventional open approach to the cyst for bone grafting if necessary.

Postoperative Rehabilitation Protocol

Postoperatively, the ankle is maintained in a soft, compressive dressing with immobilization in a posterior and stirrup splint or a removable cam walker–type boot. The patient is instructed to not bear weight for the first 6 to 10 days after surgery to ensure adequate healing of incisions. From this point forward, there is no consensus about which weight-bearing protocol produces the best results.

Our preference for any noncystic lesions undergoing curettage, drilling, or microfracture is to begin toe-touch weight bearing in a cam boot for 4 to 6 weeks, followed by progression to full weight bearing over the next 2 to 3 weeks. This is followed by weaning from the boot over a 4-week period into a protective ankle brace and supportive sneaker. An ankle brace is recommended for any athletic or exercise activity for up to 6 months postoperatively. Active ankle range of motion (ROM) is begun by the patient three to four times per day during postoperative week 2. Formal physical therapy is started after week 3 with ROM, strengthening, and low-impact activities, including pool therapy in the deep end and stationary bike riding in the boot initially and then without. Treadmill walking can be undertaken at week 10, with progression to running on the treadmill at week 12 as long as the operative ankle remains pain free. If the patient is comfortable with treadmill running and demonstrates appropriate form, formal running on a softer surface such as a flat trail or track can be initiated.

During the fourth postoperative month, the patient is allowed to begin cutting and jumping with sport-specific activities in a structured environment. Progression to increasing levels of stress on the ankle is judged by lack of pain and swelling in the ankle. In an elite athlete, a follow-up MRI at the 6-month mark is used to assess healing before return to competitive sports. Some persistent change in the articular cartilage and bone is expected at this stage, but there should be some covering fibrocartilage evident and less bone edema. Athletes should be warned to expect some degree of discomfort in the ankle on resuming competition, but this usually improves over the next 6 months as long as there is no further injury.

Postoperative rehabilitation of cystic lesions entails a slightly more conservative approach with regard to weight bearing. If bone grafting of the cystic lesion is performed, the patient is told to not bear weight for a minimum of 6 weeks. With radiographic evidence of incorporation of the bone graft into the lesion, consolidation of the bone graft donor site, and healing of any necessary osteotomies, the patient can begin progressive weight bearing in a boot over a 4-week period, followed by transition to a sneaker and brace as previously described. A patient with a cystic lesion with an intact cartilage roof that has undergone retrograde drilling is prevented from bearing weight for 2 to 4 weeks if the lesion is smaller than 1.5 cm^2 and for 4 to 6 weeks if the lesion is larger than 1.5 cm^2. Otherwise, early ROM with a therapy program as described is allowed, with the exception of a proportional delay in impact activities, walking, and running. As with noncystic lesions, healing can be assessed around the sixth postoperative month. However, CT is the more appropriate imaging modality to evaluate reconstitution of bony architecture.

PEARLS&PITFALLS

PEARLS
- The rehabilitation program is a critical part of the surgical outcome.
- The patient must understand this preoperatively.

PITFALLS
- Patients who do not expect some discomfort after surgery as they resume activity will be unhappy or fail to follow through with their rehabilitation.
- Warn patients ahead of time, and be sure that they do not persist in an activity or exercise that is creating pain or progressively worsening it.

CONCLUSIONS

OLTs continue to present a treatment challenge to the orthopedic surgeon. By following the indications from contemporary literature, an appropriate surgical treatment plan can be developed. Attention to detail in the preoperative setting allows the surgeon to strategically design the arthroscopic approach or open surgical approach, or both, that will be best suited for the lesion's location, size, and cystic characteristics. Necessary special equipment and tools for the case should be confirmed with the operating room. The postoperative rehabilitation is tailored according to the type of procedure performed. Ultimately, treatment of OLTs with the methods outlined in this chapter should yield favorable outcomes for a high percentage of patients, lead to a better quality of life, and allow return to a desired, preinjury level of activity.

REFERENCES

1. Steadman JR, Rodkey WG, Singleton SB, Briggs KK. Microfracture technique for full-thickness chondral defects: technique and clinical results. *Oper Tech Orthop*. 1997;7:300-304.
2. Chuckpaiwong B, Berkson EM, Theodore GH. Microfracture for osteochondral lesions of the ankle: outcome analysis and outcome predictors of 105 cases. *Arthroscopy*. 2008;24:106-112.
3. Robinson DE, Winson IG, Harries WJ, Kelly AJ. Arthroscopic treatment of osteochondral lesions of the talus. *J Bone Joint Surg Br*. 2003;85:989-993.
4. Kumai T, Takakura Y, Higashiyama I, Tamai S. Arthroscopic drilling for the treatment of osteochondral lesions of the talus. *J Bone Joint Surg Am*. 1999;81:1229-1235.
5. Kelberine F, Frank A. Arthroscopic treatment of osteochondral lesions of the talar dome: a retrospective study of 48 cases. *Arthroscopy*. 1999;15:77-84.
6. Smith BW, Cuttica D, Hyer CF, et al. Osteochondral lesions in the talus: predictors of outcome and treatment algorithm. Presented at the 23rd Annual Meeting of the American Orthopaedic Foot and Ankle Society, July, 2008; Denver, CO.
7. Muir D, Saltzman CL, Tochigi Y, Amendola N. Talar dome access for osteochondral lesions. *Am J Sports Med*. 2006;34:1457-1463.
8. Schimmer RC, Dick W, Hintermann B. The role of ankle arthroscopy in the treatment strategies of osteochondritis dissecans lesions of the talus. *Foot Ankle Intl*. 2001;22:895-900.
9. Choi WJ, Lee JW, Kim BS, Han SH. Correlation of defect size and clinical outcome in osteochondral lesion of the talus. Presented at the 23rd Annual Meeting of the American Orthopaedic Foot and Ankle Society, July 2008;Denver, CO.
10. Ferkel RD, Zanotti RM, Komenda GA, et al. Arthroscopic treatment of chronic osteochondral lesions of the talus: long-term results. *Am J Sports Med*. 2008;36:7150-1761.
11. Lahm A, Erggelet C, Steinwachs M, Reichlet A. Arthroscopic management of osteochondral lesion of the talus: results of drilling and usefulness of the magnetic resonance imaging before and after treatment. *Arthroscopy*. 2000;16:299-304.
12. Tol JL, Struijs PAA, Bossuyt PMM, et al. Treatment strategies in osteochondral defects of the talar dome: a systematic review. *Foot Ankle Int*. 2000;21:119-126.
13. Giannini S, Vannini F. Operative treatment of osteochondral lesions of the talar dome: current concepts review. *Foot Ankle Int*. 2004;25:168-175.
14. Baurns MH, Heidrich G, Shultz H, et al. Autologous chondrocyte transplantation for treating cartilage defects of the talus. *J Bone Joint Surg Am*. 2006;88:303-308.
15. Whittaker JP, Smith G, Makwana N, et al. Early results of autologous chondrocyte implantation in the talus. *J Bone Joint Surg Br*. 2005;87:179-183.
16. Giannini S, Buda R, Vannini F, et al. Arthroscopic autologous chondrocyte implantation in osteochondral lesions of the talus: surgical technique and results. *Am J Sports Med*. 2008;36:873-880.
17. Lee CH, Chao KH, Huang GS, Wu SS. Osteochondral autografts for osteochondritis dissecans of the talus. *Foot Ankle Int*. 2003;85:989-993.
18. Sammarco JG, Makwana NK. Treatment of talar osteochondral lesions using local osteochondral graft. *Foot Ankle Int*. 2002;22:693-698.
19. DeLee JC. Fractures and dislocations of the foot. In: Mann RA, Coughlin MJ, eds. *Surgery of the Foot and Ankle*. 6th ed. St. Louis, MO: Mosby, 1991;1465-1518.
20. Stone JW. Osteochondral lesions of the talar dome. *J Am Acad Orthop Surg* 1996;4:63-73.
21. Taranow WS, Bisignani GA, Towers JD, et al. Retrograde drilling of osteochondral lesions of the medial talar dome. *Foot Ankle Int*. 1999;20:474-480.
22. Kono M, Takao M, Naito K, et al. Retrograde drilling for osteochondral lesions of the talar dome. *Am J Sports Med*. 2006;34:1450-1456.
23. Becher C, Thermann H. Results of microfracture in the treatment of articular cartilage defects of the talus. *Foot Ankle Int*. 2005;26:583-589.
24. Mithoefer K, Williams RJ, Warren RF, et al. The microfracture technique for treatment of articular cartilage lesions of the knee: a prospective cohort study. *J Bone Joint Surg Am*. 2005;87:1911-1920.
25. Schuman L, Struijs PAA, Van Dijk CN. Arthroscopic treatment of osteochondral defects of the talus: results at follow up at 2 to 11 years. *J Bone Joint Surg Br*. 2002;84B:364-368.
26. Savva N, Jabur M, Davies M, Saxby T. Osteochondral lesions of the talus: results of repeat arthroscopic débridement. *Foot Ankle Int*. 2007;28:669-673.
27. Gobbi A, Francisco RA, Lubowitz JH, et al. Osteochondral lesions of the talus: randomized controlled trial comparing chondroplasty, microfracture, and osteochondral autograft transplantation. *Arthroscopy*. 2006;22:1085-1092.
28. Green, JP. Osteochondritis dissecans of the knee. *J Bone Joint Surg Br*. 1966;48B:82-91.
29. Green WT, Banks HH. Osteochondritis dissecans in children. *J Bone Joint Surg Am*. 1953;35A:26-47, 64.
30. Van Demark RE. Osteochondritis dissecans with spontaneous healing. *J Bone Joint Surg Am*. 1952;34A:143-148.
31. Wiberg G. Spontaneous healing of osteochondritis dissecans in the knee joint. *Acta Orthop Scand*. 1943;14:270-277.
32. Berndt AL, Harty M. Transchondral fractures (osteochondritis dissecans) of the talus. *J Bone Joint Surg Am*. 1959;41A:988-1020.
33. Canale ST, Belding RH. Osteochondral lesions of the talus. *J Bone Joint Surg Am*. 1980;62:97-102.
34. Flick AB, Gould N. Osteochondritis dissecans of the talus (transchondral fracture of the talus): review of the literature and new surgical approach for medial dome lesions. *Foot Ankle Int*. 1985;5:165-185.
35. Pettine KA, Morrey BF. Osteochondral fractures of the talus: a long-term follow-up. *J Bone Joint Surg Br*. 1987;69:89-92.
36. Van Beucken K, Barrack RL, Alexander AH, et al. Arthroscopic treatment of transchondral talar dome fractures. *Am J Sports Med*. 1989;17:350-356.
37. O'Farrell TA, Costello BG. Osteochondritis dissecans of the talus: the late results of surgical treatment. *J Bone Joint Surg Br*. 1982;64:494-497.
38. Petrella RJ, Petrella M. A prospective, randomized, double-blind, placebo-controlled study to evaluate the efficacy of intraarticular hyaluronic acid for osteoarthritis of the knee. *J Rheumatol*. 2006;33:951-956.
39. Salk RS, Chang TJ, D'Costa WF, et al. Sodium hyaluronate in the treatment of osteoarthritis of the ankle: a controlled, randomized, double-blind pilot study. *J Bone Joint Surg Am*. 2006;88:295-302.

40. Sun S, Chou Y, Hsu C, et al. Efficacy of intra-articular hyaluronic acid in patients with osteoarthritis of the ankle: a prospective study. *Osteoarthritis Cartilage*. 2006;14:867-874.

41. Mei-Dan O, Maoz G, Swatzon M, et al. Treatment of osteochondritis dissecans of the ankle with hyaluronic acid injections: a prospective study. *Foot Ankle Int*. 2008;29:1771-1178.

42. Pritsch M, Horoshovski H, Farine I. Arthroscopic treatment of osteochondral lesions of the talus. *J Bone Joint Surg Am*. 1986;68A: 862-865.

43. Mintz DN, Tashijian GS, Connell DA, et al. Osteochondral lesions of the talus: a new magnetic resonance grading system with arthroscopic correlation. *Arthroscopy*. 2003;19:353-359.

44. Bale RJ, Hoser C, Rosenberger R, et al. Osteochondral lesions of the talus: computer-assisted retrograde drilling—feasibility and accuracy in initial experiences. Radiology 2001;218:278-282.

45. Saxena A, Eakin C. Articular talar injuries in athletes. *Am J Sports Med*. 2007;35:1680-1687.

SUGGESTED READINGS

Ferkel RD. Arthroscopic surgery. In: The Foot and Ankle. Philadelphia, PA: Lippincott-Raven; 1996,

Osteochondral Lesions of the Talar Dome:
Cartilage Replacement Using Osteochondral Autogenous Transplantation and Mosaicplasty

Mark Glazebrook ● Johnny Tak-Choy Lau ● Jean-Pascal Allard

TERMINOLOGY

The term *osteochondritis dissecans* was first used in 1887, when Konig[1] described an inflammatory lesion of cartilage and underlying bone in the knee joint that resulted in loss of structural integrity, causing pain and dysfunction. Since then, it has been recognized that lesions of the bone and cartilage may appear spontaneously or may be caused by a traumatic event to the joint surface.[2] The general term *osteochondral lesion* (OCL) has gained more widespread use than osteochondritis dissecans.

ETIOLOGY, EPIDEMIOLOGY, AND CLASSIFICATION

In the ankle joint, an OCL can occur spontaneously or as the result of trauma, and there appears to be a relationship between the location of the lesion and the cause.[3,4] In a comprehensive review of the early literature that included more than 500 cases of OCL, Flick and Gould[5] found that 98% of lateral lesions and only 70% of medial lesions were associated with a traumatic event. This and other reports[2,6] led to the associations of traumatic OCLs with lateral lesions and spontaneous OCLs with medial lesions.

The incidence of OCL depends on the etiologic factors involved. In an early study, Bosien and colleagues[7] reported the incidence of OCL to be 6.5% with ankle sprains, and Hinterman and coworkers[8] and Leontaritis and associates[9] reported the incidence of OCL as 69% and 74%, respectively.

The most recognized classification system is that of Berndt and Harty,[2] which is useful for research purposes and preoperative planning. It is based on radiographic imaging or intraoperative findings. Stage I is a small, subchondral compression; stage II is partial fragment detachment; stage III is complete fragment detachment with no displacement; and stage IV is complete fragment detachment with displacement.

PATIENT EVALUATION

History and Physical Examination

Patients with an OCL usually present with the complaint of persistent pain in the ankle that is frequently localized to the side of the lesion. In acute cases, the pain is accompanied by swelling, ecchymosis, and decreased range of motion. In chronic cases, the pain is usually a dull ache in the ankle joint and is associated with stiffness. Crepitus, discomfort with weight bearing, decreased range of motion, mechanical clicking, and recurrent swelling should raise the suspicion of an OCL. If a thorough history does not elicit a traumatic event or instability, the examiner should seek factors predisposing to vascular insufficiency, including endocrine, vascular, hematologic, and coagulation disorders and any relevant family history. Patients also should be questioned about symptoms in the contralateral ankle.

Physical examination should begin with assessment of the standing alignment to identify an associated coronal plane deformity. Inspection of the ankle with an acute injury usually reveals swelling and ecchymosis, but the ankle sometimes appears completely normal, as is often the case with delayed presentations. An attempt to elicit tenderness with palpation should be made by focusing on the common OCL sites. Posteromedial lesions may be tender in response to palpation when the ankle is dorsiflexed and the region posterior to the medial malleolus is palpated. Anterolateral lesions may be tender when the joint is palpated laterally with the ankle in plantar flexion. These findings are often nonspecific because the tenderness is likely related to joint synovitis rather than the OCL itself. The joint should be taken through a range of motion to assess stiffness and to feel for crepitus and mechanical signs of clicking or locking. Ligamentous stability should be assessed to ascertain evidence of associated laxity, particularly of the lateral ligament complex. The examination is completed with a thorough neurovascular assessment and examination of the contralateral ankle for comparison.

Diagnostic Imaging

Plain radiographs are the initial investigation of a suspected OCL. Anteroposterior, lateral, and mortise views should be obtained on presentation. Radiographs in various degrees of plantar flexion and dorsiflexion may help to demonstrate posteromedial and anterolateral lesions, respectively. Plain radiographs of the opposite ankle should be obtained to exclude bilateral lesions. Radiographs are often limited in their ability to demonstrate an OCL, and with continued clinical suspicion, further diagnostic imaging may be necessary.

Bone scintigraphic results correlate with osteochondral injury, and scans can be useful for discerning which joint is causing clinical discomfort if other imaging modalities have not located the lesion. More advanced imaging has largely replaced scintigraphy, but it still provides a valuable tool in the workup of persistent ankle pain if immediate access to computed tomography (CT) or magnetic resonance imaging (MRI) is not available to the evaluating physician.

CT provides best information regarding bony architecture of the lesion, and it assists in accurately determining its dimensions. Scans in the coronal, sagittal, and axial planes should be obtained, especially when initial radiographs appear normal and the result of bone scintigraphy is positive.

MRI affords an accurate assessment of the ankle's soft tissue structures, including the articular cartilage and supporting ligaments. Multiplanar evaluation is possible with no radiation exposure to the patient. Sequences can identify the size and location, and they provide information about the stability of the lesion. DeSmet and colleagues[10] prospectively showed an excellent correlation between staging with MRI and arthroscopic results, correctly predicting stable and unstable lesions in 92% of cases. In some circumstances, MRI may overestimate the size of the OCL due to associated edema, and CT may be better suited for defining the dimensions of the defect.

TREATMENT

The use of non–weight-bearing articular surfaces as a donor site for osteochondral autogenous transplantation (OAT) grafts for the treatment of OCL began in the 1980s. Yamashita and coworkers[11] published a case report on two patients who had an OAT graft harvested from the non–weight-bearing portion of the medial femoral condyle and transplanted to an OCL of the same knee.

In 1993, Matsusue and associates[12] reported their 3-year follow-up of cases treated with a new technique that involved transplantation of multiple osteochondral plugs harvested from the same knee. They used the press-fit method of cylindrical osteochondral plugs described by Garrett[13] for allografts. They harvested two osteochondral autogenous graft (OAG) plugs from

the lateral femoral patellar groove and one from the anterolateral side of the intercondylar notch.

In 1996, Bobic[14] was the first to publish a case series (12 patients) describing multiple OAT grafts for the treatment of knee OCLs associated with anterior cruciate ligament reconstruction. In 1997, Hangody and colleagues[15] published their first report of their prospective case series. They described 44 patients with 1 to 5 years of follow-up after multiple OAG plugs were used to treat OCLs of the knee. Most patients had good or excellent outcomes. They were the first to call the procedure *mosaicplasty*. We now commonly use this term for the technique of using multiple OAT graft plugs to treat an OCL. Some surgeons make distinction between OAT and mosaicplasty, using the former to describe the use of only one graft plug and the latter to describe the use of multiple graft plugs. These terms can be used interchangeably, but for clarification, we use the term *mosaicplasty osteochondral autogenous transplantation* (MOAT) when referring to transplantation with multiple graft plugs and OAT when referring to transplantation of a single graft plug.

Evidence-Based Studies of Osteochondral Autogenous Transplantation and Mosaicplasty Osteochondral Autogenous Transplantation

Given the success of OAT and mosaicplasty in the knee, there was a logical extension of this technique to the ankle. In reviewing the literature on OAT and MOAT in the ankle before February 2009, 15 studies were identified. All articles were reviewed and assigned a classification (i.e., I through IV) using the *Journal of Bone and Joint Surgery* levels of evidence for primary research questions.[16] The 15 studies included 1 level II study, 1 level III study, and 13 level IV studies (Table 13-1).

Level IV Evidence

In 1997, Hangody and coworkers[17] were the first to report on use of MOAT for treatment of OCL of the talus. In a preliminary report of a prospective case series (level IV), MOAT was done on 11 patients with OCLs larger than 10 mm diameter. The outcome results after at least 1 year of follow-up were excellent and promising. This study included second-look arthroscopies in three patients and one cartilage biopsy. Arthroscopy showed good incorporation of the grafts, with articular surface congruency and normal cartilage appearance. Biopsy showed normal articular hyaline cartilage (i.e., collagen type II) and proteoglycans and fibrocartilage bonding at the graft-recipient junction. Donor-site morbidity was a concern, because 3 of 11 patients had occasional knee pain and 2 of 11 had knee pain with activities (one with a 10-degree extension lag).

In 2001,[18] 2003,[19] and 2008,[20] Hangody and coworkers expanded their prospective case series report (level IV) after 2 to 9 years of follow-up after MOAT for OCL of the talus. The report included 98 patients with 92% to 94% good or excellent clinical results and less than 3% had knee pain after 1 year. Further assessment included 28 MRI scans, 19 CT scans, 8 second-look arthroscopies, and 4 biopsies. CT, MRI, and arthroscopy showed good incorporation of the grafts, with articular surface congruency and normal cartilage appearance. Biopsies showed normal articular cartilage collagen (type II) and proteoglycans. Three postoperative knee arthroscopies showed a donor-site defect covered by fibrocartilage congruent with the surrounding hyaline cartilage.

TABLE 13-1   Clinical Outcome Studies of Mosaicplasty Osteochondral Autogenous Transplantation for Talar Osteochondral Lesions

Study	Study Type (Level of Evidence)	Lesion Size	Good or Excellent Outcome Rate (Sample Size)	Degree of Knee Pain	Comments
Hangody et al,[17] 1997	Prospective case series (IV)	D > 10 mm	100% (11*)	Knee pain in 36%	First published study on talus MOAT
Scranton et al,[24] 2001	Retrospective case series (IV)	D = 4 to 8 mm (graft size)	100% (10*)	No knee pain after 1 yr	Cystic lesions; only one cylindrical plug used
Hangody et al,[18] 2001	Prospective case series (IV)	Mean A = 1 cm^2 (range, 0.5-2.5 cm^2)	94% (36*)	No knee pain after 1 yr	Postoperative assessment with 28 MRI scans, 19 CT scans, and 8 second-look arthroscopies
Assenmacher et al,[26] 2001	Retrospective case series (IV)	Mean A = 0.49 cm^2	Decreased VAS: 7.7 to 3.1 (9)	No knee pain	Use of anterior tibial wedge osteotomy; 8 of 9 had only one plug
Gautier et al,[21] 2002	Retrospective case series (IV)	Mean A = 180 mm^2	91% (11)	No knee pain	
Al-Shaikh et al,[23] 2002	Retrospective case series (IV)	Mean A = 120 mm^2	83% (19)	Knee pain in 10.5%	No outcome difference between lesions larger or smaller than 1 cm^2
Sammarco et al,[28] 2002	Prospective case series (IV)	Mean A = 62 mm^2	100% (12)	No knee harvest	Local autograft, usually one plug, tibial plafond osteotomy
Hangody et al,[19] 2003	Prospective case series (IV)	Mean A = 1 cm^2 (range, 0.5-2.5 cm^2)	92% (63*)	Knee pain in 3%	Results similar to those of their previous study[18]
Lee et al,[27] 2003	Prospective case series (IV)	Mean A = 98 mm^2	100% (18)	Mild knee pain in 11%	16 second-look arthroscopies; 87.5% had cartilage continuity
Baltzer et al,[22] 2005	Prospective case series (IV)	Mean A = 1.7 cm^2	95% (43)	Knee pain in 2%	Second-look arthroscopies showed good cartilage integration
Kreuz et al,[29] 2006	Prospective case series (IV)	Mean D = 6.3 mm	91% (35)	No knee harvest	Local autograft, better outcome without osteotomy or with tibial wedge osteotomy
Scranton et al,[25] 2006	Retrospective case series (IV)	D = 8 to 20 mm	90% (50)	2% knee pain after 3 mo	Cystic lesions; advocates for fewer transplantations with larger plugs
Gobbi et al,[31] 2006	Randomized, controlled trial (II)	Mean A = 3.7 cm^2	83% (12 of 33 had OAT)	No knee pain	RCT: chondroplasty, microfracture and OAT; no differences found
Hangody et al,[20] 2008	Prospective case series (IV)	Mean A = 1 cm^2 (range, 0.5-2.5 cm^2)	93% (98)	Knee pain in 3%	Mixed joints study (1097 total; 98 talus patients)
Haasper et al,[30] 2008	Retrospective cohort study (III)	Mean A = 68.9 ± 32.2 mm^2	71% (14)	Knee pain in 64% at 1 yr	No difference between previously treated and untreated patients

Represents patients who are included in other case series published later by the same investigators.

A, area; D, CT, computed tomography; diameter; MOAT, mosaicplasty osteochondral autogenous transplantation; MRI, magnetic resonance imaging; OAT, osteochondral autogenous transplantation; RCT, randomized, controlled trial; VAS, visual analog scale.

In smaller case series (level IV), Gauthier and colleagues[21] and Baltzer and coworkers[22] described 11 (retrospective) and 43 (prospective) cases, respectively, that had MOAT for OCL of the talus. More than 90% of their patients were satisfied with the results. In another retrospective case series (level IV), Al-Shaihk and associates[23] performed MOAT on 19 patients with larger OCLs (mean area of 120 mm^2). Eighty-three percent of patients

were satisfied with the results, and two patients (10.5%) reported mild knee pain. They found no difference in outcomes between patients with lesions larger than 1 cm^2 and those with lesions smaller than 1 cm.^{2}

In 2001[24] and 2006,[25] Scranton and colleagues confirmed earlier promising results with a retrospective case series (level IV) that evaluated 50 patients. Their technique included the transplantation of only one cylindrical plug in patients having cystic lesions that were 4 to 20 mm of diameter. The results were equally impressive, and the investigators advocated arthroscopic harvesting and the use of larger and fewer plugs to minimize peripheral graft chondrocytes death and to simplify the technique. In a retrospective case study (level IV), Assenmacher and coworkers[26] reported the use of single-plug OAT in 8 of 9 patients, who had an average decrease in the visual analog scale (VAS) score of 7.7 to 3.1 after the procedure. They also described the use of an anterior tibial wedge osteotomy (i.e., plafondplasty) in five patients for lesions in the central third of the talar dome to avoid a malleolar osteotomy. Preoperative MRI showed an excellent correlation for OCL grading, and postoperative MRI showed integration of the grafts.

In a prospective case series (level IV) reported by Lee and associates,[27] 18 patients had 100% good or excellent outcomes. Two of the 18 patients (11%) had mild knee pain, and 14 (87.5%) of 16 second-look arthroscopies showed cartilage continuity with the native cartilage.

To minimize the risk of knee pain associated with violating an asymptomatic joint to harvest the OAG, Sammarco and colleagues[28] performed a local osteochondral graft for an OCL with a mean area of 62 mm,[2] and they typically used a one-plug graft. They harvested the grafts from the medial or lateral talar facet on the same side as the lesion they were treating. In the prospective case series (level IV), the investigators reported that all 12 patients were satisfied with the results and that they had no talar collapse.

In a prospective case series (level IV), Kreuz and coworkers[29] reported 91% good or excellent results using local OAT grafts harvested from the medial or lateral talar facet. They subdivided their series into four subgroups: no osteotomy, medial malleolar osteotomy, tibial wedge plafond osteotomy, and posterolateral approach. They found better outcomes in the two groups not undergoing osteotomies compared with the others and found better outcomes for the tibial wedge osteotomy group compared with the medial malleolar osteotomy group.

Level III Evidence

In a small, retrospective cohort study (level III) of 14 patients, Haasper and coworkers[30] did not find differences in outcomes between previously treated and previously untreated OCL patients receiving MOAT. The lesions were small (68.9 ± 32.2 mm^2) and a surprisingly large number of patients reported knee pain at a minimum of 1-year of follow-up.

Level II Evidence

In a randomized, controlled trial (level II), Gobbi and colleagues[31] compared chondroplasty, microfracture, and MOAT in 33 ankles. The American Orthopaedic Foot and Ankle Society (AOFAS) Hindfoot Score, the Ankle-Hindfoot Scale, and the Subjective Assessment Numeric Evaluation improved in all groups, and the investigators found no significant difference in outcomes among the three groups. There was an inverse correlation between size of the defect and outcome in the microfracture and OAT groups. To have comparable techniques, the central and posterior lesions that needed a malleolar osteotomy were excluded from the study.

Technique Advantages and Disadvantages

The advantages of using MOAT over other techniques to treat OCL are a one-step procedure with relatively fast recovery and hyaline cartilage covering more than 80% of the treated lesion, and consistently more than 80% to 90% good clinical results. Multiple, small autografts have the advantage of reduced complications at the donor site, better fit to the shape of the defect, and avoidance of screws or wires for fixation with the press-fit implantation technique.[32]

The disadvantages of MOAT are related to donor-site morbidity, fibrocartilage filling the dead space between OAT grafts, and the technical challenge of obtaining optimal success.

Indications and Contraindications

Débridement with subchondral bone penetration produced consistently good or excellent outcome results.[31] In a prospective case series that used the microfracture technique, Chuckpaiwong and associates[33] had 100% good or excellent results in patients with lesions less than 15 mm in diameter but only 3% good or excellent results in patients with lesion larger than 15 mm in diameter. The only randomized, controlled trial (level II) comparing MOAT with a form of subchondral bone penetration technique showed no difference in outcomes.[31] The only level III study of MOAT showed no difference between patients with OCLs previously treated by subchondral bone penetration and untreated patients.[30]

Given a lack of literature to support superior outcomes for OAT and mosaicplasty for the treatment of OCL and because of the procedure's inherently more invasive nature and the potential morbidity at the donor site, we feel that OAT and mosaicplasty should be reserved for failure of a prior attempt of arthroscopic débridement associated with any technique of subchondral bone penetration (i.e., curettage, drilling, or microfracture), at least for OCLs of the talus smaller than 15 mm in diameter. However, the literature does not provide direction about the primary treatment of OCLs larger than 15 mm in diameter. There may be a role for primary MOAT technique, especially for medial, deep, and cystic OCLs, which have worse results than lateral, more shallow, and wafer OCLs.[25,34-36] Even for failed prior débridement and subchondral bone penetration, there is at least one study showing 92% good results with revision using the same procedure by the same surgeon.[37]

When deciding where to harvest the OAT grafts, the surgeon should consider the fact that patellofemoral peripheries allow up to 3 to 4 cm^2 of graft plugs for harvest. That is sufficient for grafting most large, contained talar OCLs treated by MOAT.[20] However, for smaller lesions needing only one or two plugs, some surgeons advocate local graft harvest from medial or lateral non–weight-bearing talar facets. This prevents violation of a normal knee joint and avoids chronic knee pain.

Other than obvious contraindications such as infection, tumors, rheumatoid arthritis, diabetes with neuropathy, or sympathetic dystrophy, OAT and mosaicplasty should be use with caution in patients with signs of osteoarthritis other than mild osteophytes that can be removed during the same surgical procedure. Ankle instability and alignment deformity should be addressed before or at the same time to prevent failure due to higher than normal contact stress on the transplanted grafts. Hangody and colleagues[20] advise caution in treating patients older than 50 years because of their decreased repair capacity.

Surgical Technique

The procedure can be done under spinal or general anesthesia. The patient is positioned supine. A thigh tourniquet is used in most cases. Ankle arthroscopy may be carried out first, especially if it is a primary procedure, to confirm the location and grade of the OCL and to assess other cartilage and ankle pathology (Fig. 13-1). If the lesion is small and anterior, an all-arthroscopic technique can be used. Otherwise, an open technique is needed.

For medial OCLs, a medial approach with a medial osteotomy (Fig. 13-2) is usually needed because most of those OCLs are more posterior. The osteotomy may be a step cut or an oblique osteotomy to provide a good perpendicular view of the talar dome. To achieve this view, the talus must be rotated into valgus, and a pin can be inserted into the talar body[19] or a non-invasive ankle distractor can be used.[38] Some surgeons advocate an anterior tibial wedge osteotomy for smaller and middle-third lesions instead of a malleolar osteotomy,[26,28,29] but we cannot confirm this approach because we have no experience with the technique.

For lateral OCLs, an anterolateral approach is usually needed. Because these OCLs often have a more anterior location, extreme plantar flexion usually can expose the lesions. If a large, posterior lesion needs more exposure, a lateral malleolar osteotomy[21] (Fig. 13-3) or a release of the anterior talofibular ligament and calcaneofibular ligament by a periosteal flap at their origin on the distal fibula may be used.[39] A good perpendicular view (see Fig. 13-3) of OCL of the talar surface is mandatory to allow perpendicular insertion of the graft plugs.

After good exposure, débridement and removal of all diseased cartilage and bone debris with a curette or knife is done until a sharply defined, viable cartilage rim and a clean bony bed of the lesion are obtained. Using MOAT-specific instruments (various companies offer complete sets of instruments), the defect is exactly sized, and the number, diameter, depth, and location of the graft plugs and recipient holes are determined (Fig. 13-4). The intended location of the planned mosaic is marked on the recipient bed with the appropriate sizer-tamp or cutting chisels.

Larger graft plugs typically are used first to fill most of the defect, and smaller grafts are used to fill the remaining dead space not covered by the primary plugs (Fig. 13-5). Analysis of a cadaveric contact model study showed that four 4-mm-diameter graft plugs better restored joint contact area and pressure to normal levels than two 6-mm-diameter graft plugs in a talar OCL made in the center of the contact zone.[40] More grafts may also allow for better contouring to fit the original surface anatomy and minimize the unfilled space. However, the use of more grafts in transplantation is more technically demanding and may signify a larger area of nonviable hyaline cartilage because of the rate of possible peripheral graft chondrocytes death of up to 24%.[41]

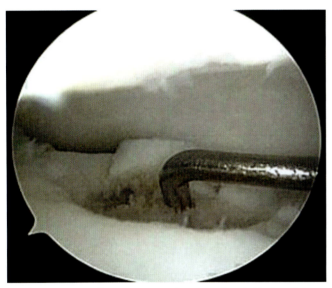

FIGURE 13-1 An arthroscopic view of an osteochondral lesion of the talar dome.

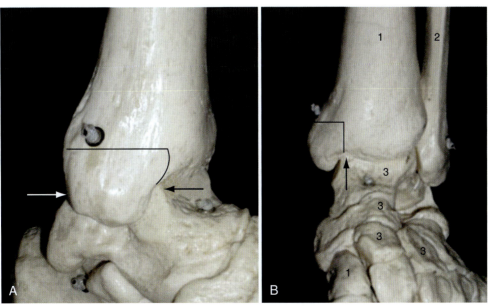

FIGURE 13-2 An open approach to the talar dome using a medial malleolar osteotomy.

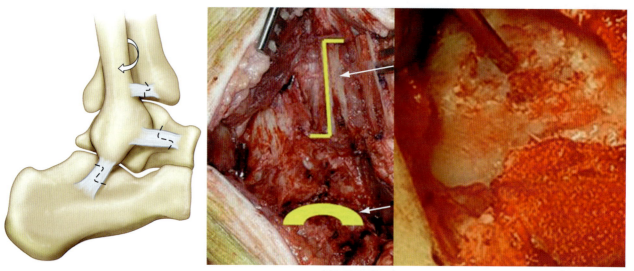

FIGURE 13-3 An open approach to the talar dome using a lateral malleolar osteotomy.

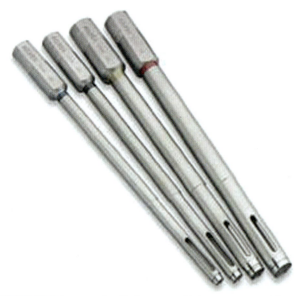

FIGURE 13-4 An example of industry-specific instruments used for osteochondral allograft transplantation. *(Courtesy of Smith & Nephew, Andover, MA.)*

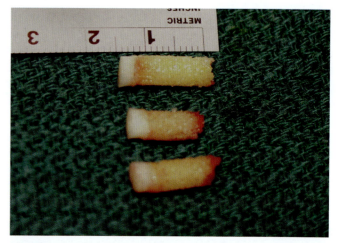

FIGURE 13-5 Intraoperative picture showing the harvest site for osteochondral allograft transplantation.

This is why some arthroscopists advocate using fewer larger graft plugs.[24,25]

OAT graft plugs may be harvested from the ipsilateral knee (see Fig. 13-5). This can be done by arthroscopy or by miniarthrotomy, depending on the number and size of grafts needed and the ability of the surgeon. We prefer the open technique. The medial, proximal, non–weight-bearing surface of the medial femoral condylar edge is our preferred donor site. Although Marymont and coworkers[42] showed with an MRI study that the best donor site for filling a medial talar lesion is the superolateral femur and although we found no literature to support our approach, we think there are more risks of patellofemoral symptoms from lateral harvesting.

For talar defects, Demirci and colleagues[43] showed that the grafts should be taken from condylar edges, where the chondral thickness is decreased. Flexing the knee allows up to four graft plugs to be harvested. For more graft plugs, the lateral femoral condylar edge can be used. The graft plugs are harvested with the appropriately sized, tubular, cutting harvester chisels. It is important to be perpendicular to the articular surface in both planes when harvesting the graft. Each graft length is recorded. Expect up to 0.2 mm of normal expansion of the cartilage plugs after removing them from the harvester.[19]

Next, the recipient bed is cleaned again. Sequential drilling, dilation, and delivery are performed for each graft using the appropriate drill guide–delivery cylinder (see Fig. 13-4). Remaining perpendicular to the articular surface is mandatory. Drilling should be 3 to 4 mm deeper than the graft plug length.[19] When delivering the grafts, care should be taken to set them as flush as possible with the surrounding articular surface of the native cartilage (Fig. 13-6). Huang and associates[44] showed that small incongruities could remodel, provided they did not exceed 1 mm in either direction. Pearce and coworkers[45] showed that grafts left 2 mm proud and

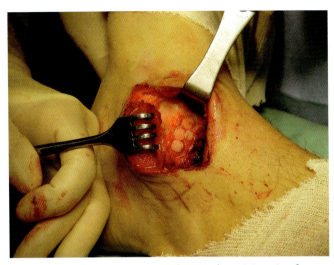

FIGURE 13-6 Intraoperative picture showing the recipient site after osteochondral allograft transplantation.

- For a lateral OCL, an anterolateral approach should be combined with plantar flexion of the ankle to expose the lesion.
- For MOAT, specific equipment is used to harvest the graft. Larger graft plugs are used first to fill most of the defect, and smaller grafts are then used to fill the remaining dead space not covered by the primary plugs.

repositioned by weight bearing caused perigraft fissuring, fibroplasia, and subchondral cavitations. They concluded these complications were caused by excessive motion between the graft and recipient site in the proud grafts. However, the graft plugs also must not be sunk too deeply. After all grafts are transplanted, the ankle is reduced and moved through its entire range of motion with slight axial compression. This ensures congruency of the MOAT.

If an osteotomy was used, it is reduced and fixed with two screws inserted through predrilled holes. If lateral ligament release was used, repair is made as in a classic Broström ligament repair.

Wound closure is made in layers, and a knee drain can be use. A well-padded Jones compression dressing with a below-knee splint is applied, and the foot is kept elevated for 1 or 2 days during the hospital stay. Patients receive standard prophylactic antibiotics and pain management.

Postoperative Management and Rehabilitation

Some surgeons advocate immediate ankle range of motion,[18,19] and others advocate no motion for 3 weeks.[24,25] We usually start controlled range of motion after stitches are removed at 10 to 14 days if the wound is clean. The patient is kept in a removable cast boot to prevent weight bearing for 6 weeks. We then allow progressive weight bearing over a 4-week period. Formal physiotherapy usually starts at 6 weeks. Unprotected weight bearing is allowed at 10 weeks, and athletic activities should be postponed until 6 months.

Complications

The most common complication and the main drawback of the technique is knee pain. In a review of the literature, we found 274 patients who have had OAT grafts harvested from the knee for the treatment of talar OCLs. Eighteen of them had some form of knee symptoms, ranging from mild and occasional pain to activity-related pain with an extension lag. The overall rate of knee pain was 6.6%. In a retrospective case series that specifically addressed knee pain, Reddy and colleagues[46] reported that 4 (36%) of 11 patients had poor knee outcomes according the Lysholm criteria, and they concluded that donor-site morbidity can be significant and interfere with daily living activities. We agree that chronic knee pain is a significant potential complication that should be considered by the surgeon and discussed with the patient.

Other complications may include neuroma, symptomatic hardware, wound healing problems, infection, incomplete relief of pain, chronic pain syndrome, degenerative osteoarthritis of the ankle or patellofemoral joint, and recurrence of the OCL.[47]

PEARLS & PITFALLS

- Lateral OCLs are more likely to be associated with trauma, and medial OCLs are more likely to be spontaneous.
- The routine imaging workup of an OCL consists of plain radiography, CT, and MRI. If CT or MRI is not available, a bone scan is useful to identify an OCL.
- It is not clear what to conclude from the published literature about the primary treatment of OCLs larger than 15 mm in diameter. There may be a role for primary MOAT technique, especially for medial, deep, and cystic OCLs, which have worse results than lateral, more shallow, and wafer OCLs.
- For an OCL of the talus that is less than 15 mm in diameter, OAT and mosaicplasty should be reserved for failure of a prior attempt of arthroscopic débridement associated with any technique of subchondral bone penetration (i.e., curettage, drilling, or microfracture).
- Arthroscopic débridement is possible for lateral OCLs, but medial OCLs may require a medial malleolar osteotomy.
- For a medial OCL, a medial malleolar osteotomy should be predrilled to facilitate open reduction and internal fixation, and it should be performed high enough to obtain access to the OCL.

REFERENCES

1. Barrie HJ. Osteochondritis dissecans 1887.1987. A centennial look at Konig's memorable phrase. *J Bone Joint Surg Br* 1987;69:693-695.
2. Berndt AL, Harty M. Transchondral fractures (osteochondritis dissecans) of the talus. *J Bone Joint Surg Am.* 1959;41A:988-1020.
3. Anderson IF, Crichton KJ, Grattan-Smith T, et al. Osteochondral fractures of the dome of the talus. *J Bone Joint Surg Am.* 1989;71:1143-1152.
4. Bruns J, Rosenbach B, Kahrs J. [Etiopathogenetic aspects of medial osteochondrosis dissecans tali.] *Sportverletz Sportschaden.* 1992;6:43-49.
5. Flick AB, Gould N. Osteochondritis dissecans of the talus (transchondral fractures of the talus): review of the literature and new surgical approach for medial dome lesions. *Foot Ankle.* 1985;5:165-185.
6. Canale ST, Belding RH. Osteochondral lesions of the talus. *J Bone Joint Surg Am.* 1980;62:97-102.
7. Bosien WR, Staples OS, Russell SW. Residual disability following acute ankle sprains. *J Bone Joint Surg Am.* 1955;37A:1237-1243.
8. Hintermann B, Regazzoni P, Lampert C, et al. Arthroscopic findings in acute fractures of the ankle. *J Bone Joint Surg Br.* 2000;82:345-351.
9. Leontaritis N, Hinojosa L, Panchbhavi VK. Arthroscopically detected intra-articular lesions associated with acute ankle fractures. *J Bone Joint Surg Am.* 2009;91:333-339.

10. De Smet AA, Fisher DR, Burnstein MI, et al. Value of MR imaging in staging osteochondral lesions of the talus (osteochondritis dissecans): results in 14 patients. *AJR Am J Roentgenol.* 1990;154:555-558.
11. Yamashita F, Sakakida K, Suzu F, Takai S. The transplantation of an autogeneic osteochondral fragment for osteochondritis dissecans of the knee. *Clin Orthop Relat Res.* 1985;(201):43-50.
12. Matsusue Y, Yamamuro T, Hama H. Arthroscopic multiple osteochondral transplantation to the chondral defect in the knee associated with anterior cruciate ligament disruption. *Arthroscopy.* 1993;9:318-321.
13. Garrett JC. Osteochondral allografts. *Instr Course Lect.* 1993;42:355-358.
14. Bobic V. Arthroscopic osteochondral autograft transplantation in anterior cruciate ligament reconstruction: a preliminary clinical study. *Knee Surg Sports Ttraumatol Arthrosc.* 1996;3:262-264.
15. Hangody L, Kish G, Kárpáti Z, et al. Arthroscopic autogenous osteochondral mosaicplasty for the treatment of femoral condylar articular defects. A preliminary report. *Knee Surg Sports Ttraumatol Arthrosc.* 1997;5:262-267.
16. Wright JG, Swiontkowski MF, Heckman JD. Introducing levels of evidence to the journal. *J Bone Joint Surg Am.* 2003;85A:1-3.
17. Hangody L, Kish G, Kárpáti Z, et al. Treatment of osteochondritis dissecans of the talus: use of the mosaicplasty technique—a preliminary report. *Foot Ankle Int.* 1997;18:628-634.
18. Hangody L, Kish G, Modis L, et al. Mosaicplasty for the treatment of osteochondritis dissecans of the talus: two to seven year results in 36 patients. *Foot Ankle Int.* 2001;22:552-558.
19. Hangody L. The mosaicplasty technique for osteochondral lesions of the talus. *Foot Ankle Clin.* 2003;8:259-273.
20. Hangody L, Vásárhelyi G, Hangody LR, et al. Autologous osteochondral grafting—technique and long-term results. *Injury.* 2008;39(Suppl 1):S32-S39.
21. Gautier E, Kolker D, Jakob RP. Treatment of cartilage defects of the talus by autologous osteochondral grafts. *J Bone Joint Surg Br.* 2002;84:237-244.
22. Baltzer AW, Arnold JP. Bone-cartilage transplantation from the ipsilateral knee for chondral lesions of the talus. *Arthroscopy.* 2005;21:159-166.
23. Al-Shaikh RA, Chou LB, Mann JA, et al. Autologous osteochondral grafting for talar cartilage defects. *Foot Ankle Int.* 2002;23:381-389.
24. Scranton PE, McDermott JE. Treatment of type V osteochondral lesions of the talus with ipsilateral knee osteochondral autografts. *Foot Ankle Int.* 2001;22:380-384.
25. Scranton PE, Frey CC, Feder KS. Outcome of osteochondral autograft transplantation for type-V cystic osteochondral lesions of the talus. *J Bone Joint Surg Br.* 2006;88:614-619.
26. Assenmacher JA, Kelikian AS, Gottlob C, Kodros S. Arthroscopically assisted autologous osteochondral transplantation for osteochondral lesions of the talar dome: an MRI and clinical follow-up study. *Foot Ankle Int.* 2001;22:544-551.
27. Lee CH, Chao KH, Huang GS, Wu SS. Osteochondral autografts for osteochondritis dissecans of the talus. *Foot Ankle Int.* 2003;241:815-822.
28. Sammarco GJ, Makwana NK. Treatment of talar osteochondral lesions using local osteochondral graft. *Foot Ankle Int.* 2002;23:693-698.
29. Kreuz PC, Steinwachs M, Erggelet C, et al. Mosaicplasty with autogenous talar autograft for osteochondral lesions of the talus after failed primary arthroscopic management: a prospective study with a 4-year follow-up. *Am J Sports Med.* 2006;34:55-63.
30. Haasper C, Zelle BA, Knobloch K, et al. No mid-term difference in mosaicplasty in previously treated versus previously untreated patients with osteochondral lesions of the talus. *Arch Orthop Trauma Surg.* 2008;128:499-504.
31. Gobbi A, Francisco RA, Lubowitz JH, et al. Osteochondral lesions of the talus: randomized controlled trial comparing chondroplasty, microfracture, and osteochondral autograft transplantation. *Arthroscopy.* 2006;22:1085-1092.
32. Giannini S, Vannini F. Operative treatment of osteochondral lesions of the talar dome: current concepts review. *Foot Ankle Int.* 2004;25:168-175.
33. Chuckpaiwong B, Berkson EM, Theodore GH. Microfracture for osteochondral lesions of the ankle: outcome analysis and outcome predictors of 105 cases. *Arthroscopy.* 2008;24:106-112.
34. Robinson DE, Winson IG, Harries WJ, Kelly AJ. Arthroscopic treatment of osteochondral lesions of the talus. *J Bone Joint Surg Br.* 2003;85:989-993.
35. Kelberine F, Frank A. Arthroscopic treatment of osteochondral lesions of the talar dome: a retrospective study of 48 cases. *Arthroscopy.* 1999;15:77-84.
36. Schimmer RC, Dick W, Hintermann B. The role of ankle arthroscopy in the treatment strategies of osteochondritis dissecans lesions of the talus. *Foot Ankle Int.* 2001;22:895-900.
37. Savva N, Jabur M, Davies M, Saxby T. Osteochondral lesions of the talus: results of repeat arthroscopic débridement. *Foot Ankle Int.* 2007;28:669-673.
38. Dela Cruz EL, Brockbank GR. Use of the noninvasive ankle distractor with talar dome osteochondral graft transplantation. *J Foot Ankle Surg.* 2005;44:311-312.
39. Kish G, Modis L, Hangody L. Osteochondral mosaicplasty for the treatment of focal chondral and osteochondral lesions of the knee and talus in the athlete. Rationale, indications, techniques, and results. *Clin Sports Med* 1999;18:45-66, vi.
40. Choung D, Christensen JC. Mosaicplasty of the talus: a joint contact analysis in a cadaver model. *J Foot Ankle Surg.* 2002;41:65-75.
41. Huntley JS, Bush PG, McBirnie JM, et al. Chondrocyte death associated with human femoral osteochondral harvest as performed for mosaicplasty. *J Bone Joint Surg Am.* 2005;87:351-360.
42. Marymont JV, Shute G, Zhu H, et al. Computerized matching of autologous femoral grafts for the treatment of medial talar osteochondral defects. *Foot Ankle Int.* 2005;26:708-712.
43. Demirci S, Jubel A, Andermahr J, Koebke J. Chondral thickness and radii of curvature of the femoral condyles and talar trochlea. *Int J Sports Med.* 2008;29:327-330.
44. Huang FS, Simonian PT, Norman AG, Clark JM. Effects of small incongruities in a sheep model of osteochondral autografting. *Am J Sports Med.* 2004;32:1842-1848.
45. Pearce SG, Hurtig MB, Clarnette R, et al. An investigation of 2 techniques for optimizing joint surface congruency using multiple cylindrical osteochondral autografts. *Arthroscopy.* 2001;17:50-55.
46. Reddy S, Pedowitz DI, Parekh SG, et al. The morbidity associated with osteochondral harvest from asymptomatic knees for the treatment of osteochondral lesions of the talus. *Am J Sports Med.* 2007;35:80-85.
47. Nakagawa Y, Suzuki T, Matsusue Y, et al. Bony lesion recurrence after mosaicplasty for osteochondritis dissecans of the talus. *Arthroscopy.* 2005;21:630.

SUGGESTED READING

Tol JL, Struijs PAA, Bossuyt PM, et al. Treatment strategies in osteochondral defects of the talar dome: a systematic review. *Foot Ankle Int.* 2000;21:119-126.

Osteochondral Lesions of the Talar Dome:
Cartilage Replacement Using Autologous Chondrocyte Implantation and Allografts

Gregory C. Berlet ● Eric R. Giza

Osteochondral lesions of the talus (OLTs) are rare, representing only about 4% of all such lesions in the body.[1] This lesion also has been called osteochondritis dissecans, transchondral fracture, talar dome fracture, and osteochondral defect. OLTs consist of a focal cartilage deficit with associated reactive bone edema.

Several staging systems have evolved since Berndt and Harty proposed the first system based on radiographic imaging of the talus in 1959 (Table 14-1).[2] Loomer and colleagues[3] reviewed computed tomographic (CT) data of 92 patients with OLTs and found a previously unclassified lesion—the radiolucent lesion—in 77% of the patients in their series. In 1999, Hepple and coworkers,[4] using magnetic resonance imaging (MRI) added another characteristic to the original classification system—stage 5, subchondral cyst formation.

For clarity, most investigators prefer the simplicity of the Berndt and Harty classification system. However, MRI is the imaging modality of choice instead of the plain radiographs used in the original classification description.

NORMAL AND PATHOLOGIC ANATOMY

The talar dome is trapezoidal, and its anterior surface averages 2.5 mm wider than the posterior surface. The medial and lateral articular facets of the talus articulate with the medial and lateral malleoli. The articular surface of these facets is contiguous with the superior articular surface of the talar dome. Approximately 60% of the dome of the talus is covered by the trochlear articular cartilage, which is incapable of supporting intrinsic repair. The cartilage is largely avascular and incapable of healing through the typical inflammatory phase. Because the chondrocytes are contained in a thick extracellular matrix, they are unable to migrate from uninjured matrix to the zone of injury.

The talus has no muscular or tendinous attachments. Most of the blood supply of the talus enters by the neck through the sinus tarsi. The dorsalis pedis artery supplies the head and neck of the talus. The artery of the sinus tarsi is formed from branches of the peroneal and dorsalis pedis arteries. The artery of the tarsal canal branches from the posterior tibial artery. The sinus tarsi artery and the tarsal canal artery join to form an anastomotic sling inferior to the talus, from which branches enter the talar neck.

The articular cartilage of the talus is inconsistent with the posteromedial corner, having a greater depth of cartilage than the anterolateral. This manifests in geographic mechanical properties and may influence the rate and type of articular injury.[5-7]

TABLE 14-1	Staging System Proposed by Berndt and Harty
Stage	**Description**
Stage 1	Compression of the border of the talus
Stage 2	Incomplete detachment of fragment
Stage 3	Complete detachment, no displacement
Stage 4	Displaced fragment or loose body

From Berndt AL, Harty M. Transchondral fractures (osteochondritis dissecans) of the talus. J Bone Joint Surg Am. 1959;41A:988-1020.

PATIENT EVALUATION

History and Physical Examination

Patients typically present with chronic ankle pain and various degrees of swelling, catching, stiffness, and instability. Ligamentous instability may be a predisposing factor, and joint laxity should be assessed with the anterior drawer test and with varus and valgus stress. Strength should be assessed by comparison with the contralateral ankle. Palpation may reveal tenderness behind the medial malleolus when the ankle is dorsiflexed, indicating a posteromedial lesion. Anterolateral lesions may be tender when the anterolateral ankle joint is palpated with the joint in maximal plantar flexion. An effusion in a chronically painful joint usually indicates intra-articular pathology, which can include an OLT.

A history of trauma is documented in more than 85% of patients.[8-12] In most cases, the mechanism of injury is an inversion injury to the lateral ligamentous complex. Although the cause of nontraumatic OLTs is unknown, a primary ischemic event may be responsible. Nontraumatic OLTs can also be familial, multiple lesions can occur in the same patient, and identical medial talar lesions have occurred in identical twins.[13]

Diagnostic Imaging

Patients with an acute ankle injury with hemarthrosis or substantial tenderness should first undergo weight-bearing plain radiography (i.e., anteroposterior, lateral, and mortise views). Radiographs in various degrees of plantar flexion and dorsiflexion may help in diagnosing posteromedial and anterolateral lesions, respectively.[14] Plain radiographs of the contralateral ankle should be obtained, because there is a 10% to 25% incidence of a contralateral lesion.[15]

MRI can identify occult injuries of the subchondral bone and cartilage that may not be detected with routine radiographs.[16,17] Classic MRI findings include areas of low signal intensity on T1-weighted images, which suggests sclerosis of the bed of the talus and indicates a chronic lesion.[18,19] T2-weighted images reveal a rim that represents instability of the osteochondral fragment.[18,20] After treatment, MRI should reveal a reduction or disappearance of the low signal intensity on T1-weighted images and the rim on T2-weighted images.

TREATMENT

Indications and Contraindications

Symptomatic patients with negative findings on plain radiographs should undergo an initial period of immobilization followed by physical therapy. Patients whose plain radiographic images indicate OLTs and patients who remain symptomatic after 6 weeks should undergo additional evaluation with MRI.

Surgical repair of OLTs is contraindicated when the risks outweigh the perceived benefits. Risks include active infection in the operative area, the likelihood of patient noncompliance, and patients who are medically unstable. Relative contraindications include degenerative changes of the ankle involving more than an isolated OLT. Studies have shown that a trial of conservative therapy does not adversely affect surgery performed after conservative therapy has failed.[1,21]

Treatment Options

The goals of cartilage repair are to restore the articular cartilage surface, match the biochemical and biomechanical properties of normal hyaline cartilage, improve the patient's symptoms and function, and prevent or slow progression of focal chondral injury.

The approach to the OLT can be facilitated through open or arthroscopic approaches. Most primary interventions are performed with the assist of the arthroscope (i.e., microfracture). Open approaches are indicated for lesions unable to be accessed through the arthroscope or when the selected therapy requires direct access to the lesion.

Arthroscopy of the Ankle

Anterior Ankle Arthroscopy. Arthroscopic surgery of the anterior ankle allows the direct visualization of intra-articular structures of the anterior ankle joint without an arthrotomy or malleolar osteotomy. The congruency of the distal tibia and talar dome makes arthroscopic visualization difficult through a single portal. The distal tibia is concave in the sagittal plane and convex in the coronal plane. The anterior tibial plafond is slightly convex with a medial notch (i.e., notch of Harty) that recedes approximately 4 mm near the junction of the plafond with the medial malleolus. This is an ideal location for introduction of the arthroscopic instruments. The medial malleolus is approximately 2 cm anterior to the lateral malleolus. Anatomic studies have shown that the tibial plafond covers only two thirds of the talar dome in any position.

Anteromedial and anterolateral portals are the standard approach for anterior ankle arthroscopy. The anteromedial portal is located at the level of the joint line just medial to the anterior tibialis tendon. The notch of Harty allows passage of the arthroscope posteriorly. The saphenous vein and nerve run along the anterior border of the medial malleolus. The saphenous nerve and its branches are usually located lateral to the vein and are at risk with this approach. Staying close to the tibialis anterior tendon minimizes the risk of damage to the saphenous structures.

The anterolateral portal is found just lateral to the peroneus tertius, entering the joint between the fibula and the talus just distal to the joint line. In this location, the lateral and medial branches of the superficial peroneal nerve may be injured if their locations are not carefully identified before a skin incision is made.

Distraction techniques facilitate the placement of the arthroscope and instruments into the tightly configured ankle joint (Fig. 14-1). Noninvasive techniques involving straps, harnesses, and outriggers are distraction methods used most commonly. These techniques minimize the risk of neurovascular injury and other complications.[22]

Posterior Ankle Arthroscopy. Occasionally, posterior lesions are not accessible from the anterior ankle. In these cases, a posterior arthroscopic approach is favored. Through the posterior scope, 54% of the talar dome surface can be visualized and treated.[23]

Arthroscopic Débridement with Microfracture. Arthroscopic treatment of OLTs involves three principles: removing loose bod-

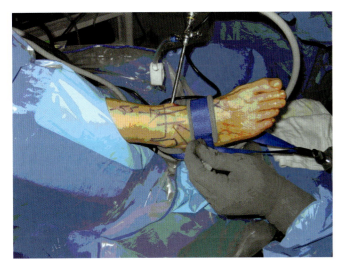

FIGURE 14-1 Ankle arthroscopic setup.

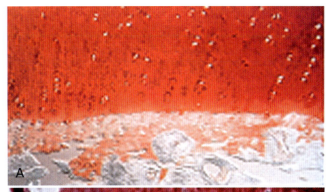

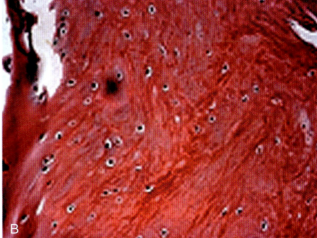

FIGURE 14-3 A, Hyaline cartilage is made up of proteoglycan aggregate; collagen types II, IX, and XI; and collagen fiber in an organized orientation. **B,** Fibrocartilage consists of proteoglycan, collagen type I, and collagen fiber in an unorganized orientation.

ies, securing the OLT to the talar dome (i.e., open reduction with internal fixation), and stimulating development of fibrocartilage. Open reduction with internal fixation is reserved for large, acute OLTs. More often, the lesion is débrided to a stable articular rim, and marrow stimulation techniques are used to create the healing cartilage.

The microfracture technique for OLTs is based on the success of similar techniques in the knee (Fig. 14-2).[24,25] Using awls, microfractures (i.e., perforations) are made approximately 3 to 4 mm apart in the subchondral bone while maintaining the integrity of the bone plate. The microfracture technique promotes new tissue formation by releasing substances such as mesenchymal stem cells, growth factors, and healing proteins.[24] Ultimately, cartilage-like cells (i.e., fibrocartilage) form and fill the original defect.

Tol and associates[26] reviewed 32 studies that reported the results of treatment for OTL. Nonoperative treatment had an average success rate of 45%, whereas the best success rate of 85% was achieved with excision, curettage, and drilling. Posteromedial

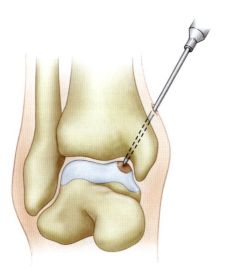

FIGURE 14-2 An osteochondral lesion of the talus was drilled to create a fibrocartilage cap.

lesions are difficult to access with this technique. The size of the lesion also plays a role in the success or failure of this procedure. In the meta-analysis by Tol and colleagues,[26] the lesion size averaged 0.7 cm; currently, lesions larger than 1 cm are thought to have a less predictable outcome with microfracture.

The limitation of microfracture is that fibrocartilage is created to fill the defect. This is predominantly type I cartilage, which lacks the organized structure of normal hyaline cartilage and therefore has inferior wear characteristics (Fig. 14-3).

We retrospectively reviewed the results of arthroscopy and microfracture in 189 patients; MRI was used to determine the size of the lesion.[27] Good results were achieved in 132 patients with an average lesion size of 0.67 cm²; 22 patients with an average lesion size of 0.76 cm² had fair results; and 36 patients with an average lesion size of 1.09 cm² had poor results (Fig. 14-4).

Open Approaches to the Ankle: Malleolar Osteotomies

The tibiotalar articular surface can be accessed through arthrotomies and arthroscopically. For techniques in which an articular graft must be delivered to the articular defect, an open approach is often favored. Muir and colleagues[28] studied nine cadavers to evaluate the accessibility of the talar dome by various approaches about the ankle. They used four arthrotomies and three osteotomies and characterized the percentage of the talar dome that

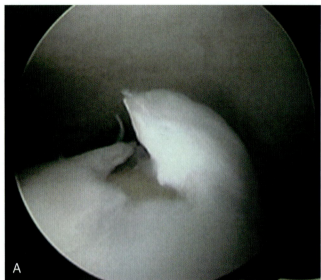

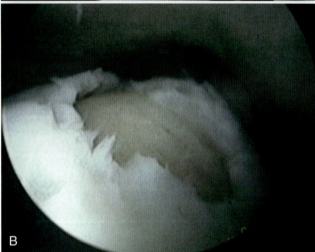

FIGURE 14-4 A and **B,** MRI shows the results of arthroscopy and microfracture.

could be accessed in a perpendicular fashion with respect to the articular surface. They found that without an osteotomy, up to 24% of the medial talar dome (average, 17%) and 25% of the lateral talar dome (average, 20%) could not be accessed. Osteotomies add an average of 22% exposure, although there remains a central 15% that is inaccessible in a perpendicular manner.[28]

Chevron Medial Malleolar Osteotomy. The chevron medial malleolar osteotomy is advantageous for many reasons. It is a reproducible technique that is familiar to most orthopedic surgeons, it provides good perpendicular access to the medial talar dome, it can be adjusted for the location of the lesions, it is vertically stable, and it is performed in the metaphyseal bone, which provides reliable healing.

When planning a medial malleolar osteotomy, careful preoperative identification of the exact location of the lesion on CT or MRI is important to ensure that the osteotomy cut will allow access to the lesion. The location of the osteotomy cut can be confirmed intraoperatively through a small arthrotomy before making the definitive bone cut.

The patient is placed in a supine position, and a thigh tourniquet is applied. A central incision is created over the medial malleolus, and careful dissection is performed to identify and protect the posterior tibial tendon. The anteromedial aspect of the joint is identified, and a small arthrotomy is performed to assist in visualizing the angle of the osteotomy.

Drill holes for two 4.5-mm screws are placed across the planned osteotomy site before making the cut. The holes are drilled and tapped to ensure anatomic reduction of the osteotomy. The chevron is oriented with the apex proximal, which facilitates a perpendicular approach to the medial talus. The periosteum is divided sharply along the proposed osteotomy.

The bone cut is performed with an oscillating saw along two thirds of its length and finished with an osteotome. Care is taken to ensure the talar cartilage is not disturbed. Passing a suture through the drill holes enables the surgical assistant to provide atraumatic retraction of the medial osteotomy fragment inferiorly. The posterior portion of the flexor retinaculum must be divided to allow adequate retraction.

Anterolateral Tibial Osteotomy for Lateral Talar Dome Access. Unlike access to the medial talus, full access to the lateral talus requires a limited fibular osteotomy with dislocation of the ankle or an osteotomy of the tibia and the fibula. The latter provides for superior visualization of the lateral talus, and it can be incorporated to access central lesions previously believed to be inaccessible.[29,30]

The patient is positioned supine with a bump under the ipsilateral hip. The incision is centered over the anterolateral aspect of the distal fibula and extended to the dorsum of the foot. The dissection interval carries the superficial peroneal nerve, extensor digitorum longus, and peroneus tertius medially.

For the final fixation, transverse screws are placed across the tibia through holes that are predrilled and tapped before the osteotomy is cut. These screws run parallel to the joint line, with the option of adding another screw perpendicular to the osteotomy. The fibula is stabilized with a one-third tubular plate at the completion of the operation.

An anterior starting point for the osteotomy is guided by the location of the lesion on the talus. The osteotomy has an approximate angle of 45 degrees from the lateral tibial plafond, with its proximal extension carrying through the fibula. The syndesmotic membrane is left intact.

The tibial osteotomy is divided with a saw but finished with an osteotome. The anterior talofibular ligament is sectioned to allow posterolateral retraction of the osteotomy.

Biologic Articular Resurfacing Options

Autologous Chondrocyte Implantation. Autologous chondrocyte implantation (ACI) of the talus involves placing cultured chondrocytes underneath a periosteal patch that is placed over the OLT.[31] Chondrocytes are harvested during a prior surgery from the knee or ankle (Fig. 14-5). Often, the damaged area of chondral tissue can be used for the biopsy, which obviates the need for damaging healthy tissue.[32] The biopsy typically yields 2 to 3 million cells that can be stored for more than 1 year. When required, the cells are then expanded in culture for 6 to 8 weeks,

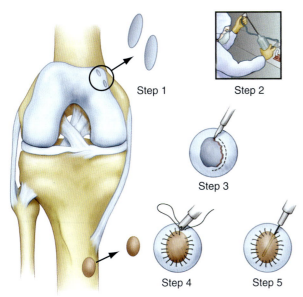

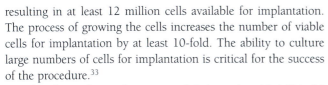

FIGURE 14-5 Cell preparation for autologous chondrocyte implantation.

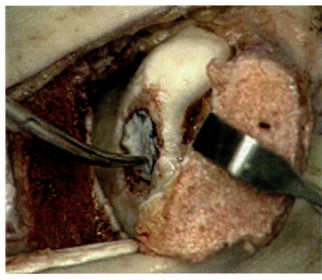

FIGURE 14-6 Cell implantation with a periosteal graft.

resulting in at least 12 million cells available for implantation. The process of growing the cells increases the number of viable cells for implantation by at least 10-fold. The ability to culture large numbers of cells for implantation is critical for the success of the procedure.[33]

Whittaker and coworkers reported their results with ACI in 10 patients at 4 years' follow-up.[34] Eight of the 10 patients had failed prior arthroscopic treatment. At a mean follow-up of 24 months, 90% were "pleased" or "extremely pleased" with the surgical result. Full-thickness biopsies were obtained in five patients requiring repeat arthroscopy; two showed hyaline cartilage, and three showed fibrocartilage. The results confirmed some donor-site morbidity. The Lysholm knee score returned to normal in three patients at 1 year but remained reduced by 15% in seven patients.[34]

Other surgeons have found similar results.[35,36] Baums and associates[37] reported the results for 12 patients treated with ACI at a mean follow-up of 63 months. There were six medial and six lateral lesions with an average size of 2.3 cm^2. At 63 months' follow-up, all patients were very satisfied or satisfied with the result. Based on the Hannover score, there were seven excellent, four good, and one satisfactory results. The preoperative American Orthopaedic Foot and Ankle Society (AOFAS) Hindfoot Score was 43.5 and the 63-month follow-up score was 88.4. MRI showed congruent graft incorporation in seven patients, and four had irregularity of the articular surface.[37]

Autologous Chondrocyte Implantation: Surgical Technique. After the lesion is exposed, it is curetted to a stable border, and a template is created using the foil sleeve from a suture package. Care is taken not to disturb the subchondral bone under the lesion, because bleeding from the bone can disrupt the periosteal patch and chondrocytes. Epinephrine-soaked pledgets are placed on the lesion, and the tourniquet is deflated. Next, the periosteal patch is harvested from the tibia approximately 4 cm distal to the tibial tubercle.

Careful dissection is carried out to remove the subcutaneous fat overlying the tibia without disturbing the periosteum. Next, the template is centered on the tibia, and the periosteum is cut with an extra 2-mm border around the template using a no. 15 scalpel.

The periosteum is removed carefully using a periosteal elevator, and the cambium layer (closest to the bone) is identified because it will be placed facing the subchondral bone over the lesion (Fig. 14-6). The tibial incision is closed in a standard fashion. The periosteal patch is then sutured to the lesion using 6-0 Vicryl that has been lubricated with sterile mineral oil. Before placing the final suture at the distal portion of the lesion, the perimeter is sealed with fibrin glue, and an angiocatheter is used to place some saline in the patch to ensure that the construct is sealed.

Cultured chondrocytes are injected into the lesion, and the final suture is placed. The medial malleolus is reduced and then stabilized with two 4.5-mm screws. A drain is placed in the anterior aspect of the joint, and the incision is closed in a layered fashion. The drain is removed after 24 hours, and a splint is used until the incision has healed. The patient is encouraged to start gentle range-of-motion exercises 2 weeks postoperatively. Weight bearing is restricted for 6 weeks and then is increased gradually over the next 6 weeks in a cast boot. Full weight bearing without a boot is permitted after 12 weeks.

Matrix-Based Chondrocyte Implantation. Matrix-based chondrocyte implantation (MACI) is similar to ACI; however, the chondrocytes are not placed under a periosteal patch but are embedded in a type I/III bilayer collagen membrane (Fig. 14-7). As with ACI, the cells are first harvested from the ankle or knee and then cultured to produce 15 to 20 million cells. Similar to ACI, the MACI technique allows the surgeon to increase by at least 10-fold the cells available for implantation into the defect. A second-stage operation is used to implant the membrane over the talar defect.[38,39]

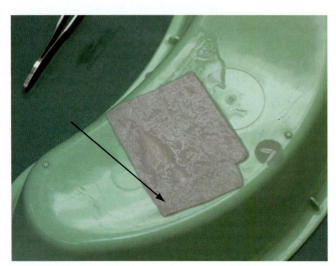

FIGURE 14-7 In matrix-based chondrocyte implantation, a collagen or hyaluronan membrane is seeded with chondrocytes.

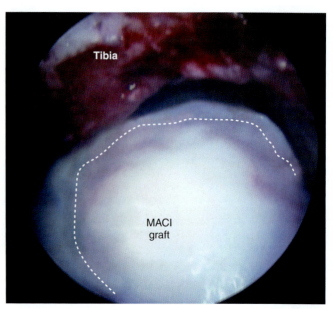

FIGURE 14-8 In matrix-based chondrocyte implantation, the graft is sealed with fibrin tissue sealant.

MACI is technically easier than ACI, and no tibial or malleolar osteotomy is required. Two operations are required, and the cells can be stored for more than 1 year after initial harvest. Cherubino and colleagues[40] reported on 13 patients with short-term follow-up (i.e., 6 to 12 months) for knee osteochondral defects. No complications were reported, and repeat MRIs at 6 months demonstrated the presence of hyaline-like cartilage at the site of implantation.

Ronga and colleagues[41] described six patients who were treated with the MACI technique for chondral defects in the ankle. The follow-up averaged 33.8 months, and the average age of the patients was 28.6 years. All defects were medial except for one "kissing" lesion. At the 2-year follow-up assessment, five ankles had improved AOFAS scores. All ankles had a second-look arthroscopy, and the five with improved scores had hyaline-like cartilage that was stable to probing. The ankle that did not improve had no detectable cartilage.[41]

Giza and coworkers reviewed 10 patients with full-thickness defects who underwent MACI. At the 2-year follow-up assessment, there were significant clinical improvements in the AOFAS ($P <$ .05) and SF-36 ($P <$ .001) scores.

Talus Matrix-Based Chondrocyte Implantation: Surgical Technique. The size and location of the chondral defect are assessed by ankle arthroscopy, and talar articular cartilage is harvested. The harvested chondrocytes are placed in a nutrient medium tube and sent to a cell laboratory (Genzyme Biosurgery, Boston, MA) along with 100 mL of autologous blood divided among 10 tubes. The cells are enzymatically separated from the matrix and cultured for 6 to 8 weeks to produce 15 to 20 million dedifferentiated cells. These cells are embedded in a type I/III collagen membrane bilayer and returned to the surgeon for implantation.[33]

The implantation procedure is performed in a tourniquet-controlled, bloodless field. The joint is exposed with a small anterolateral or anteromedial incision, and the use of a malleolar osteotomy usually is not required. The use of a limited plafondplasty, as described by Assenmacher and associates,[42] can improve access. The defect is prepared to stable margins using a curette, and a template of the lesion is prepared. The graft is cut from the MACI membrane and placed into the defect on top of a layer of fibrin tissue sealant (Fig. 14-8). The graft stability is tested with range of motion of the ankle joint.

The postoperative protocol involves no weight bearing for 6 weeks. A splint is used until the incision is healed, and gentle range-of-motion exercises are then permitted. Partial weight bearing is allowed after 6 weeks, full weight bearing after 12 weeks, higher joint loading (e.g., jogging) after 6 months, and return to sports after 12 months.

Autologous Osteochondral Grafting: Osteochondral Autograft Transplantation and Mosaicplasty. The osteochondral autograft transplantation (OAT) procedure grafts a single plug from the femoral trochlea or condyle into the OLT on the talar dome (Fig. 14-9),[43] whereas the mosaicplasty procedure transplants multiple plugs.[44] The OAT procedure results in reduced ingrowth of the fibrocartilage, although donor-site morbidity may be greater because of harvesting a single, larger plug. The placement of multiple plugs with the mosaicplasty technique more accurately matches the contour of the talar dome and the surface area of the defect, and it enables approximately 20% to 40% of the defect to be filled with fibrocartilage (Fig. 14-10).[45]

Al-Shaikh and colleagues[45] reported 19 patients who underwent mosaicplasty for lesions that averaged 12 × 10 mm. Plugs were harvested from the trochlear border of the ipsilateral femoral condyle. The postoperative AOFAS Ankle Score at 16 months

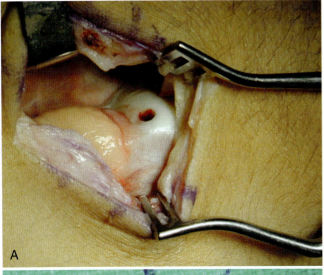

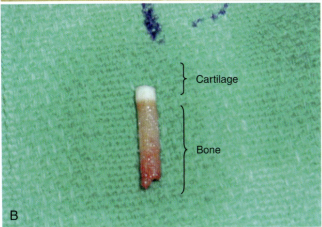

FIGURE 14-9 A, The site is prepared to receive a single graft plug for osteochondral autogenous transplantation (OAT). **B,** The OAT graft theoretically addresses the bone and cartilage injuries.

averaged 88. Most patients had occasional mild pain but excellent function; there were no adverse effects in the knee.[45]

Another study reported that 94% of 36 patients undergoing mosaicplasty had good or excellent results, with follow-up ranging from 2 to 7 years.[46] Prior surgical procedures had failed in 29 of the patients. Gautier and coworkers[47] also reported good or excellent results for 11 patients, with an average follow-up of 24 months. Those grafts were harvested from the ipsilateral knee without adverse effects on the knee.

In another study, plugs were harvested from the ipsilateral medial or lateral articular facet of the talus in 12 patients. Significant improvement in AOFAS scores was reported ($P < .0001$), and no structural failures occurred in the graft or donor site.[48]

Synthetic Scaffolds. The OsteoCure synthetic bone graft plugs, a poly-DL-lactic-coglycolic acid (PLGA) mixed with calcium sulfate scaffold, have been used as a synthetic osteochondral graft. This product was developed as a void filler in the donor hole when autogenous osteochondral grafts were harvested. The use of synthetic osteochondral grafts has been introduced as a means

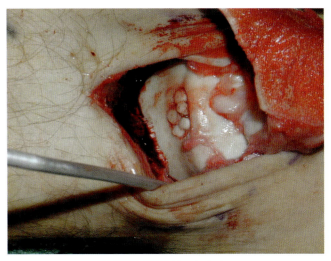

FIGURE 14-10 Mosaicplasty.

to avoid the autologous donor-site morbidity or the financial and supply issues of the allograft. Preclinical testing using a goat model showed integration of the OsteoCure into the osteochondral defect at 12 months postoperatively.[49]

Our experience, however, has shown various rates of resorption, with some radiographs showing radiolucent defects indicative of calcium absorption.[50] There are no published reports of the use of OsteoCure, but pathologic analysis of a failed OsteoCure specimen was performed after the case was revised to an osteochondral plug. The specimen showed a central focus where the cartilage and underlying bone were disrupted and replaced by fibrous tissue containing multinucleated giant cells. There was no bony ingrowth into this focus, and there was no evident ingrowth of hyaline cartilage, although there was some fibrocartilage at the periphery of the defect, which could represent some ingrowth of chondrocytes into fibrous tissue.[50]

Fresh Osteochondral Allograft Transplantation

The treatment strategies of microfracture, ACI, MACI, synthetic plugs, and OAT all share the same limitation: they require a contained lesion. These treatment strategies depend on circumferential support of the repair technique. For microfracture, the fibrocartilage is inherently unstable and will shear off in an uncontained lesion. Cartilage cells—whether contained in a sponge or under a periosteal membrane—cannot adequately restore the contour of the talar shoulder, and osteochondral plugs require a circumferential press-fit to stay in the transplanted position.

To address which OLTs are inappropriate for the use of these techniques, a modification to the classification system has been recommended to include the additional anatomic details of location and containment. Using the classification of Raikin,[51] which divides the talus into nine geographic locations, an additional notation of contained or uncontained is appropriate for shoulder lesions. The most common lesion found in Raikin's study was a midtalar medial lesion (zone 4). If this lesion extended to the

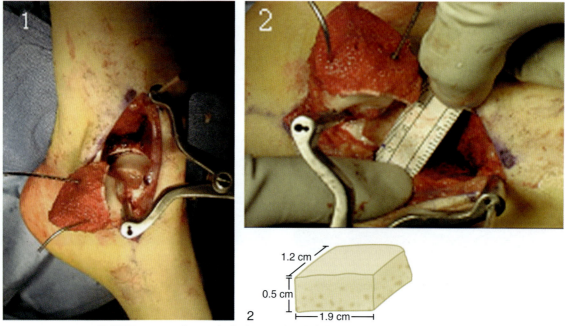

FIGURE 14-11 Technique for fresh osteochondral allograft transplantation (FOCAT).

shoulder with no medial wall intact, it would more appropriately be referred to as a zone 4, uncontained lesion.

For the uncontained shoulder lesions, fresh talus allografts have a role. These grafts have the potential to deliver living chondrocytes in a matrix that has little immunologic response from the host. At 21 days after harvest, the average chondrocyte viability is 50%. In the knee, osteochondral grafts can survive for 25 years, with phenotyping proving viable chondrocytes from the original donor.[52]

Grafts are matched for size and side, with a low tolerance for any mismatch (<2 mm). The osteochondral defect is excised with curettes and an osteotome to create a block defect. The donor graft is prepared with careful measurements from the host. The size of the graft can be large enough to include a full hemitalus, although this is rarely necessary. The average graft size is 2 cm². Grafts are press-fit and secured with bioabsorbable compression screws recessed below the articular surface.

We conducted a prospective study of the use of fresh osteochondral allografts in 17 patients who had failed arthroscopic excision, microfracture, and débridement (Fig. 14-11).[53] Preoperatively, all patients were assessed with plain radiographs, MRI, and a AOFAS Hindfoot Score. Postoperative assessment consisted of the AOFAS Hindfoot Score, radiographic assessment of osteotomy healing, graft subsidence, and radiolucency, followed by MRI assessment annually thereafter. The mean defect area was 2.0 cm². Postoperatively, patients were allowed motion at 4 weeks and did not bear weight on the affected extremity for 6 weeks. All patients had statistically significantly higher AOFAS scores, pain subscores ($P < .001$), and improved function subscores. Fifteen osteotomies healed within 3 months, and the remaining two healed by 1 year.[53] Radiolucencies around the transplanted graft were evaluated to reflect graft healing and the potential for later collapse. There were three cases with persistent radiolucencies at 2 years' follow-up. Five cases had graft subsidence averaging 3.8 mm (range, 2 to 9 mm),

with persistent radiolucency of the graft on the inferior surface confirmed as a substantial risk factor for later collapse. However, clinical outcomes were only slightly associated with graft subsidence. The only revision in this case series was one graft that collapsed 1 year postoperatively. The graft survival rate is 94.1% (16 patients) at the 2-year follow-up assessment.[53]

PEARLS & PITFALLS

- MRI is the modality of choice for identifying and staging OLTs.
- Conservative treatment should be tried first; failed conservative treatment has no adverse effects on the outcome of subsequent surgical procedures.
- Knowledge and awareness of adjacent venous and neural anatomy are crucial to avoid injury to these structures during an arthroscopic approach to the lesion.
- Microfracture results in the development of fibrocartilage to fill the defect.
- Fibrocartilage is inferior to normal hyaline cartilage and has inferior wear characteristics.
- Chondrocyte harvesting and culture yields at least 12 million cells for implantation after approximately 6 to 8 weeks.

POSTOPERATIVE REHABILITATION PROTOCOL

The postoperative protocol is individualized for the approach and the techniques used to re-establish the articular surface. Patients who undergo arthroscopic débridement with microfracture do not bear weight for 4 weeks. Non–weight-bearing motion is started at 2 weeks to promote molding of the joint surface and synovial lubrication. Boot walker ambulation is begun at 4 weeks, with transfer into a shoe with a protective brace occurring at 6 to 8 weeks. Physical therapy, including manual joint mobilizations, is very helpful and is begun 2 months postoperatively. An ankle effusion is an indication that the joint requires additional time and less mechanical stress, and it should be used to guide physical therapy and the patient's return to sports or other activities. The time for return to activity after arthroscopy and microfracture was 15.1 ± 4 weeks for stage 2 to 4 osteochondral defects of the talus.[54] Seijas and associates[55] found that 93.5 % of soccer players had returned to full athletic participation by 3.5 years postoperatively and played at the same level they enjoyed before injury.

Osteochondral grafting (e.g., autograft, allograft, synthetic), chondrocyte transplantation (i.e., ACI or MACI), and fresh bulk allografts all share a similar postoperative regimen. Patients are instructed not to bear weight for an average of 6 weeks to allow the osteotomy to heal. Patients without osteotomies also are instructed not to bear weight for 6 weeks. Protected ambulation in a boot walker is permitted until the patient feels comfortable, and then the patient is transferred to a shoe with an ankle brace. Physical therapy guidelines are similar to those for microfracture, with the addition of tendon mobilization around osteotomy sites. In a study of 12 patients with ACI for talar osteochondral defects, 6 patients were involved in competitive athletics, and all patients returned to full participation after treatment.[37]

CONCLUSIONS

Articular defects in the ankle consist primarily of lesions of the talus. The surgical treatment for talar OLT lesions has historically consisted of arthroscopy and microfracture, with anticipation of good results. However, poorer outcomes have been associated with lesions that are larger than 1 cm². For these larger lesions and for those that have failed primary management with microfracture, there is good evidence to support the successful treatment with the evolving techniques of osteochondral grafting, chondrocyte transplantation, and bulk fresh allograft transplantation. Synthetic grafts, although attractive in theory, have not shown great promise.

The future includes continued development of scaffolds for chondrocyte transplantation, better systems for cartilage graft preparation and transplantation, and perhaps a synthetic prosthetic replacement for focal cartilage defects.

REFERENCES

1. Alexander AH, Lichtman DM. Surgical treatment of transchondral talar-dome fractures (osteochondritis dissecans). Long-term follow-up. *J Bone Joint Surg Am.* 1980;62:646-652.
2. Berndt AL, Harty M. Transchondral fractures (osteochondritis dissecans) of the talus. *J Bone Joint Surg Am.* 1959;41A:988-1020.
3. Loomer R, Fisher C, Lloyd-Smith R, et al. Osteochondral lesions of the talus. *Am J Sports Med.* 1993;21:13-19.
4. Hepple S, Winson IG, Glew D. Osteochondral lesions of the talus: a revised classification. *Foot Ankle Int.* 1999;20:789-793.
5. Wan L, de Asla RJ, Rubash HE, Li G. Quantification of ankle articular cartilage topography and thickness using a high resolution stereophotography system. *J Orthop Res.* 2008;26:1081-1089.
6. Millington SA, Grabner M, Wozelka R, et al. Osteoarthritis. *Cartilage.* 2007;15:205-211.
7. Sugimoto K, Takakura Y, Tohno Y, et al. Cartilage thickness of the talar dome. *Arthroscopy.* 2005;21:401-404.
8. Anderson IF, Crichton KJ, Grattan-Smith T. Osteochondral fractures of the dome of the talus. *J Bone Joint Surg Am.* 1989;71:1143-1152.
9. Baker CL, Andrews JR, Ryan JB. Arthroscopic treatment of transchondral talar dome fractures. *Arthroscopy.* 1986;2:82-87.
10. Parisien JS. Arthroscopic treatment of osteochondral lesions of the talus. *Am J Sports Med.* 1986;14:211-217.
11. Pettine KA, Morrey BF. Osteochondral fractures of the talus. A long-term follow-up. *J Bone Joint Surg Br.* 1987;69:89-92.
12. Van Buecken K, Barrack RL, Alexander AH. Arthroscopic treatment of transchondral talar dome fractures. *Am J Sports Med.* 1989;17:350-355.
13. Woods K, Harris I. Osteochondritis dissecans of the talus in identical twins. *J Bone Joint Surg Br.* 1995;77:331.
14. Stroud CC, Marks RM. Imaging of osteochondral lesions of the talus. *Foot Ankle Clin.* 2000;5:119-133.
15. Stone JW. Osteochondral lesions of the talar dome. *J Am Acad Orthop Surg.* 1996;4:63-73.
16. Loredo R, Sanders TG. Imaging of osteochondral injuries. *Clin Sports Med.* 2001;20:249-278.
17. Elias I, Jung JW, Raikin SM, et al. Osteochondral lesions of the talus: change in MRI findings over time in talar lesions without operative intervention and implications for staging systems. *Foot Ankle Int.* 2006;27:157-166.
18. Higashiyama I, Kumai T, Takakura Y. Follow-up study of MRI for osteochondral lesion of the talus. *Foot Ankle Int.* 2000;21:127-133.
19. Mesgarzadeh M, Sapega AA, Bonakdarpour A, et al. Osteochondritis dissecans: analysis of mechanical stability with radiography, scintigraphy, and MR imaging. *Radiology.* 1987;165:775-780.
20. De Smet AA, Fisher DR, Burnstein MI. Value of MR imaging in staging osteochondral lesions of the talus (osteochondritis dissecans): results in 14 patients. *AJR Am J Roentgenol.* 1990;154:555-558.
21. Flick AB, Gould N. Osteochondritis dissecans of the talus (transchondral fractures of the talus): review of the literature and new surgical approach for medial dome lesions. *Foot Ankle.* 1985;5:165-185.
22. Frey C. Foot and ankle arthroscopy and endoscopy. In: Myerson MS, ed. *Foot and Ankle Disorders.* Philadelphia, PA: WB Saunders; 2000; 1477-1511.
23. Sitler DF, Amendola A, Bailey CS, et al. Posterior ankle arthroscopy: an anatomic study. *J Bone Joint Surg Am.* 2002;84A:763-769.
24. Steadman JR, Rodkey WG, Rodrigo JJ. Microfracture: surgical technique and rehabilitation to treat chondral defects. *Clin Orthop* 2002;391(Suppl):S362-S369.
25. Sledge SL. Microfracture techniques in the treatment of osteochondral injuries. *Clin Sports Med.* 2001;20:365-377.
26. Tol JL, Struijs PAA, Bossuyt PM, et al. Treatment strategies in osteochondral defects of the talar dome: a systematic review. *Foot Ankle Int.* 2000;21:119-126.
27. Berlet GC, Smith. Successful use of fresh-frozen osteochondral allograft for the management of osteochondral lesions of the talus: a prospective study. Paper presented at the 2008 Summer Meeting of the American Orthopaedic Foot and Ankle Society, June 26, 2008; Denver, CO.
28. Muir D, Saltzman CL, Tochigi Y, Amendola N. Talar dome access for osteochondral lesions. *Am J Sports Med.* 2006;34:1457-1463.
29. Bluman EM, Antosh IJ. Technique tip: tibiofibular osteotomy for increased access to the lateral ankle joint. *Foot Ankle Int.* 2008;29:735-738.
30. Tochigi Y, Amendola A, Muir D, Saltzman C. Surgical approach for centrolateral talar osteochondral lesions with an anterolateral osteotomy. *Foot Ankle Int.* 2002;23:1038-1039.
31. Peterson L, Minas T, Brittberg M, Nilsson A. Two to nine year outcome after autologous chondrocytes transplantation of the knee. *Clin Orthop Relat Res.* 2000;(374):212-234.
32. Giannini S, Buda R, Grigolo B, et al. The detached osteochondral fragment as a source of cells for autologous chondrocytes implantation (ACI) in the ankle joint. *Osteoarthritis Cartilage.* 2005;13:601-607.
33. Williams K, Genzyme Corporation, Perth, Australia. Personal communication. 2001.
34. Whittaker JP, Smith G, Makwana N, et al. Early results of autologous chondrocytes implantation in the talus. *J Bone Joint Surg Br.* 2005;87:179-183.
35. Giannini S, Buda R, Grigolo B, et al. Autologous chondrocyte transplantation in osteochondral lesions of the ankle joint. *Foot Ankle Int.* 2001;22:513-517.
36. Koulalis D, Schultz W, Psychogios B, Papagelopoulos PJ. Articular reconstruction of osteochondral defects of the talus through autologous chondrocyte transplantation. *Orthopedics.* 2004;27:559-561.
37. Baums MH, Heidrich G, Schultz W, et al. Autologous chondrocyte transplantation for treating cartilage defects of the talus. *J Bone Joint Surg Am.* 2006;88:303-308.
38. Marlovits S, Striessnig G, Kutscha-Lissberg F, et al. Early postoperative adherence of matrix-induced autologous chondrocyte implantation for the treatment of full-thickness cartilage defects of the femoral condyle. *Knee Surg Sports Traumatol Arthrosc.* 2005;13:451-457.

39. Zheng MH, Willers C, Kirilak L, et al. Matrix-induced autologous chondrocyte implantation (MACI): biological and histological assessment. *Tissue Eng.* 2007;13:737-746.

40. Cherubino P, Grassi FA, Bulgheroni P, Ronga M. Autologous chondrocyte implantation using a bilayer collagen membrane: a preliminary report. *J Orthop Surg.* 2003;11:10-15.

41. Ronga M, Grassi FA, Montoli C, et al. Treatment of deep cartilage defects of the ankle with matrix-induced autologous chondrocyte implantation (MACI). *Foot Ankle Surg.* 2005;11:29-33.

42. Assenmacher JA, Kelikian AS, Gottlob C, Kodros S. Arthroscopically assisted autologous osteochondral transplantation for osteochondral lesions of the talar dome: an MRI and clinical follow-up study. *Foot Ankle Int.* 2001;22:544-551.

43. Gobbi A, Francisco RA, Lubowitz JH, et al. Osteochondral lesions of the talus: randomized controlled trial comparing chondroplasty, microfracture, and osteochondral autograft transplantation. *Arthroscopy.* 2006; 22:1085-1092.

44. Haasper C, Zelle BA, Knobloch K, et al. No mid-term difference in mosaicplasty in previously treated versus previously untreated patients with osteochondral lesions of the talus. *Arch Orthop Trauma Surg.* 2008; 128:499-504.

45. Al-Shaikh RA, Chou LB, Mann JA. Autologous osteochondral grafting for talar cartilage defects. *Foot Ankle Int.* 2002;23:381-389.

46. Hangody L, Kish G, Modis L. Mosaicplasty for the treatment of osteochondritis dissecans of the talus: two to seven year results in 36 patients. *Foot Ankle Int.* 2001;22:552-558.

47. Gautier E, Kolker D, Jakob RP. Treatment of cartilage defects of the talus by autologous osteochondral grafts. *J Bone Joint Surg Br.* 2002;84:237-244.

48. Sammarco GJ, Makwana NK. Treatment of talar osteochondral lesions using local osteochondral graft. *Foot Ankle Int.* 2002;23:693-698.

49. Sharma B, Fermanian S, Cascio B. Chondral lesion repair in a goat model using an integrated hydrogel scaffold and marrow stimulation. Poster presented at the American Academy of Orthopaedic Surgeons, 2006; xxxx, xx.

50. Berlet GC, Penney N, Hyer C, et al. Microscopic analysis of a failed synthetic osteochondral graft of the talar dome: a case presentation. Presented at the 2009 Summer Meeting of the American Orthopaedic Foot and Ankle Society, July 2009; Vancouver, Canada.

51. Elias I, Zoga AC, Morrison WB, et al. Osteochondral lesions of the talus: localization and morphologic data from 424 patients using a novel anatomical grid scheme. *Foot Ankle Int.* 2007;28:154-161.

52. Gross AE, Kim W, Las Heras F, et al. Fresh osteochondral allografts for posttraumatic knee defects: long-term followup. *Clin Orthop Relat Res.* 2008;(466):1863-1870.

53. Berlet GC, Hyer CF, Philbin TM, et al. Successful management of talar osteochondral lesions using fresh osteochondral allograft. Presented at the 2009.Summer Meeting of the American Orthopaedic Foot and Ankle Society, July 2009; Vancouver, Canada.

54. Saxena A, Eakin C. Articular talar injuries in athletes: results of microfracture and autogenous bone graft. *Am J Sports Med.* 2007;35:1680-1687.

55. Seijas R, Alvarez P, Ares O, et al. Osteocartilaginous lesions of the talus in soccer players. *Arch Orthop Trauma Surg.* 2008; Dec 3 [Epub ahead of print].

Osteochondral Lesions of the Talar Dome:
New Horizons in Cartilage Replacement

Stephen P. Abelow ● Pedro Guillen ● Marta Guillen ● Isabel Guillen

Osteochondral lesions of the talar dome larger than 2.5 to 3.0 cm^2 pose a special problem in the young and middle-aged population (Figs. 15-1 to 15-3). These lesions affect the articular cartilage of the talar dome and the underlying subchondral bone.[1] If encountered acutely or if a large fragment exists, some of these lesions can be stabilized and internally fixed with metallic or bioabsorbable implants. Success rates of 78% (range, 40% to 100%) have been reported with reduction and fixation of the osteochondral fragments.[2] Most of the acute lesions suitable for internal fixation are laterally located and are usually anterior on the talar dome, making them relatively easy to access using a small, anterolateral arthrotomy incision or arthroscopic techniques.

Unfortunately, patients with these lesions represent a small proportion of those who present for treatment of symptomatic osteochondral lesions of the talar dome. Most have chronic, medial lesions, which tend to occur more posteriorly on the talar dome. They are more difficult to access and usually require a medial

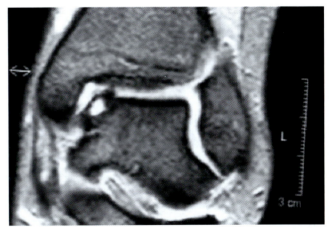

FIGURE 15-2 Anteroposterior magnetic resonance imaging shows an osteochondral lesion of the medial talus.

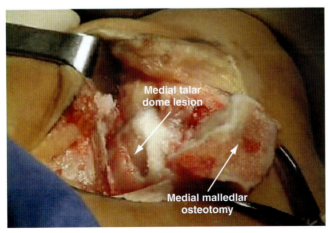

Medial talar dome lesion

Medial malledlar osteotomy

FIGURE 15-1 Grade IV lesion of the talar dome.

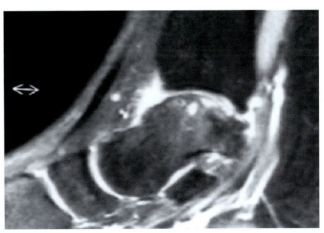

FIGURE 15-3 Lateral view of an osteochondral lesion of the talus.

malleolar osteotomy for open exposure. The posteromedial lesions more commonly manifest as chronic lesions that have greater depth than their lateral counterparts and that demonstrate degenerated articular cartilage with necrotic supporting subchondral bone.

Most chronic lesions of the posteromedial talar dome may be treated with conventional arthroscopic techniques, including débridement of the major fragments of bone and articular cartilage, establishment of a stable articular cartilage margin with perpendicular edges, and some type of marrow stimulation of the bony base, such as abrasion, drilling, or microfracture. This technique can produce good or excellent results in approximately 80% of patients.

Patients who fail conventional treatment or who have lesions known to have a poor prognosis with conventional treatment may be treated with some type of articular cartilage replacement technique. Large lesions (>1.5 to 2 cm in diameter) and lesions associated with large subchondral cysts (stage V lesions) are thought to have a poor prognosis with standard débridement procedures and may be considered for articular cartilage replacement. The indications for surgical cartilage replacement are symptomatic, deep lesions classified by the International Cartilage Repair Society (ICRS) as grade 3 (i.e., greater than 50% cartilage depth and down to but not through subchondral bone) or grade 4 (i.e., subchondral bone exposed, with lesions extending through the subchondral bone plate or deeper into the trabecular bone). There should be no uncorrected malalignment or instability and no significant osteoarthritis.

When considering the appropriate treatment for a talar dome lesion, it is important to separate the short-term from the long-term goals. In the short term, the goal is to eliminate or reduce pain to improve function. In the long term, the goal is to forestall the development of degenerative arthritis in the ankle joint while maintaining pain relief. In evaluating the various types of articular cartilage replacement techniques presented in this and previous chapters discussing autologous osteoarticular transplant techniques and autologous chondrocyte implantation (ACI) techniques, it is important to understand that there has been no level 1 study that has prospectively evaluated a randomized group of patients to compare techniques in the ankle.

Autologous osteochondral implantation techniques using plugs obtained from the knee joint or ACI using cultured chondrocytes implanted beneath a layer of periosteum using open techniques are approved for use in the United States. Orthopedic surgeons in other countries are using various types of articular cartilage implantation techniques that are potentially more amenable to arthroscopic surgery but are not approved for use in the United States. They represent a promising avenue of research for treatment of these lesions and are described in this chapter.

COLLAGEN-COVERED AUTOLOGOUS CHONDROCYTE IMPLANTATION

The technique of harvesting and suturing a periosteal patch in ACI is technically demanding and time consuming. Problems such as periosteal patch quality, symptomatic periosteal hypertrophy, and delamination have stimulated the development of biocompatible and bioabsorbable membranes to cover the chondral defect. A bi-

layer, absorbable, porcine collagen I/III membrane (Chondro-Gide, Geistlich Biomaterial, Wolhuser, Switzerland) has been used in European studies instead of a periosteal patch. The membrane is degraded by enzymatic division (i.e., collagenase), and the resultant collagen fragments denature at 37° C to gelatin.

In a prospective study presented at the ICRS meeting in 2004, Steinwachs[17] described 163 patients treated for chondral defects in the knee with ACI using a periosteal flap or the Chondro-Gide membrane instead of the periosteal patch. At approximately 3 years of follow-up, 78% of patients in the periosteal group reported good or excellent results, and 88% of patients in the Chondro-Gide group reported good or excellent results. Statistical significance was not discussed by the investigator. There were no cases of membrane hypertrophy.[17]

MATRIX/MEMBRANE-INDUCED AUTOLOGOUS CHONDROCYTE IMPLANTATION

Matrix/membrane-induced autologous chondrocyte implantation (MACI) is a second-generation chondrocyte implantation process. MACI is a new biotechnology in which cultured autologous chondrocytes are impregnated onto a highly purified, porcine collagen I/III membrane (Verigen AG, Genzyme Corp., Cambridge, MA) (Fig. 15-4). The MACI implant can be fixed to the chondral defect by fibrin glue (with little or no suture necessary), suture, or bioabsorbable pins or tacks. The procedure can be performed arthroscopically or by mini-arthrotomy. No periosteal graft is needed.

Open Technique

Chondrocytes are harvested arthroscopically from a non–weight-bearing area of the ipsilateral knee (200 to 300 mg of healthy cartilage). The chondrocytes are then cultured and expanded in

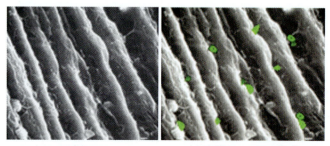

Matrix (collagen)

Autologous chondrocytes seeded on membrane (electron microscopy)

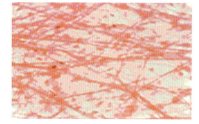

Collagen membrane and chondrocytes (light microscopy H/E)

FIGURE 15-4 Chondrocytes (green) seeded on a collagen membrane.

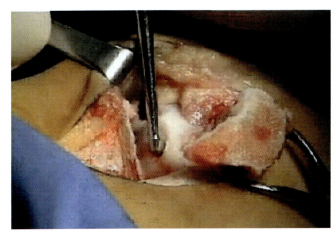

FIGURE 15-5 The defect is curetted to create a stable cartilage rim with sharply vertical walls.

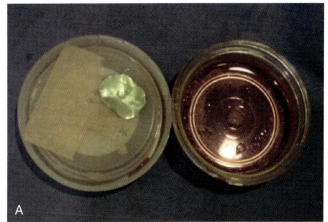

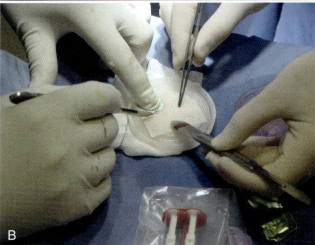

FIGURE 15-7 Templating (**A**) and cutting (**B**) the matrix-based chondrocyte implant.

vitro (3 to 5 weeks) and then impregnated on an absorbable, three-dimensional, bilayered, purified, porcine collagen I/III membrane. The bilayer structure has a smooth side that acts as a natural barrier and faces the joint. Chondrocytes are seeded on the porous side of the matrix. The membrane is tear resistant and can be templated and cut to shape. The membrane is nonantigenic (i.e., telopeptides are split during the manufacturing process), and it is bioabsorbable. The bioabsorbable membrane can be fixed to the ankle cartilage defect with fibrin glue, pins, or suture.

The talar dome lesion may be approached using a simple arthrotomy for an anterior lesion, or a malleolar osteotomy may be required to expose a middle to posterior talar lesion. The osteochondral defect is débrided, and the base is curetted to remove the calcified cartilage layer (Fig. 15-5). A stable cartilage rim with sharp vertical walls of healthy cartilage is created, and the chondral defect is templated for size and shape (Fig. 15-6). The MACI membrane is cut to the proper shape with a scalpel or scissors (Fig. 15-7). The membrane is then fixed with fibrin glue (Tisucol, Baxter, Spain) (Fig. 15-8). Suture or bioabsorbable pins, or both, may be used, but fibrin glue by itself is usually all that is needed (Figs. 15-9 and 15-10).[18,19]

Postoperatively, the patient is placed into a soft dressing, and continuous passive motion is initiated for 8 weeks, during which time the patient does not bear weight on the extremity. Patients with larger and more central lesions are not allowed to bear weight for 12 weeks.

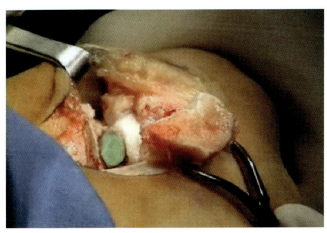

FIGURE 15-6 Templating the defect.

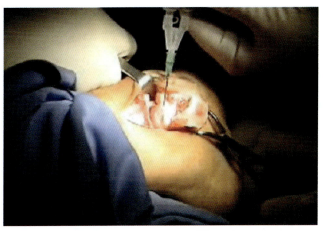

FIGURE 15-8 Application of fibrin glue.

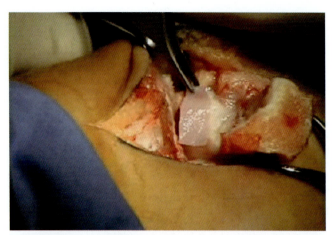

FIGURE 15-9 The matrix-based chondrocyte implantation membrane is placed on the talus.

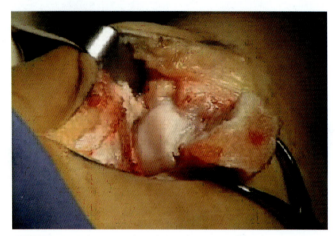

FIGURE 15-10 The matrix-based chondrocyte implantation membrane is implanted on the talus.

Arthroscopic Technique

Chondrocytes for culture are obtained from the knee joint as described previously. After the chondrocyte population has been expanded in vitro and impregnated on the membrane, standard ankle arthroscopy is performed through a specially designed arthroscopic cannula, and the cartilage defect is curetted using sharp ring curettes to remove the calcified cartilage layer. The surgeon creates a stable articular cartilage rim with sharp vertical walls of healthy cartilage. Using a flexible ruler, a standard probe, and a specially designed arthroscopic caliper, the size of the lesion is calculated. A template is created using packaging from a suture pack or a rubber drain, and it is placed in the cartilage defect to test for size.

Placement of the graft is performed using a dry scope technique, which is done without fluid in the joint. Two small anchors with 5-0 absorbable sutures are then placed at opposite sides of the periphery of the cartilage lesion (i.e., 3 and 9 o'clock or 12 and 6 o'clock). The sutures are then passed through the MACI membrane outside the joint at points corresponding to the cartilage lesion (Figs. 15-11 to 15-13).

The membrane is guided down the suture to the cartilage defect using the specially designed articulated passer. The mem-

brane is then smoothed out using an articulated T smoother or tamper. Fibrin glue (Tisucol) is then placed under the membrane. The membrane over the grafted area is smoothed out to the contours of the cartilage defect. The articulated inserter is used to hold the graft in place, and the T smoother is used to remove the excess glue and ensure that the periphery of the graft is well fitted and securely glued in place. The two sutures are then tied over the graft using arthroscopic knot-tying technique. Pressure is applied for 6 or 7 minutes to allow the fibrin glue to fully set. The joint is taken through ranges of motion to ensure the graft is stable. For easily accessible lesions, the membrane can be pushed down the canula and held in place by fibrin glue and bioabsorbable pins (Figs. 15- 14 to 15-18).

We have developed new instrumentation that allows the membrane to be pierced in its center and then placed in the center of the cartilage defect. The membrane is then pushed down the canula with a slotted articulated inserter and held in place by the arthroscopic skewer. Fibrin glue is then placed under the membrane, and the membrane is smoothed out. The excess glue is removed, and the membrane contours to the cartilage defect while the fibrin glue is setting (see Figs. 15-16 and 15-17).

Cherubino and colleagues[20] reported six patients with deep chondral defects of the ankle averaging 3.4 cm^2 (range, 2.5 to 4 cm^2) treated using the MACI technique. At an average follow-up of 42.1 months, the American Orthopaedic Foot and Ankle Society (AOFAS) clinical-functional scores improved for five of the six patients. No complications were observed in the postoperative period. Second-look arthroscopy in the five successful ankles revealed the defect to be completely filled by hyaline-like tissue as determined by probing the surface, but biopsy of the regenerated surface was not performed. In five ankles, postoperative magnetic resonance imaging (MRI) demonstrated the presence of hyaline-like cartilage in the site of the defect according to the MRI criteria.[20]

MACI procedures have been used to treat 131 knees and 19 ankles at the Clinica CEMTRO in Madrid, Spain. The first 50 cases (42 knees, 8 ankles) were evaluated and reported in a level IV nonrandomized study with no control group.[19] Defects were large, ICRS grade 3 (i.e., severely abnormal, 50% cartilage depth) or ICRS grade 4 (i.e., severely abnormal, extending into the subchondral bone). The size of the lesion varied from 3 to 6 cm.^{2} in the combined knee and ankle groups. Two years postoperatively, 88% of the patients reported no or little pain. All patients returned to their previous level of work activity. MRI showed a change in signal intensity postoperatively with a progressive decrease of subchondral edema. Biopsy of knee lesions has shown immature chondrocytes and immature cartilage. Second-look arthroscopy revealed good reparative tissue when probed (Fig. 15-19).

The biomedical unit at the Clinica CEMTRO in Madrid, Spain, is investigating the use of allogenic chondrocytes seeded onto a membrane to offer an "off-the-shelf MACI" and "instantaneous MACI" in which the chondrocytes are harvested and seeded on a matrix in one surgical setting. The use of various polypeptides applied to the membrane to upregulate anabolic growth factors and downregulate catabolic growth factors is being investigated.

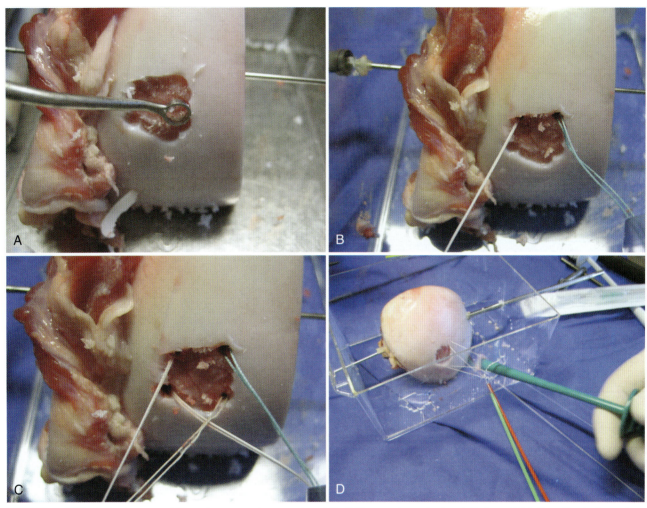

FIGURE 15-11 The lesion is curetted (**A**), and suture anchors are placed (**B, C**). The membrane is placed (**D,** *lower right*). *(From Chu C, ed. Articular cartilage surgery. Oper Tech Orthop. 2006;16:217-292.)*

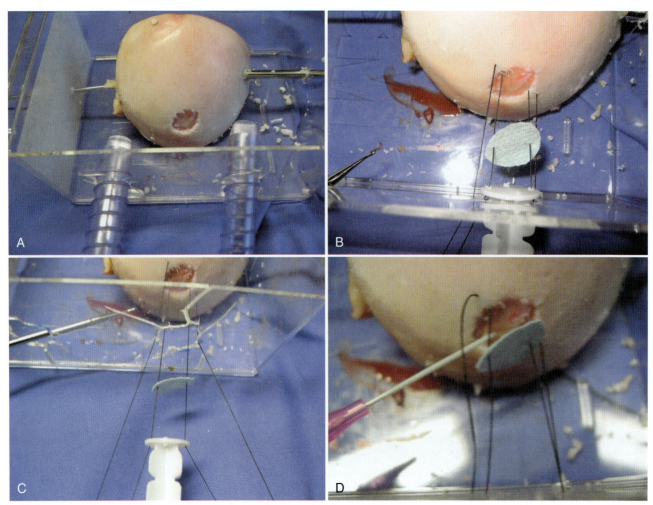

FIGURE 15-12 Placement of the membrane (**A, B, C**) and fibrin glue (**D**). *(From Chu C, ed. Articular cartilage surgery.* Oper Tech Orthop. *2006;16:217-292.)*

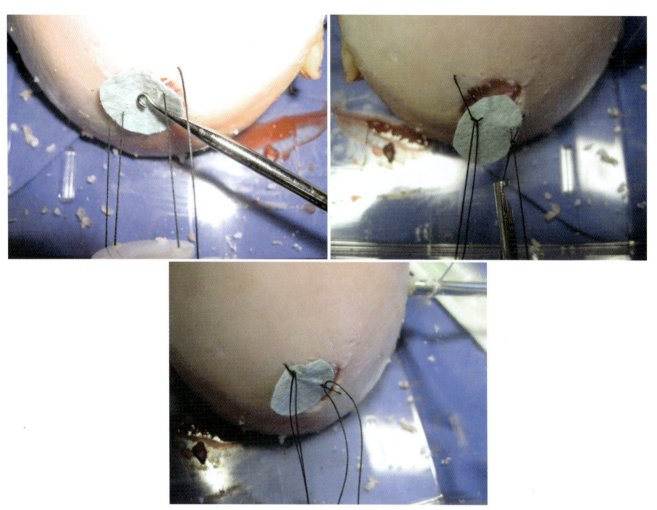

FIGURE 15-13 The membrane is secured by suture as well as fibrin glue. *(From Chu C, ed. Articular cartilage surgery.* Oper Tech Orthop. *2006;16:217-292.)*

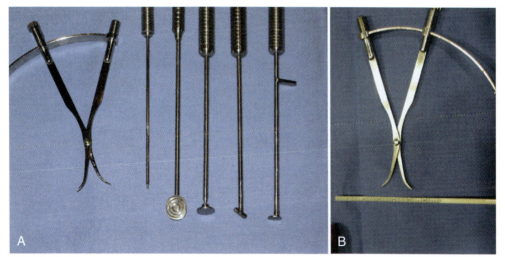

FIGURE 15-14 Arthroscopic instrumentation for matrix-based chondrocyte implantation. (**A**) Arthroscopic membrane inserter, articulated T smoother and articulated membrane tamp. (**B**) Arthroscopic caliper and flexible ruler. *(From Chu C, ed. Articular cartilage surgery.* Oper Tech Orthop. *2006;16:217-292.)*

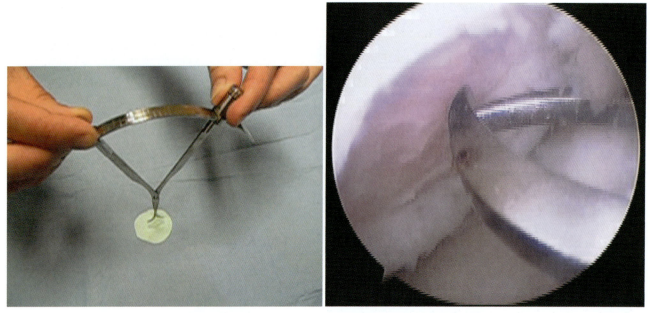

FIGURE 15-15 Arthroscopic caliper. *(From Chu C, ed. Articular cartilage surgery. Oper Tech Orthop. 2006;16:217-292.)*

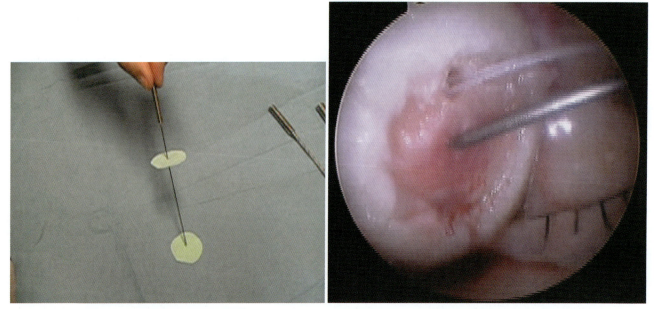

FIGURE 15-16 The graft for matrix-based chondrocyte implantation is inserted into cartilage defect. *(From Chu C, ed. Articular cartilage surgery. Oper Tech Orthop.2006;16:217-292.)*

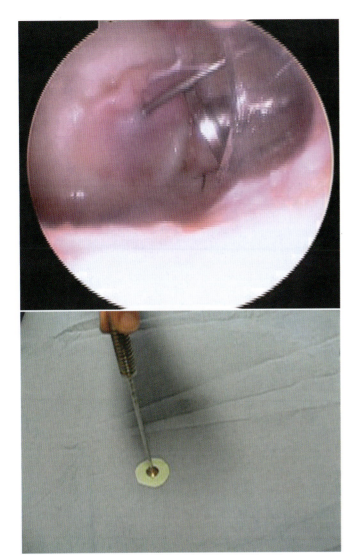

FIGURE 15-17 The graft for matrix-based chondrocyte implantation is held in place while the glue is setting. *(From Chu C, ed. Articular cartilage surgery.* Oper Tech Orthop. *2006;16:217-292.)*

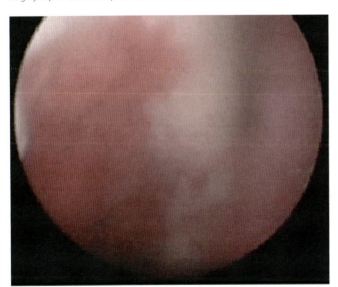

FIGURE 15-18 Autologous chondrocyte implant for matrix-based chondrocyte implantation. *(From Chu C, ed. Articular cartilage surgery.* Oper Tech Orthop. *2006;16:217-292.)*

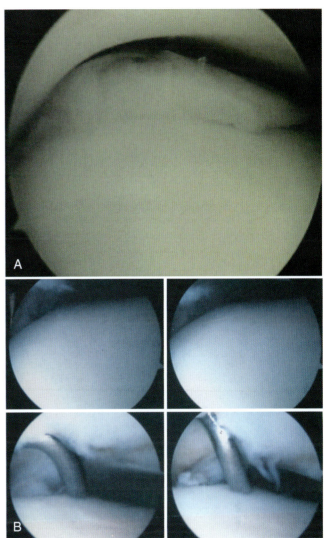

FIGURE 15-19 The arthroscopic view shows a full-thickness cartilage defect (**A**) *(upper)*. Follow-up at 2 years and 4 months postoperatively shows the results of matrix-based chondrocyte implantation (**B**).

OTHER SCAFFOLDS AND BIOMATERIALS

Various scaffolds of a synthetic nature and hybrid materials in a variety of fibers, meshes, and gels have been applied to cartilage tissue engineering. Hyalograft C is a tissue-engineered graft consisting of autologous chondrocytes expanded in vitro and seeded onto a three-dimensional, nonwoven, hyaluronic acid scaffold, which is a benzyl ester of hyaluronic acid. The membrane is auto-adhesive and is amenable to arthroscopic implantation. This graft material has been extensively studied in the knee by Marcacci and colleagues[21] at Instituti Rizzoli in Bologna, Italy, with encouraging preliminary results. A large, multicenter study in Italy of 129 patients demonstrated 91.5% improvement in their knee symptoms, functionality, and activity level. Giannini and colleagues[22] reported 35 patients with osteochondral lesions of the talus treated with Hyalograft C ACI. There was no control group in the study. All patients were satisfied with their results. The AOFAS scores were improved from 50.8 ± 12 points preoperatively to 92.2 ± 9 points at 12 months' follow-up. Three of the lesions in patients who remained symptomatic were biopsied at 1 year postoperatively. The histologic appearance was described as hyaline-like tissue with some evidence of type II collagen present.[23]

Chondrocelect® is a membrane-based, autologous chondrocyte implant using a set of molecular markers that predict the outcome of the in vivo cartilage-forming capacity. The chondrocytes are characterized to yield a phenotypically stable cartilage-forming cell population. By using a higher concentration of better-quality chondrocytes, a higher-quality structural repair is anticipated.[24] In a multicenter, prospective, randomized study of patients with symptomatic chondral defects of the knee femoral condyle, Saris and coworkers[25] compared treatment with microfracture to characterized chondrocyte implantation. They found that at short-term follow-up 1 year after treatment, characterized chondrocyte implantation resulted in regenerated tissue that was superior to that seen after microfracture in biopsy specimens. However, clinical results at 1 year of follow-up were similar for both treatments.[25]

Several other materials are in early phases of clinical testing. Bioseed-C® is a polyglactin/poly-p-dioxanone fleece (Biotissue Technologies, Freiberg, Germany) in which autologous chondrocytes are seeded. This can be inserted arthroscopically. Cartipatch® is a hydrogel composed of agarose and alginate for the matrix. It can be mixed with a cell suspension and can be molded. The alginate provides matrix elasticity, making it easy to handle. Hyaline cartilage with collagen II immunostaining was observed in one uncontrolled, level IV study.[28] Arthromatrix® (Orthogen/Arthrex Biosystems) is an equine collagen I/III membrane seeded with chondrocytes, and Novocart 3D® is a collagen-based, biphasic carrier onto which autologous chondrocytes are seeded.[30]

Co.don® chondrosphere[31] is a proprietary material in which chondrocytes that are processed and cultured in the presence of autologous serum form in vitro a three-dimensional chondrogenic tissue by generating their own extracellular matrix, which is similar to the matrix of hyaline cartilage. These autologous, engineered chondrospheroids serve as a basis for cartilage repair. The procedure can be performed using minimally invasive techniques. Preliminary pilot studies in humans are being conducted in Europe.

Autologous Matrix-Induced Chondrogenesis

Autologous matrix-induced chondrogenesis (AMIC) is a one-step procedure in which microfracture of the cartilage defect is performed (allowing bone marrow stem cells and growth factors to be released into the defect area), and the base is covered with a porcine collagen I/III matrix (Chondro-Gide matrix®) to stabilize the defect area and provide a suitable environment for the generation of new cartilage tissue. The membrane is fixed with fibrin glue and 10 mL of autologous patient serum. In a level IV, retrospective, uncontrolled case series, Behrens[32] reported 25 patients with improvement of the ICRS and Cincinnati knee scores.

Platelet-Rich Plasma

Platelet-rich plasma is plasma that is rich in growth factors. These growth factors have a recognized influence on cellular activity. Autologous platelet-rich plasma can be used by itself or mixed with allograft or autograft to aid in cartilage regeneration.[33]

In vitro, plasma-rich growth factors (PRGFs) have been shown to increase the total glycosaminoglycans synthesis produced by the chondrocytes and to decrease its degradation, increase the matrix collagen II content, and stimulate chondrogenesis, thereby increasing proliferation, differentiation, and adhesion of the chondrocytes. The PRGFs counteract the molecular effects that encourage the cartilage degeneration (e.g., nitrous oxide, metalloproteinases, interleukins).

In a level IV, retrospective, uncontrolled case series, Cugat[33] reported a rate of 78.2% for excellent or good results in the reduction or disappearance of pain and a rate of 77.7% for excellent or good results in improvement of function in cases of osteoarthritis. The follow-up time was short. The experience at Clinica CEMTRO in Madrid, Spain, using PRP for osteoarthritis was not encouraging.

Stem Cells

The results of ACI have shown that we are still a long way from regenerating articular cartilage. Because the chondrocyte is a rather quiescent cell, researchers are trying to develop alternative cell types, including mesenchymal stem cells (MSCs)[34] to repair and regenerate tissues. An embryonic stem cell (ESC) is capable of differentiating into many tissue types, whereas differentiation of adult stem cells usually is restricted to the tissue type in which it resides. A MSC is potentially a multilineage progenitor cell that retains its capacity to divide and whose progeny can differentiate into mesodermal tissue cells such as cartilage, bone muscle, fat, tendon, and ligament.[35]

In principle, the goals of using stem cells are to induce and expand a group of multipotent cells down a signaled pathway into an end-stage phenotype or one that is capable of further development after implantation; to deliver the cells to the repair site using a scaffold; and to bind them to the edges of the defect.[35]

With current methods, autologous chondrocytes are essentially aged chondrocytes. Perhaps using stem cells may result in a higher-quality biologic and mechanical repair of cartilage tissue. MSCs have been shown to result in good repair of chondral tissue.[36,37] ESCs may have offer the best repair of regenerated cartilage, but ethical and scientific issues regarding the use of ESCs in humans limits their application.

CONCLUSIONS

Full-thickness cartilage lesions pose a problem. Of the second- and third-generation autologous cultured chondrocyte technologies, none of them provides complete biomechanical or histologic restoration of native hyaline cartilage. There has not been a randomized, prospective, double-blind, statistically significant study documenting the true superiority of these tissue-engineered or bioengineered constructs in the ankle. However, promising research is occurring in one-stage MACI procedures, allogenic cartilage repair technologies, and progenitor cell and stem cell applications to cartilage regeneration.

REFERENCES

1. Berndt AC, Harty M. Transchondral fractures (osteochondritis dissecans) of the talus. *J Bone Joint Surg Am.* 1959;41:988-1020.
2. Verhagen RA, Struijs PA, Bossmyt PM, Van Dijk CN. Systemic review of treatment strategies for osteochondral defects of the talar dome. *Foot Ankle Clin.* 2003;8:233-243.
3. Williams SK, Amiel D, Bull S, et al. Prolonged storage effects on the articular cartilage of fresh human osteochondral allograft. *J Bone Joint Surg Am.* 2003;85:2111-2120.
4. Ryan J, Jamali AA, Bugbee W. Fresh osteochondral all grafting. In: Zansi S, Brittberg M, Marcacci M, eds. *Basic Science, Clinical Repair, and Reconstruction of Articular Cartilage Defects: Current Status and Prospects.* Bologna, Italy: Timeo Editore; 2006:212-229.
5. Gross AE, Aguids Z, Hutchinson CR. Osteochondritis defects of the talus treated with fresh osteochondral allograft transplantation. *Foot Ankle Int.* 2001;22:385-391.
6. Kim CW, Jamali A, Tontz WL, et al. Treatment of posttraumatic ankle arthrosis with bipolar tibiotalar osteochondral shell allografts. *Foot Ankle Int.* 2002;23:1091-1102.
7. Brittberg M, Lindahal A, Nilson A, et al. Treatment of deep cartilage defects in the knee with autologous cartilage transplantation. *N Engl J Med.* 1994;331:889-895.
8. Peterson L. ACI surgical techniques and results at 2-10 years. In: Zansi S, Brittberg M, Marcacci M, eds. *Basic Science, Clinical Repair, and Reconstruction of Articular Cartilage Defects: Current Status and Prospects.* Bologna, Italy: Timeo Editore; 2006:325-332.
9. Peterson L, Minas T, Brittberg M, et al. Two to nine year outcome after autologous chondrocyte transplantation of the knee. *Clin Orthop.* 2000;(374):212- 234.
10. Peterson L, Brittberg M, Lindahal A. Autologous chondrocyte transplantation of the ankle. *Foot Ankle Clin.* 2003;8:291-303.
11. Nan EK, Ferkel RD. Autologous chondrocytes implantation of the ankle: two to five year follow up. Presented at the American Orthopaedic Society for Sports Medicine Meeting, March 13, 2004; San Francisco, CA.
12. Ferkel RD, Hommen JP. Arthroscopy of the foot and ankle. In: Coughlin MJ, Mann RA, Saltzman CL, eds. *Surgery of the Foot and Ankle.* Philadelphia, PA: Mosby; 2007:1667-1677.
13. Koulalis D, Schultz W, Heydu M. Autologous chondrocyte transplantation for osteochondritis dissecans of the talus. *Clin Orthop.* 2002; (395):286-292.
14. Brittberg M. Talus cartilage lesions treated with autologous chondrocyte implantation. In: Zansi S, Brittberg M, Marcacci M, eds. *Basic Science, Clinical Repair, and Reconstruction of Articular Cartilage Defects: Current Status and Prospects.* Bologna, Italy: Timeo Editore; 2006:333-340.
15. Giannini S, Buda R, Grigolo B, Vannini F. Autologous chondrocyte transplantation in osteochondral lesions of the ankle joint. *Foot Ankle Int.* 2001;22:513-517.
16. Whittaker JP, Smith G, Makwana N, et al. Early results of autologous chondrocyte implantation in the talus. *J Bone Joint Surg Br.* 2005;87B:179-183.
17. Steinwachs MR. ACI and resorbable collagen membrane: Chondro-Gide surgical technique and results. In: Zansi S, Brittberg M, Marcacci M, eds. *Basic Science, Clinical Repair, and Reconstruction of Articular Cartilage Defects: Current Status and Prospects.* Bologna, Italy: Timeo Editore; 2006:389-392.
18. Abelow SP, Guillen P, Ramos T. Arthroscopic techniques for matrix-induced autologous chondrocyte implantation for treatment of large chondral defects in the knee and ankle. *Oper Tech Orthop.* 2006;16: 257-261.
19. Abelow SP, Guillen P, Fernandez T, Guillen I. Autologous chondrocyte implantation for the treatment of large chondral defects in the knee and ankle. Presented at the Arthroscopy Association of North America Annual Meeting, 2005; Vancouver, BC.
20. Cherubino P, Ronga M, Grassi FA, et al. Clinical results with MACI. In: Zansi S, Brittberg M, Marcacci M, eds. *Basic Science, Clinical Repair, and Reconstruction of Articular Cartilage Defects: Current Status and Prospects.* Bologna, Italy: Timeo Editore; 2006:565-569.
21. Marcacci M, Kon E, Zaffagnini S, Iacono F. Surgical transplantation of autologous chondrocytes: simple procedure by arthroscopic technique, In: Zansi S, Brittberg M, Marcacci M, eds. *Basic Science, Clinical Repair, and Reconstruction of Articular Cartilage Defects: Current Status and Prospects.* Bologna, Italy: Timeo Editore; 2006:457-461.
22. Kon E, Reggiani LM, Delcogliano M, Filardo G. Multicentric study and results in Italy. In: Zansi S, Brittberg M, Marcacci M, eds. *Basic Science, Clinical Repair, and Reconstruction of Articular Cartilage Defects: Current Status and Prospects.* Bologna, Italy: Timeo Editore; 2006:509-514.
23. Giannini S, Buda R, Vannini F, Grigolo B. Treatment of ankle defects with Hyalograft C. In: Zansi S, Brittberg M, Marcacci M, eds. *Basic Science, Clinical Repair, and Reconstruction of Articular Cartilage Defects: Current Status and Prospects.* Bologna, Italy: Timeo Editore; 2006:475-480.
24. Vanlauwe J, Bijlstra A, Bellemans J, Luyten F. Chondrocelct, an improved ACI product. In: Zansi S, Brittberg M, Marcacci M, eds. *Basic Science, Clinical Repair, and Reconstruction of Articular Cartilage Defects: Current Status and Prospects.* Bologna, Italy: Timeo Editore; 2006:369-386.
25. Saris D, Vanlauwe J, Victor J, et al. Characterized chondrocyte implantation results in better structural repair when treating symptomatic cartilage defects of the knee in a randomized controlled trial versus microfracture. *Am J Sports Med.* 2008;36:235-246.
26. Mrosek EH, Erggelet C. Autologous chondrocyte implantation with a resorbable 3D polymer matrix (Bioseed-C). In: Zansi S, Brittberg M, Marcacci M, eds. *Basic Science, Clinical Repair, and Reconstruction of Articular Cartilage Defects: Current Status and Prospects.* Bologna, Italy: Timeo Editore; 2006:413-417.
27. Erggelet C, Sittinger M, Lahm A. The arthroscopic implantation of autologous chondrocytes for the treatment of full-thickness cartilage defects in the knee joint. *Arthroscopy.* 2003;19:108-110.
28. Selmi TAS. Barnouin L, Bussiere C, Neyret P. Cartipatch. In: Zansi S, Brittberg M, Marcacci M, eds. *Basic Science, Clinical Repair, and Reconstruction of Articular Cartilage Defects: Current Status and Prospects.* Bologna, Italy: Timeo Editore; 2006:431-438.
29. Braun K, Imhoff AB. Arthromatrix (Orthagen/Arthrex). In: Zansi S, Brittberg M, Marcacci M, eds. *Basic Science, Clinical Repair, and Reconstruction of Articular Cartilage Defects: Current Status and Prospects.* Bologna, Italy: Timeo Editore; 2006:403-405.
30. Gaissmaier C, Fritz J, Schewe B, et al. Development of NOVOCART 3D, a novel system for scaffold augmented transplantation of autologous chondrocytes. In: Zansi S, Brittberg M, Marcacci M, eds. *Basic Science, Clinical Repair, and Reconstruction of Articular Cartilage Defects: Current Status and Prospects.* Bologna, Italy: Timeo Editore; 2006:573-585.
31. Libera J, Luethi U, Alasevic OJ. Co.don chondrosphere (Co.don AG) autologous matrix engineered cartilage transplantation. In: Zansi S, Brittberg M, Marcacci M, eds. *Basic Science, Clinical Repair, and Reconstruction of Articular Cartilage Defects: Current Status and Prospects.* Bologna, Italy: Timeo Editore; 2006:591-600.
32. Behrens P, Rogan IM. AMIC, autologous matrix induced chondrogenesis. In: Zansi S, Brittberg M, Marcacci M, eds. *Basic Science, Clinical Repair, and Reconstruction of Articular Cartilage Defects: Current Status and Prospects.* Bologna, Italy: Timeo Editore; 2006:767-770.
33. Cugat R, Carrillo JM, Serra I, Soler C. Articular cartilage defects reconstruction by plasma rich growth factors. In: Zansi S, Brittberg M, Marcacci M, eds. *Basic Science, Clinical Repair, and Reconstruction of Articular Cartilage Defects: Current Status and Prospects.* Bologna, Italy: Timeo Editore; 2006:801-807.
34. Derbies A, Magalia M, Mastrogiacomo M, Cancedda R. Human mesenchymal stem/progenitor cells: isolation, characterization and chondrogenic differentiation. In: Zansi S, Brittberg M, Marcacci M, eds. *Basic Science, Clinical Repair, and Reconstruction of Articular Cartilage Defects: Current Status and Prospects.* Bologna, Italy: Timeo Editore; 2006:773-780.
35. Lee EH, Hui JH. Stem cells in the treatment of partial and full thickness cartilage defects. In: Zansi S, Brittberg M, Marcacci M, eds. *Basic Science, Clinical Repair, and Reconstruction of Articular Cartilage Defects: Current Status and Prospects.* Bologna, Italy: Timeo Editore; 2006:791-798.
36. Wakitani S, Goto T, Young RG, et al. Mesenchymal cell-based repair of large full thickness defects of articular cartilage. *J Bone Joint Surg Am.* 1994;76A:579.
37. Hue JH, Lee EH. Stem cells in the treatment of partial and full thickness cartilage defects. In: Zansi S, Brittberg M, Marcacci M, eds. *Basic Science, Clinical Repair, and Reconstruction of Articular Cartilage Defects: Current Status and Prospects.* Bologna, Italy: Timeo Editore; 2006:791-798.

SUGGESTED READINGS

Chu C, ed. Articular cartilage surgery. *Oper Tech Orthop.* 2006;16:217-292.
Zansi S, Brittberg M, Marcacci M, eds. *Basic Science, Clinical Repair, and Reconstruction of Articular Cartilage Defects: Current Status and Prospects.* Bolgna, Italy: Timeo Editore; 2006.

Tendoscopy

C. Niek van Dijk • Peter A.J. de Leeuw • Maayke N. van Sterkenburg

In the past 3 decades, arthroscopy has become the preferred technique to treat intra-articular ankle pathology. Extra-articular problems of the ankle have traditionally demanded open surgery, which has been associated with some serious complications. The rate of complications reported with open surgery for posterior ankle impingement varies between 15% and 24%, and the incidence of these complications has stimulated the development of extra-articular endoscopic techniques. Endoscopic surgery offers advantages related to any minimally invasive procedure, such as fewer wound infections, less blood loss, smaller wounds, and less morbidity. Surgery is performed on an outpatient basis, and subsequent care focuses on regaining function.

To become familiar with the endoscopic techniques used in foot and ankle surgery, surgeons can train in a cadaveric setting through international courses that are offered annually.[1,2] Tendoscopy can be performed for the diagnosis and treatment of pathologic conditions of the peroneal tendons, the posterior tibial tendon, and the flexor hallucis longus (FHL) tendon. These endoscopic procedures and their indications are discussed in this chapter.

TENDOSCOPY OF THE PERONEAL TENDONS

Peroneal tendon pathology frequently coexists with or results from chronic lateral ankle instability. These disorders often cause chronic ankle pain in runners and ballet dancers.[3] Post-traumatic lateral ankle pain is common, but peroneal tendon pathology is not always recognized as a cause of these symptoms. In a study by Dombek and coworkers, only 60% of peroneal tendon disorders were accurately diagnosed at the first clinical evaluation.[4]

Pathology consists of tenosynovitis, tendon dislocation or subluxation, and (subtotal) rupture or snapping of one or both of the peroneal tendons. It accounts for most symptoms at the posterolateral aspect of the ankle. Other causes of posterolateral ankle pain are rheumatoid synovitis, bony spurs, calcifications or ossicles, pathology of the posterior talofibular ligament (PTFL), or disorders of the posterior compartment of the subtalar joint. Posterior ankle impingement can manifest as posterolateral ankle pain.[5]

The primary indication for treating pathology of the peroneal tendons is pain.[6] If conservative treatment fails, the surgical intervention involves débridement of the tendons, fibular groove deepening in case of recurrent peroneal tendon dislocation, and an adequate and precise determination of the location and extent of tendon ruptures. Van Dijk introduced a tendoscopic approach to treat a wide variety of peroneal tendon disorders, and the subsequent patient follow-up was published in 2006.[7] The tendoscopic technique is safe and produces good or excellent clinical outcomes, making it a good alternative to open surgical approaches.

Anatomy

The peroneal muscles are located in the lateral compartment of the leg, also known as the peroneal compartment. Both muscles are innervated by the superficial peroneal nerve and the peroneal, and medial tarsal arteries supply the muscles with blood through separate vinculae.[8,9] The peroneus brevis tendon is situated dorsomedial to the peroneus longus tendon from its proximal aspect up to the fibular tip, where it is relatively flat. Just distal to this lateral malleolus tip, the peroneus brevis tendon becomes rounder and crosses the round peroneus longus tendon. The distal posterolateral part of the fibula forms a sliding channel for the two peroneal tendons. This malleolar groove is formed by a periosteal cushion of fibrocartilage that covers the bony groove.[10] Posterolaterally, the tendons are held into position by the superior peroneal retinaculum.[7,11]

The peroneal tendons act as lateral ankle stabilizers. In chronic ankle instability, more strain is put on these tendons, resulting in hypertrophic tendinopathy, tenosynovitis, and ultimately in tendon tears.[7]

In 1803, Monteggia was the first to describe peroneal tendon dislocation in a female ballet dancer.[12] These tendons dislocate if the superior peroneal retinaculum ruptures, frequently because of an inversion or dorsiflexion trauma of the foot with the muscles contracted, or if it is congenitally absent or weak.[11] A non-concave fibular groove predisposes to dislocation. The cartilaginous rim, located laterally from the fibular groove, adds to the overall depth of the groove.[13] If this rim is absent or flat, the tendons are more likely to dislocate.[14]

Patient Evaluation

History and Physical Examination

Tendinopathy of the peroneal tendons often coexists with a lateral ankle sprain, and the diagnosis of peroneal tendon pathology in a patient with lateral ankle pain can be difficult.[15] The anterior drawer test and varus stress test are applied routinely to detect laxity of the ankle ligaments. In acute cases, the detailed history should include reconstruction of the trauma mechanism. The presence of associated conditions such as rheumatoid arthritis, psoriasis, hyperparathyroidism, diabetic neuropathy, calcaneal fracture, fluoroquinolone use, and local steroid injections is important, because they can increase the degree of peroneal tendon dysfunction.[16] The differential diagnosis includes fatigue fractures or fractures of the fibula, posterior impingement of the ankle, and lesions of the lateral ligament complex. Post-traumatic or postoperative adhesions and irregularities of the posterior aspect of the fibula (i.e., peroneal groove) also can be responsible for symptoms in this region.

Patients with tendinopathy have crepitus and recognizable tenderness over the tendons on palpation. Swelling, tendon dislocation, and signs of tenosynovitis can be found at the lateral aspect of the posterior ankle.

Patients with peroneal tendon dislocation typically complain of lateral instability, giving way, and sometimes a popping or snapping sensation over the lateral aspect of their ankle. On physical examination, the tendons can be subluxated by active dorsiflexion and eversion, which provokes the pain.[17]

Diagnostic Imaging

If the Ottowa ankle rules do not indicate abnormalities, applying diagnostics in the acute phase after an inversion trauma should be questioned. However, when peroneal tendon pathology is suspected, additional diagnostics should be applied, and when posterolateral ankle pain persists after the initial trauma, diagnostic imaging should be considered. Routine weight-bearing radiographs in the anteroposterior and lateral directions are advised in these cases to rule out avulsion fractures, spurs, calcifications, or ossicles.

Peroneal tendon dislocation is a clinical diagnosis, and it is frequently accompanied by a tendon rupture. Additional investigations such as magnetic resonance imaging (MRI) and ultrasonography may be helpful in diagnosing partial tears of the tendon of peroneus brevis or longus.[18] Both modalities are considerably accurate and precise, although ultrasonography is more cost effective.[19]

Treatment

Conservative Management

Conservative management should be attempted first. This includes activity modification, footwear changes, temporary immobiliza-

tion, and corticosteroid injections. Lateral heel wedges can take the strain off the peroneal tendons, which may allow healing.[16]

Surgical Technique

The patient is placed in the lateral decubitus position. Alternatively, the patient can be placed in the supine position with the foot in endorotation. A support can be placed under the leg, allowing the ankle to be moved freely. Before anesthesia is administered, the patient is asked to evert the foot so that the peroneal tendons can be visualized clearly. Their course is drawn on the skin, and the locations of the portals are marked (Fig. 16-1). The surgery can be performed under local, regional, epidural, or general anesthesia. After exsanguination, a tourniquet is inflated around the thigh of the affected leg.

A distal portal is made 2 to 2.5 cm distal to the posterior edge of the lateral malleolus. An incision is made through the skin, and the tendon sheath is penetrated with an arthroscopic shaft with a blunt trocar. A 2.7-mm, 30-degree arthroscope is then introduced.

The inspection starts approximately 6 cm proximal to the posterior tip of the fibula, where a thin membrane splits the tendon compartment into two separate tendon chambers. More distally, the tendons lie in one compartment. A second portal is made 2 to 2.5 cm proximal to the posterior edge of the lateral malleolus under direct vision by placing a spinal needle directly over the tendons (Fig. 16-2). Through the distal portal, a complete overview of both tendons can be obtained.

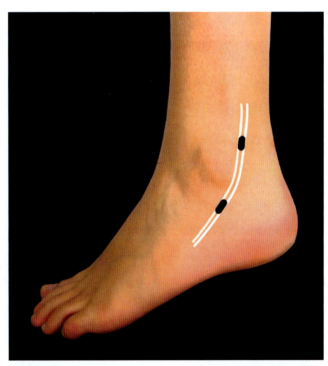

FIGURE 16-1 The patient is placed in the lateral decubitus position. Alternatively, the patient can be placed in the supine position with the foot in endorotation. A support can be placed under the leg, allowing the ankle to move freely. The patient is asked to evert the foot, which usually allows the peroneal tendons to be visualized clearly. Its course is drawn on the skin *(white line),* and the location of the portals is marked *(black areas).*

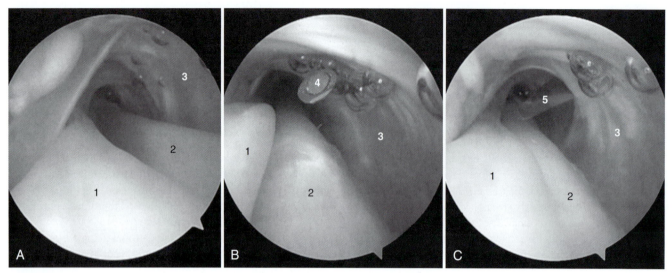

FIGURE 16-2 A, Peroneal tendoscopic image shows a left ankle with the arthroscope in the distal portal, and both tendons are clearly visualized. Peroneus longus tendon (1), peroneus brevis tendon (2), tendon sheath (3). **B,** Peroneus longus tendon (1), peroneus brevis tendon (2), tendon sheath (3), the location of the proximal portal is determined under direct vision with a spinal needle (4). **C,** Peroneus longus tendon (1), peroneus brevis tendon (2), tendon sheath (3), the definite portal is created with a retrograde knife directly over the tendons (5).

By rotating the arthroscope over and between both tendons, the entire compartment can be inspected (Fig. 16-3). When a total synovectomy of the tendon sheath has to be performed, it is advisable to make a third portal more distal or more proximal than the portals described previously. When a rupture of one of the tendons is seen, endoscopic synovectomy is performed, and the rupture is repaired through a mini-open approach.

In patients with recurrent dislocation of the peroneal tendon, endoscopic fibular groove deepening can be performed through this tendoscopic approach. It is a time-consuming procedure because of the limited working area. Groove deepening is performed from within the tendon sheath, with the risk of iatrogenic damage to the tendons. We therefore prefer an approach based on the two-portal hindfoot technique, with an additional portal located 4 cm proximal to the posterolateral portal.[20]

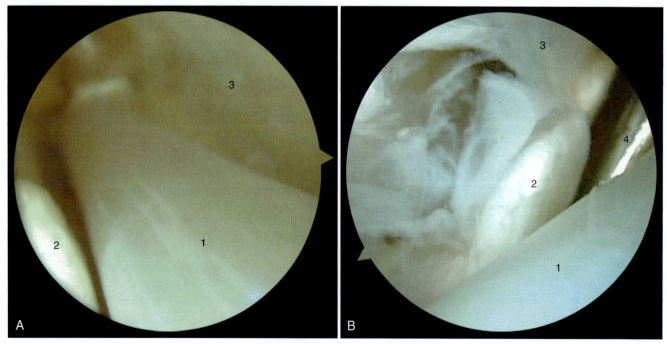

FIGURE 16-3 A 28-year-old woman with persistent pain over the peroneal tendons behind the lateral malleolus of the left ankle did not respond to conservative treatment. Magnetic resonance imaging did not show a partial-length rupture of the tendons. Excessive fluid was present in the tendon sheath. Immunohistopathologic examination of the loose body showed giant cell proliferation. **A,** The tendoscopic image shows the peroneal tendon. Inside the tendon sheath, a calcified deposit recognized (1, peroneal tendon; 2, semi-loose body; 3, tendon sheath). **B,** By changing the visualization angle, the loose body is more clearly visualized. It has partially been detached from the tendon sheath (1, peroneal tendon; 2, semi-loose body; 3, tendon sheath; 4, probe).

At the end of the procedure, the portals are sutured to prevent sinus formation, and a compressive dressing is applied. Antibiotics are not routinely given.

Postoperative Rehabilitation Protocol

Postoperative management consists of a pressure bandage and partial weight bearing for 2 to 3 days. Full weight bearing is allowed as tolerated, and active range-of-motion exercises should be started immediately after surgery.

TENDOSCOPY OF THE POSTERIOR TIBIAL TENDON

In the absence of intra-articular ankle pathology, posteromedial ankle pain is most often caused by disorders of the posterior tibial tendon. Incompetence of the posterior tibial tendon due to an inflammatory process or partial- or full-thickness tearing gives rise to midtarsal instability and is the most common cause of adult-onset flatfoot deformity. The relative strength of this tendon is more than twice that of its primary antagonist, the peroneus brevis tendon. Without the activity of the posterior tibial tendon, there is no stability at the midtarsal joint, and the forward propulsive force of the gastrocnemius-soleus complex acts at the midfoot instead of at the metatarsal heads. Total dysfunction eventually leads to a flatfoot deformity.

These disorders can be divided in two groups: the younger group of patients, who had dysfunction of the tendon caused by some form of systemic inflammatory disease (e.g., rheumatoid arthritis), and an older group of patients, whose tendon dysfunction is mostly caused by chronic overuse.[21] After trauma, surgery, and fractures, adhesions and irregularity of the posterior aspect of the tibia can be responsible for symptoms in this region.

A dysfunctional posterior tibial tendon usually evolves to painful tenosynovitis. Tenosynovitis is also a common extra-articular manifestation of rheumatoid arthritis, in which hindfoot problems are a significant cause of disability. Tenosynovitis in rheumatoid patients eventually leads to a ruptured tendon.[22]

The precise cause is unknown. The condition is classified on the basis of clinical and radiographic findings.

Anatomy

The posterior tibial muscle arises from the interosseous membrane and the proximal adjacent surfaces of the tibia and fibula, and it is part of the deep posterior compartment of the calf. The tendon forms in the distal third of the calf and passes behind the medial malleolus, where it changes direction.[23] The posterior tibial tendon is the most superficial structure coursing directly behind the medial malleolus.

Pain complaints are often localized in the relative hypovascular zone immediately distal to the medial malleolus, beginning 4 cm proximal to the insertion of the tendon.[24] This hypovascular zone may contribute to the development of degenerative changes and consequently to ruptures.[25]

The posterior tibial tendon is held in the retromalleolar groove by a strong fibro-osseous tunnel and the flexor retinaculum originating from the tip of the medial malleolus and inserting into the calcaneus. Distally, the retinaculum blends with the sheath of the tendon and the superficial deltoid ligament.[23] The anterior, major slip of the tendon inserts primarily into the tuberosity of the navicular, the inferior capsule of the medial naviculocuneiform joint, and the inferior surface of the medial cuneiform. A second slip extends to the plantar surfaces of the cuneiforms and the bases of the second, third, and fourth metatarsals.[23]

A tendon sheath surrounds the posterior tibial tendon, and both structures are connected by a vincula, which carries part of the blood supply to the tendon. A vincula can become symptomatic when damaged, causing thickening, shortening, and scarring of the distal free edge. In these patients, a painful local thickening can be palpated posterior and just proximal to the tip of the medial malleolus.[25]

Coursing laterally through the tarsal tunnel, the flexor digitorum longus and FHL tendons can be found. Between the flexor digitorum longus and FHL tendons are the posterior tibial nerve, artery, and veins.

Patient Evaluation

History and Physical Examination

In the early stage of dysfunction, patients complain of persistent ankle pain medially along the course of the tendon, fatigue, and aching on the medial plantar aspect of the ankle. Tenosynovitis commonly is associated with swelling.[23,25] A typical observation is abnormal wear of the medial sides of the shoes. Walking increases pain, and participation in sports activities becomes difficult.

Careful clinical examination is important, and both feet should be examined. Valgus angulation of the hindfoot is frequently seen with accompanying abduction of the forefoot (i.e., too many toes sign).[23] The sign is positive when inspecting the patient's foot from behind; in the case of significant forefoot abduction, three or more toes are visible lateral to the calcaneus, whereas normally, only one or two toes are seen. With the patient seated, the strength of the tendon and location of pain

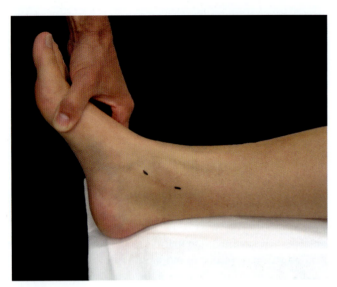

FIGURE 16-4 Before anesthesia is administered, the patient is asked to actively invert the affected foot so the tendon can be palpated. Its location is drawn onto the skin for preparing the location of the portals.

are evaluated by asking the patient to invert the foot against resistance (Fig. 16-4).

Intra-articular lesions such as a posteromedial impingement syndrome, subtalar pathology, calcifications in the dorsal capsule of the ankle joint, loose bodies, or osteochondral defects should be excluded. Entrapment of the posterior tibial nerve in the tarsal canal is commonly known as a tarsal tunnel syndrome. Clinical examination is normally sufficient to adequately differentiate these disorders from an isolated posterior tibial tendon disorder.

Diagnostic Imaging

After initial history taking and physical examination, the diagnosis can be confirmed or rejected using radiography. Conventional radiographs may show abnormal alignment such as flattening of the plantar arch or bony changes such as irregularity and hypertrophic change at the navicular attachment, providing an important clue to long-standing problems with the posterior tibial tendon.[26] However, pathology of this soft tissue structure is easier to identify using ultrasound or MRI. Ultrasound imaging is a cost-effective and accurate method for evaluating disorders of the posterior tibial tendon.[27] Thickening of the tendon or peritendinous soft tissue, hypoechoic texture, ill-definition of the fibrillar pattern, associated hypervascularity on color Doppler, thinning, splitting, and rupture may be useful clues.[26] In our practice, MRI is the method of choice because the images can be interpreted by the orthopedist, in contrast to ultrasound images, and it is therefore more helpful for preoperative planning. It is also considered the gold standard for assessing tibialis posterior dysfunction and related soft tissue injuries.[26] A major advantage is the ability to detect bony edema. Findings may include fluid or synovitis around the tendon, hypertrophy of the tendon, intrasubstance tears showing increased signal intensity, longitudinal tears, and complete tendon tears.[26]

Treatment

Conservative Management

Initially, conservative management is indicated, with rest combined with nonsteroidal anti-inflammatory drugs (NSAIDs), immobilization using a plaster cast or tape, or orthotic shoe modifications. There is no consensus about whether to use corticosteroid injections, and cases of tendon rupture after corticosteroid injections have been described.[28]

Surgery is indicated if conservative management for 3 to 6 months does not resolve the complaints.[29] It can be performed by an open or endoscopic procedure. An open synovectomy is performed by sharp dissection of the inflamed synovium while preserving the blood supply to the tendon. Postoperative management consists of plaster cast immobilization for 3 weeks, with the possible disadvantage of formation of new adhesions, followed by wearing a functional brace with controlled ankle movement for another 3 weeks and physical therapy.

Endoscopic synovectomy is indicated when access allows radical removal of inflamed synovium.[30] Several published studies have described successful endoscopic synovectomy and the advantages related to minimally invasive surgery.[9,31,32]

Surgical Technique

The procedure can be performed on an outpatient basis under local, regional, or general anesthesia. The patient is placed in the supine position. A tourniquet is placed around the upper leg. Before anesthesia, the patient is asked to actively invert the foot, so that the posterior tibial tendon can be palpated and the portals can be marked. Access to the tendon can be obtained anywhere along its course.

We prefer to make the two main portals directly over the tendon: 2 to 3 cm distal and 2 to 3 cm proximal to the posterior edge of the medial malleolus (Fig. 16-5). The distal portal is

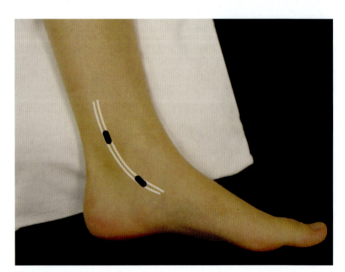

FIGURE 16-5 The patient is in the supine position. The two main portals (black areas) are made directly over the posterior tibial tendon (white lines) 2 to 3 cm distal and 2 to 3 cm proximal to the posterior edge of the medial malleolus.

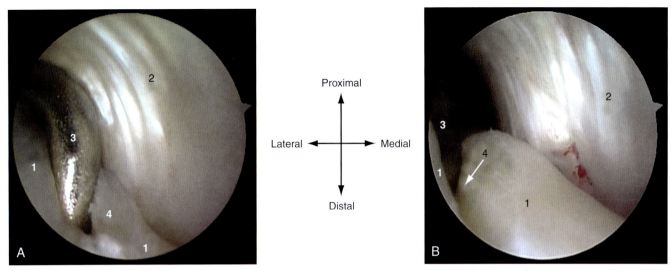

FIGURE 16-6 A 48-year-old woman had persistent pain over the posterior tibial tendon of the left foot. She sustained direct trauma to the posterior tibial tendon 1 year earlier. Physical examination revealed a normal range of motion, no signs of tendon insufficiency, but pain and swelling over the posterior tibial tendon just behind the medial malleolus. **A,** The tendoscopic image shows the arthroscope in the anterolateral portal looking proximally (1, posterior tibial tendon; 2, tendon sheath; 3, arthroscopic probe; 4, tear in posterior tibial tendon). **B,** The image shows a partial-length rupture (4) of the posterior tibial tendon (1). Repair of the rupture was performed through a mini-open repair (2, tendon sheath; 3, arthroscopic probe). •

made first; the incision is made through the skin, and the tendon sheath is penetrated by the arthroscopic shaft with a blunt trocar. A 2.7-mm, 30-degree arthroscope is introduced, and the tendon sheath is filled with saline. Irrigation is performed using gravity flow.

Under direct vision, the proximal portal is made by introducing a spinal needle, and an incision is made into the tendon sheath. Instruments such as a retrograde knife, a shaver system, blunt probes, and scissors can be used. For synovectomy in patients with rheumatoid arthritis, a 3.5-mm shaver can be used. The complete tendon sheath can be inspected by rotating the arthroscope around the tendon. Synovectomy can be performed with a complete overview of the tendon from the distal portal over the insertion of the navicular bone to approximately 6 cm above the tip of the medial malleolus.

While inspecting the tendon sheath, special attention should be given to the posterior aspect of the medial malleolar surface and the posterior ankle joint capsule. The tendon sheath between the posterior tibial tendon and the flexor digitorum longus is relatively thin, and inspection of the correct tendon should always be checked. This can be accomplished by passively flexing and extending the toes; if the tendon sheath of the flexor digitorum longus tendon is entered, the tendon will move up and down.

When remaining in the posterior tibial tendon sheath, the neurovascular bundle is not in danger. When a rupture of the posterior tibial tendon is seen, endoscopic synovectomy is performed (Fig. 16-6) ,and the rupture is repaired through a mini-open approach. Magnifying the tendon endoscopically enhances localization and extent of the rupture, and it minimizes the incision required for repair. At the end of the procedure, the portals are sutured to prevent sinus formation.

PEARLS & PITFALLS

PEARLS

- It is important to identify the location of the posterior tibial tendon before creating the portals. After asking the patient to actively invert the foot, identify the tendon, and mark the location of the portals on the skin.
- When the tendon sheath of the flexor digitorum longus is entered, you can see tendons move up and down when you passively flex and extend the toes.

PITFALLS

- The tendon sheath between the posterior tibial tendon and the flexor digitorum longus is quite thin. Always ensure that you are inspecting the correct tendon.
- Remaining in the tendon sheath of the posterior tibial tendon keeps the neurovascular bundle out of danger.
- Surgeons not familiar with endoscopic surgery are advised to train themselves in a cadaveric setting.[1,2]

Postoperative Rehabilitation Protocol

Postoperative management consists of a pressure bandage and partial weight bearing for 2 to 3 days. Active range-of-motion exercises are encouraged from the first day.

ENDOSCOPIC FLEXOR HALLUCIS LONGUS RELEASE

FHL tenosynovitis is a well-recognized cause of posteromedial ankle pain. In ballet dancers, this entity has been described as *dancer's tendinitis.*[33] Athletes performing repetitive forceful push-offs are at risk for developing FHL tendinitis.[34]

FHL tendinitis and posterior ankle impingement based on the os trigonum syndrome are distinct entities, but they frequently coexist because of their close anatomic orientation.[5,35,36] If conservative management fails, surgical intervention involves removal of the os trigonum, tendon débridement, and a release of the flexor retinaculum and tendon sheath at the level of the posterior talar process. In 2000, van Dijk introduced a two-portal endoscopic hindfoot approach that provided excellent access to the posterior aspect of the ankle and subtalar joint.[37,38] Extra-articular structures of the hindfoot, such as the os trigonum and FHL tendon, can be assessed.[38] This minimally invasive technique has been anatomically and clinically demonstrated to be safe and reliable, and it compares favorably with open surgery in terms of less morbidity and a quicker recovery.[39-42]

Anatomy

The FHL is the most laterally located bipennate muscle of the human calf. At the level of the ankle and subtalar joint complex, the FHL tendon runs distally in a fibro-osseous gliding channel located between the posteromedial and lateral talar processes. At this level, the tendon is kept in place by the flexor retinaculum. The FHL tendon passes distally and medially underneath the sustentaculum tali to eventually insert in the distal phalanx of the hallux.[43]

Isolated FHL tendon pathology is almost exclusively located behind the medial malleolus at the level of the fibro-osseous tunnel.[10,35,36,44] Hypertrophy, a nodule, or a low-riding muscle belly can cause the musculotendinous junction to be pulled inside the narrow tunnel, producing stenosing tenosynovitis, also referred to as triggering of the great toe or hallux saltans.[45] Maximal tendon tension (i.e., hyper-dorsiflexion of the ankle and great toe) can cause tendinopathy of the FHL. Tendon degeneration and ruptures most frequently occur in the region of this fibro-osseous tunnel. This can be explained by the relative incongruity between the FHL and its tunnel in a fully plantar-flexed or dorsiflexed position.[35] Another hypothesis is an avascular zone at this level of the tendon, as described by Petersen and colleagues.[46]

Posterior ankle impingement, caused by a soft tissue or bony impediment, is frequently associated with FHL tenosynovitis at the level of the fibro-osseous tunnel. Displacement of an os trigonum, a Cedell fracture, and a hypertrophic posterior talar process are examples of posterior bony ankle impingement that can cause associated tenosynovitis. Scar tissue around the tendon can provide local irritation. Posteromedially located talar osteochondral defects have been mentioned as a cause of FHL tendinopathy.[47] During the stance phase of walking, the ankle joint is in dorsiflexion, and the talar dome is in closest contact with the FHL tendon. In the push-off phase, the toes are actively flexed, moving the tendon in an opposite direction compared with the talar movement. The tendon shreds against the osteochondral defect and becomes irritated and inflamed.

Patient Evaluation

History and Physical Examination

Patients typically complain of pain located at the posteromedial aspect of the ankle that worsens with ankle motion and hallux dorsiflexion and that diminishes at rest. The tendon can be palpated behind the medial malleolus at the level of the subtalar joint. Asking the patient to repetitively flex the big toe with the

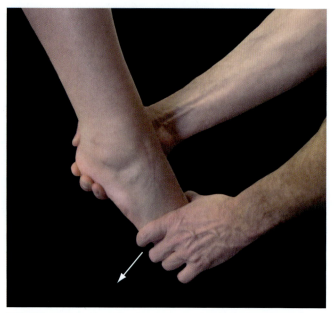

FIGURE 16-7 The forced hyper-plantar flexion test is performed with the patient sitting with the knee flexed in 90 degrees. The test is performed with repetitive, quick, passive hyper-plantar flexion movements. The test can be repeated in slight external rotation or slight internal rotation of the foot relative to the tibia. The investigator can apply this rotational movement on the point of maximal plantar flexion *(arrow)*, thereby "grinding" the (enlarged) posterior talar process or os trigonum in between tibia and calcaneus.

ankle in 10 to 20 degrees of plantar flexion increases the ability to palpate the tendon in its gliding channel. This maneuver also differentiates the FHL from posterior tibial tendon pathology. The FHL tendon glides up and down under the palpating finger of the examiner. In the case of stenosing tendinitis or chronic inflammation, crepitus and recognizable tenderness can be provoked. In some patients, a nodule can be palpated moving up and down with active movement of the great toe.

In patients with associated posterolateral ankle pain, a posterior impingement syndrome must be ruled out by means of a hyper-plantar flexion test (Fig. 16-7). The forced passive hyper-plantar flexion test result is positive when the patient experiences recognizable posterior ankle pain. A negative test result rules out a posterior ankle impingement syndrome. A positive test result is followed by a diagnostic infiltration of lidocaine in the posterior ankle compartment. Disappearance of pain after infiltration confirms the diagnosis.

Diagnostic Imaging

After performing a thorough history and physical examination, the diagnosis can be confirmed or rejected by the use of available imaging techniques. If the history and physical examination do not reveal abnormalities, additional diagnostics can be used to search for or to rule out pathology (i.e., for medicolegal reasons). Close consultation between the orthopedic surgeon and the radiologist is necessary to decide on optimal radiographic diagnostics.[48]

In patients without a history of trauma but with isolated, recognizable posteromedial ankle pain during flexion of the great toe while palpating the tendon at the level of the gliding channel,

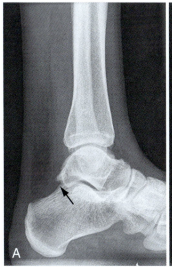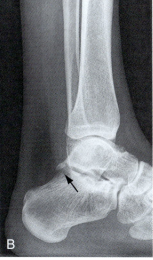

FIGURE 16-8 A 27-year-old man presented with posterior left ankle pain during plantar-flexed movements of the foot. The hyper-plantar flexion test result was positive. **A,** The standard lateral radiograph shows a possible prominent posterior talar process *(arrow)*. **B,** The lateral radiograph with the foot in 25 degrees exorotation allows an os trigonum to be more easily recognized *(arrow)*.

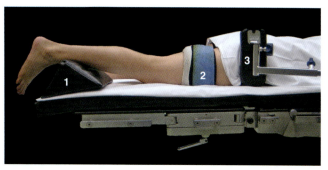

FIGURE 16-9 For posterior ankle arthroscopy, the patient is placed in a prone position. A tourniquet is applied around the upper leg (2), and a small support is placed under the lower leg (1), making it possible to move the ankle freely. A support is placed at the ipsilateral side of the pelvis to safely rotate the operating table slightly when needed (3).

no additional diagnostic tests are needed. If conservative treatment options fail, intervention demands a release regardless of the pathology. MRI can be valuable to rule out tendon ruptures.

For patients with posteromedial ankle pain associated with a positive hyper-planter flexion test result, standard weight-bearing radiographs must be obtained with anteroposterior and lateral views. If differentiation of hypertrophy of the posterior talar process from an os trigonum is difficult, a lateral hindfoot radiograph with the foot in 25 degrees of exorotation in relation to the standard lateral ankle is advised (Fig. 16-8).[49] For ballet dancers, a lateral radiograph with the foot in maximal plantar flexion can be useful to determine whether a bony posterior ankle impingement is present. In post-traumatic cases, spiral computed tomography (CT) can help to ascertain the extent of the injury or location of the osteochondral defect and the exact location of calcifications or fragments.

Treatment

Conservative Management

Nonoperative treatment options include rest, activity modification, ice therapy, NSAIDs, and physical therapy, such as stretching exercises.[35,36] Infiltration of a corticosteroid around the tendon at the level of the tunnel can be performed as a next step. Avoid iatrogenic neurovascular bundle and tendon lesions.

Conservative treatment options often do not completely resolve the complaints. An active professional ballet dancer with a competitive attitude is not likely to remain inactive for several months, and in these cases, release of the tendon and resection of the posteriorly located bony or soft tissue impediment is indicted.

Posterior Ankle Arthroscopy

The procedure is carried out as outpatient surgery under general anesthesia or spinal anesthesia. The patient is placed in a prone position. The involved leg is marked with an arrow to avoid surgery on the wrong side. A tourniquet is inflated around the thigh for hemostasis. A small support is placed under the lower leg, making it possible to move the ankle freely (Fig. 16-9). We use a soft tissue distraction device when indicated.[50]

Normal saline or lactated Ringer's solution is used. A 4.0-mm arthroscope with an inclination angle of 30 degrees is routinely used for posterior ankle arthroscopy.

The anatomic landmarks on the ankle are the lateral malleolus, medial and lateral border of the Achilles tendon, and the foot's sole. The ankle is kept in a neutral, 90-degree position. An endoscopic probe can be used to determine the exact location of the posterolateral portal. The hook is secured under the tip of the lateral malleolus. The hook is placed parallel to the foot's sole (with the foot in a 90-degree position). A straight line is drawn from the tip of the lateral malleolus to the Achilles tendon, parallel to the sole.

The posterolateral portal is made just above the line from the tip of the lateral malleolus and 1 cm anterior to the Achilles tendon (Fig. 16-10). After making a vertical stab incision, the subcutaneous layer is split by a mosquito clamp. The mosquito clamp is directed anteriorly, pointing toward the interdigital web space between the first and second toes. When the tip of the clamp touches the bone, it is exchanged for a 4.5-mm arthroscopic shaft, with the blunt trocar pointing in the same direction. By palpating the bone in the sagittal plane, the level of the ankle joint and subtalar joint can often be distinguished, because the prominent posterior talar process or os trigonum can be felt as a posterior prominence in between the two joints. The trocar is situated extra-articularly at the level of the ankle joint. The trocar is exchanged for the 4-mm arthroscope with the direction of view 30 degrees to the lateral side.

The posteromedial portal is made at the same level, just above the line of the tip of the lateral malleolus but just anterior to the medial aspect of the Achilles tendon (Fig. 16-11). After making a vertical stab incision, a mosquito clamp is introduced and directed toward the arthroscope shaft in a 90-degree angle. When the mosquito clamp touches the shaft of the arthroscope, the shaft is used as a guide to "travel" anteriorly in the direction of the ankle joint, all the way down while contacting the arthroscope shaft until it reaches the bone. The arthroscope is pulled slightly backward, sliding over the mosquito clamp until the tip of the mosquito clamp comes into view. The clamp is used to

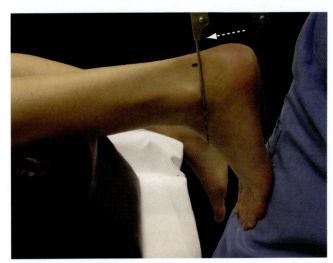

FIGURE 16-10 For marking the anatomic landmarks that are needed for portal placement, the ankle is kept in a neutral, 90-degree position. An endoscopic probe can be used to determine the exact location of the posterolateral portal. The hook is secured under the tip of the lateral malleolus. The hook is placed parallel to the foot sole, with the foot in a 90-degree position. A straight line is drawn from the tip of the lateral malleolus to the Achilles tendon, parallel to the foot's sole. The posterolateral portal *(arrow)* is made just above the line from the tip of the lateral malleolus and 1 cm anterior to the Achilles tendon.

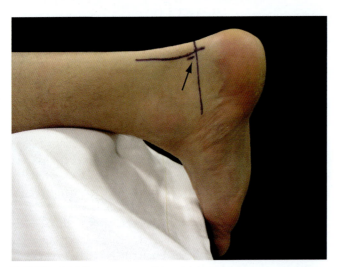

FIGURE 16-11 The posteromedial portal *(arrow)* is located at the same level as the posterolateral portal and just anterior to the Achilles tendon. An imaginary line can be drawn from the level of the posterolateral portal over the Achilles tendon to determine the location of the posteromedial portal.

spread the extra-articular soft tissue in front of the tip of the lens. When scar tissue or adhesions are present, the mosquito clamp is exchanged for a 5-mm bone-cutter shaver. The tip of the shaver is directed in a lateral and slightly plantar direction toward the lateral aspect of the subtalar joint.

The joint capsule and fatty tissue overlying the posterolateral aspect of the subtalar joint are removed, and the posterior compartment of the subtalar joint is inspected. At the level of the ankle joint, the posterolateral talar prominence and the PTFL are recognized. Just proximal to the PTFL, the intermalleolar liga-

ment, or tibial slip, is recognized, and more proximal and deeper, the tibiofibular ligament can be assessed. The cranial part of the posterior talar process is freed from scar tissue, and the medial side the FHL tendon is identified.

Removal of a symptomatic os trigonum, a fracture nonunion of the posterior talar process, or a symptomatic, large, posterior talar prominence involves partial detachment of the PTFL, detachment of the talocalcaneal ligament, and a release of the flexor retinaculum. All of these structures attach to the posterior talar prominence or os trigonum. After releasing these structures, the os trigonum can be detached with a chisel or small osteotome and removed with a grasper.

In the case of isolated tendinitis of the FHL tendon, the flexor retinaculum can be released by detaching it from the posterior talar process or os trigonum with an arthroscopic punch. Subsequently, the tendon sheath can be opened distally up to the level of the sustentaculum tali. The tendon sheath can be entered with the scope, allowing accurate tendon inspection and, if necessary, a further release can be performed (Fig. 16-12). Partial-thickness longitudinal tears are débrided. The proximal part of the tendon and the distal part of the muscle belly are inspected and débrided if inflamed, thickened, or if nodules are present. Adhesions and excessive scar tissue are removed.

By applying manual distraction to the calcaneus, the posterior compartment of the ankle opens up, and instruments can be introduced. We prefer to apply a soft tissue distractor at this point.[50] When indicated, a synovectomy or capsulectomy, or both, can be performed. The talar dome can be inspected over almost its entire surface along with the complete tibial plafond. Osteochondral defects can be débrided, and drilling or microfracture can be performed.

Bleeding is controlled by electrocautery at the end of the procedure. To prevent sinus formation, the skin incisions are closed with 3-0 nylon suture. The incisions and surrounding skin are injected with 10 mL of a 0.5 % bupivacaine/morphine solution. A sterile compressive dressing is applied. Prophylactic antibiotics are not routinely given.

PEARLS & PITFALLS

PEARLS

- Create the posterolateral portal just proximal and lateral to the imaginary intersection of the horizontal line that is perpendicular to the foot's sole, from the tip of the lateral malleolus to the Achilles tendon with the ankle in the neutral position.
- The posteromedial portal is located at the same level as the posterolateral portal, just medial to the Achilles tendon.
- Use the arthroscopic shaft, which is inserted through the posterolateral portal and directed toward the interdigital web space between the first and second toe, as a guide to travel anteriorly, with the instruments inserted through the posteromedial portal.
- Use an arthroscopic punch to detach the flexor retinaculum from the posterior talar process and to release the tendon sheath in case of tendinopathy of the FHL.
- Sufficiently release the tendon sheath all the way down to the sustentaculum tali in the case of isolated tendinopathy of the FHL.

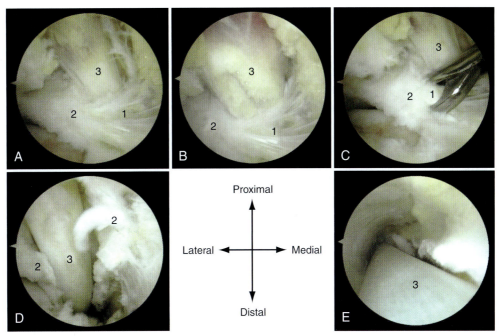

FIGURE 16-12 A 23-year-old, female ballet dancer presented with posteromedial left ankle pain that occurred during plié and relevé. On active flexion of the great toe, palpation just behind the medial malleolus over the flexor hallucis longus tendon elicited tenderness. A painful nodule could be palpated to move up and down at the level of the flexor retinaculum. Magnetic resonance imaging confirmed flexor hallucis longus tendinitis with local swelling of and fluid around the tendon. **A,** Endoscopic image displays stenosing flexor hallucis longus tenosynovitis (3). The flexor hallucis longus tendon is located just medial to the posterolateral talar process (1) and is fixed by the flexor retinaculum (2) between the posteromedial and posterolateral talar processes. **B,** By passive maximal dorsiflexion of the great toe, the muscle belly becomes entrapped behind inside the retinaculum in the tunnel. **C,** The flexor retinaculum is released by means of a punch. **D,** The endoscopic image shows complete release of the flexor hallucis longus tendon. **E,** It is possible to enter the tendon sheath distally with the arthroscope to inspect the tendon up to the level of the sustentaculum tali. Further release of the tendon sheath up to this level can be performed, when indicated.

PITFALLS
- The crural fascia (i.e., ligament of Rouvière) can be quite thick.. This ligament must be partially excised or sectioned using an arthroscopic punch or scissors to reach the level of the subtalar joint or ankle joint.
- Stay lateral from the FHL tendon to prevent damage to the neurovascular bundle.
- Be cautious while removing a hypertrophic posterior talar process with a chisel.
- Remove only the inferoposterior part, and remove the remnant with the bone cutter shaver to prevent removing too much bone at the level of the subtalar joint.
- Surgeons not familiar with endoscopic surgery are advised to train themselves in a cadaveric setting.[1,2]

Postoperative Rehabilitation Protocol

The patient can be discharged the same day of surgery, and weight bearing is allowed as tolerated. The patient is instructed to elevate the foot when not walking to prevent edema. The dressing is removed 3 days postoperatively, after which the patient is permitted to shower. Performing active range-of-motion exercises for at least three times each day for 10 minutes each is encouraged. Patients with limited range of motion are directed to a physiotherapist.

REFERENCES
1. Arthroscopy Association of North America. Master courses: foot/ankle. Available at http://www.aana.org/cme/MastersCourses/descriptions.aspx# Foot/Ankle (accessed November 2009).
2. Amsterdam Foot & Ankle Platform. Available at http://www.ankleplatform.com/page.php?id=854 (accessed November 2009).
3. Bassett FH III, Speer KP. Longitudinal rupture of the peroneal tendons. *Am J Sports Med.* 1993;21:354-357.
4. Dombek MF, Lamm BM, Saltrick K, et al. Peroneal tendon tears: a retrospective review. *J Foot Ankle Surg.* 2003;42:250-258.
5. van Dijk CN. Hindfoot endoscopy for posterior ankle pain. *Instr Course Lect.* 2006;55:545-554.
6. Selmani E, Gjata V, Gjika E. Current concepts review: peroneal tendon disorders. *Foot Ankle Int.* 2006;27:221-228.
7. Scholten PE, van Dijk CN. Tendoscopy of the peroneal tendons. *Foot Ankle Clin.* 2006;11:415-420, vii.
8. Sobel M, Geppert MJ, Hannafin JA, et al. Microvascular anatomy of the peroneal tendons. *Foot Ankle.* 1992;13:469-472.
9. van Dijk CN, Kort N. Tendoscopy of the peroneal tendons. *Arthroscopy.* 1998;14:471-478.
10. Benjamin M, Qin S, Ralphs JR. Fibrocartilage associated with human tendons and their pulleys. *J Anat.* 1995;187(Pt 3):625-633.
11. Kumai T, Benjamin M. The histological structure of the malleolar groove of the fibula in man: its direct bearing on the displacement of peroneal tendons and their surgical repair. *J Anat.* 2003;203:257-262.
12. Monteggi GB. *Instituzini Chirurgiche.* Part III. Milan, Italy: xxxx; 1803:336-341.
13. Edwards ME. The relations of the peroneal tendons to the fibula, calcaneus and cuboideum. *Am J Anat.* 1928;42:213-253.
14. Eckert WR, Davis EA Jr. Acute rupture of the peroneal retinaculum. *J Bone Joint Surg Am.* 1976;58:670-672.

15. Molloy R, Tisdel C. Failed treatment of peroneal tendon injuries. *Foot Ankle Clin*. 2003;8:115-129, ix.
16. Heckman DS, Reddy S, Pedowitz D, et al. Operative treatment for peroneal tendon disorders. *J Bone Joint Surg Am*. 2008;90:404-418.
17. Safran MR, O'Malley D Jr, Fu FH. Peroneal tendon subluxation in athletes: new exam technique, case reports, and review. *Med Sci Sports Exerc*. 1999;31:S487-S492.
18. Rosenberg ZS, Bencardino J, Astion D, et al. MRI features of chronic injuries of the superior peroneal retinaculum. *AJR Am J Roentgenol*. 2003;181:1551-1557.
19. Rockett MS, Waitches G, Sudakoff G, Brage M. Use of ultrasonography versus magnetic resonance imaging for tendon abnormalities around the ankle. *Foot Ankle Int*. 1998;19:604-612.
20. de Leeuw PAJ, Golano P, van Dijk CN. A 3-portal endoscopic groove deepening technique for recurrent peroneal tendon dislocation. *Tech Foot Ankle Surg*. 2008;7:250-256.
21. Myerson MS. Adult acquired flatfoot deformity: treatment of dysfunction of the posterior tibial tendon. *Instr Course Lect*. 1997;46:393-405.
22. Michelson J, Easley M, Wigley FM, Hellmann D. Posterior tibial tendon dysfunction in rheumatoid arthritis. *Foot Ankle Int*. 1995;16:156-161.
23. Trnka HJ. Dysfunction of the tendon of tibialis posterior. *J Bone Joint Surg Br*. 2004;86:939-946.
24. Frey C, Shereff M, Greenidge N. Vascularity of the posterior tibial tendon. *J Bone Joint Surg Am*. 1990;72:884-888.
25. Bulstra GH, Olsthoorn PG, Niek van DC. Tendoscopy of the posterior tibial tendon. *Foot Ankle Clin*. 2006;11:421-427, viii.
26. Kong A, Van d, V. Imaging of tibialis posterior dysfunction. *Br J Radiol* 2008;81:826-36.
27. Miller SD, Van HM, Boruta PM, et al. Ultrasound in the diagnosis of posterior tibial tendon pathology. *Foot Ankle Int*. 1996;17:555-558.
28. Porter DA, Baxter DE, Clanton TO, Klootwyk TE. Posterior tibial tendon tears in young competitive athletes: two case reports. *Foot Ankle Int*. 1998;19:627-630.
29. Lui TH. Endoscopic assisted posterior tibial tendon reconstruction for stage 2 posterior tibial tendon insufficiency. *Knee Surg Sports Traumatol Arthrosc*. 2007;15:1228-1234.
30. Paus AC. Arthroscopic synovectomy. When, which diseases and which joints. *Z Rheumatol*. 1996;55:394-400.
31. van Dijk CN, Kort N, Scholten PE. Tendoscopy of the posterior tibial tendon. *Arthroscopy*. 1997;13:692-698.
32. van Dijk CN, Scholten PE, Kort N. Tendoscopy (tendon sheath endoscopy) for overuse tendon injuries. *Oper Tech Sports Med*. 1997;5:170-178.
33. Hamilton WG. Tendonitis about the ankle joint in classical ballet dancers. *Am J Sports Med*. 1977;5:84-88.
34. Leach RE, DiIorio E, Harney RA. Pathologic hindfoot conditions in the athlete. *Clin Orthop Relat Res*. 1983;(177):116-121.
35. Hamilton WG, Geppert MJ, Thompson FM. Pain in the posterior aspect of the ankle in dancers. Differential diagnosis and operative treatment. *J Bone Joint Surg Am*. 1996;78:1491-1500.
36. Sammarco GJ, Cooper PS. Flexor hallucis longus tendon injury in dancers and nondancers. *Foot Ankle Int*. 1998;19:356-362.
37. van Dijk CN, van Bergen CJA. Advancements in ankle arthroscopy. *J Am Acad Orthop Surg*. 2008;16:635-646.
38. van Dijk CN, Scholten PE, Krips R. A 2-portal endoscopic approach for diagnosis and treatment of posterior ankle pathology. *Arthroscopy*. 2000;16:871-876.
39. Lijoi F, Lughi M, Baccarani G. Posterior arthroscopic approach to the ankle: an anatomic study. *Arthroscopy*. 2003;19:62-67.
40. Scholten PE, Sierevelt IN, van Dijk CN. Hindfoot endoscopy for posterior ankle impingement. *J Bone Joint Surg Am*. 2008;90:2665-2672.
41. Sitler DF, Amendola A, Bailey CS, et al. Posterior ankle arthroscopy: an anatomic study. *J Bone Joint Surg Am*. 2002;84A:763-769.
42. Willits K, Sonneveld H, Amendola A, et al. Outcome of posterior ankle arthroscopy for hindfoot impingement. *Arthroscopy*. 2008;24:196-202.
43. Sarrafian SK. *Anatomy of the Foot and Ankle: Descriptive, Topographic, Functional*. Philadelphia, PA: JB Lippincott; 1983.
44. Solomon R, Brown T, Gerbino PG, Micheli LJ. The young dancer. *Clin Sports Med*. 2000;19:717-739.
45. McCarroll JR, Ritter MA, Becker TE. Triggering of the great toe. A case report. *Clin Orthop Relat Res*. 1983;(175):184-185.
46. Petersen W, Pufe T, Zantop T, Paulsen F. Blood supply of the flexor hallucis longus tendon with regard to dancer's tendinitis: injection and immunohistochemical studies of cadaver tendons. *Foot Ankle Int*. 2003;24:591-596.
47. van Dijk CN, de Leeuw PAJ, Krips R. Diagnostic and operative ankle and subtalar joint arthroscopy. In: Porter DA, Schon LC, eds. *Baxter's The Foot and Ankle in Sport*. 2nd ed. Philadelphia, PA: Mosby-Elsevier; 2008:355-382.
48. van Dijk CN, de Leeuw PA. Imaging from an orthopaedic point of view. What the orthopaedic surgeon expects from the radiologist? *Eur J Radiol*. 2007;62:2-5.
49. van Noek DC. Anterior and posterior ankle impingement. *Foot Ankle Clin*. 2006;11:663-683.
50. van Dÿk CN, Verhagen RA, Tol HJ. Technical note: resterilizable noninvasive ankle distraction device. *Arthroscopy*. 2001;17:E12.

Fusion for Degenerative Arthritis of the Ankle

Troy M. Gorman ● Florian Nickisch ● Timothy C. Beals ● Charles L. Saltzman

Post-traumatic degeneration of the ankle is the principal cause of end-stage arthritis, and unlike arthritis of the hip or knee, it often affects younger patients. In addition to post-traumatic arthritis, other conditions that lead to degeneration of the ankle joint include rheumatoid arthritis, primary osteoarthritis, osteochondritis and osseous necrosis of the talus, postinfectious arthritis, crystalline arthropathies, hemachromatosis, and neuropathic degenerative disease.

Unlike hip and knee arthritis, primary ankle osteoarthritis is rare, and most degenerative ankle arthritis is post-traumatic in nature. Autopsy studies demonstrate that degenerative changes are about three times more prevalent in the knee than the ankle and that degenerative changes in both joints increase with increasing age.[1,2] Radiographic studies that aim to quantify the prevalence of ankle osteoarthritis are of limited value because of the low correlation between the identification of osteophytes on plain films and the development of symptomatic osteoarthritis.[3] Clinical studies suggest that knee and hip osteoarthritis is 8 to 10 times more common than ankle osteoarthritis.[1,4]

Because ankle arthritis is primarily post-traumatic, it affects a younger and more active patient population than hip and knee osteoarthritis. This fact demands a durable surgical option when nonoperative interventions have failed. The use of total ankle replacement is evolving, and new designs are being developed, but the gold standard for most cases of end-stage ankle arthritis has been open ankle arthrodesis. During the past 2 decades, arthroscopic ankle arthrodesis has become a viable alternative to the open procedure and has shown encouraging results.[5-8] Proposed advantages of arthroscopic techniques are less postoperative pain and morbidity, decreased blood loss, and shorter hospital stay. One important advantage of arthroscopic ankle arthrodesis is that it can be performed in patients with a poor soft tissue envelope (Fig. 17-1).

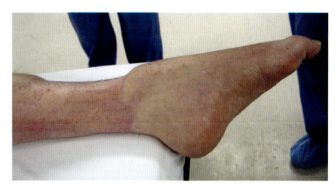

FIGURE 17-1 A patient with a poor soft tissue envelope after a burn injury went on to have a successful arthroscopic ankle arthrodesis.

ANATOMY AND PATHOGENESIS

The ankle joint is formed by the interaction of the tibia, the talus, and the fibula. The distal tibia and the medial and lateral malleoli form the ankle mortise, which contains the talus. The ankle mortise offers inherent bony stability due to its congruency, and it is further stabilized by soft tissue structures. These structures include the ligaments of the syndesmosis, the ankle capsule, the anterior talofibular ligament, the calcaneofibular ligament, the posterior talofibular ligament, the intermalleolar ligament, and medially, the deltoid ligament complex.

The ankle is relatively resistant to primary degenerative osteoarthritis, possibly because of the properties of ankle cartilage, including relatively better retention of tensile fracture stress and tensile stiffness with age, as described by Kempson and colleagues.[9] The cartilage in the ankle is metabolically different from that in the knee. Ankle cartilage appears to be less affected by the catabolic cytokine interleukin 1 (IL-1) and deleterious collagenases that are produced in response to IL-1.[10]

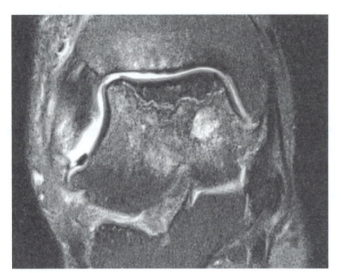

FIGURE 17-2 Magnetic resonance imaging of a patient's ankle with osseous necrosis of the talus shows collapse of subchondral bone.

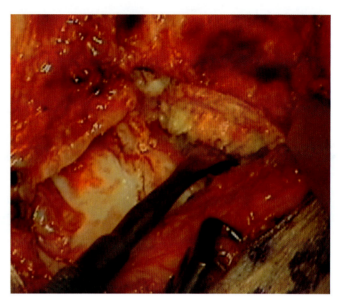

FIGURE 17-3 An intraoperative photograph demonstrates fragmentation of the talus due to osseous necrosis.

Secondary osteoarthritis of the ankle can develop after fracture or ligamentous injury. Rotational ankle fractures and ligamentous injury with recurrent instability are the most common causes.[11-15] In Saltzman's practice during 13 years, 445 (70%) of 639 patients with Kellgren-Lawrence grade 3 or 4 ankle arthritis were post-traumatic cases, and only 46 patients (7.2%) had primary oseteoarthritis.[13] Other recorded causes in this study of ankle arthritis included neuropathic disease (e.g., Charcot neuroarthropathy), inflammatory arthropathies (e.g., rheumatoid arthritis), crystalline arthropathies (e.g., pseudogout), osteochondritis, osseous necrosis, and postinfectious arthropathy.

The relative resistance of the ankle joint to primary osteoarthritis is likely a combination of its congruency, which results in inherent stability and restrained motion; unique tensile properties; and distinctive metabolic characteristics. Unfortunately, the ankle is quite susceptible to post-traumatic arthritis, and this may be related to its thinner and stiffer articular cartilage not being able to accommodate articular step-offs or the stresses of improperly constrained motion. Step-offs lead to increased local contact stresses that the thin cartilage of the ankle may not be able to accommodate as well as the thicker cartilage in the hip and knee.[16,17] These increased localized contact stresses likely contribute to the degeneration of articular cartilage that is seen after trauma. Other disease processes, such as Charcot arthropathy and osteochondritis, with large osteochondral defects can lead to step-offs or incongruity in the articular surface and result in increased contact stresses (Figs. 17-2 and 17-3).

PATIENT EVALUATION

History and Physical Examination

The first step in evaluating the patient with ankle pain is to obtain a proper history, particularly any history of trauma. One major ankle sprain can result in a significant injury to ankle joint cartilage or persistent instability, with the eventual development of degenerative changes.[13] Inquiring about other joint pain is important because multiple joint involvement may indicate sys-

temic causes, such as inflammatory arthropathy. Ankle arthritis is not usually the first manifestation of a systemic disease process. Ascertaining a diabetic history is important, because diabetes is a risk factor for Charcot neuroarthropathy and related to perioperative morbidity in those with end-stage organ disease.

It is helpful to identify what activities exacerbate or alleviate the pain. Pain with uphill walking can point to anterior impingement. Alternatively, pain at the back of the ankle with downhill walking may suggest a symptomatic os trigonum, posterior osteochondral defect, or posterior impingement. Discomfort resulting from walking on uneven ground suggests subtalar pathology or ankle instability. Lateral hindfoot pain can be caused by subfibular impingement, peroneal tendon problems (i.e., subluxating peroneals or tendinopathy), and fractures of the lateral process of the talus. Posteromedial pain is often associated with posterior tibial tendon pathology. A general sense of instability with recurrent swelling can suggest medial, lateral, and combined chronic ligament insufficiency. Because all of these pathologies may coexist, careful evaluation is essential.

Examination begins with observation, especially when the examiner has the opportunity to watch the patient walk into the examination room. Having the patient walk as part of the examination is informative, and observing overall lower extremity alignment and gait pattern is critical. Restricted ankle motion leads to early heel rise and a bent knee gait. The posture of the forefoot when it strikes the ground should be observed, because excessive forefoot varus or valgus is important to consider in surgical planning. On standing, the position of the hindfoot should be recorded. External rotation of the lower extremity is a common feature of patients with ankle arthritis.

The seated examination includes evaluation of range of motion in the ankle, hindfoot, midfoot, and forefoot. Ankle stability should be assessed by drawer testing, with the foot in plantar flexion and neutral position, which investigates the competence of the anterior talofibular ligament and calcaneofibular ligament, respectively. Talar tilt should be assessed. Foot alignment is important because deformity in the foot may cause secondary ankle disease. For example, pes planus with medial column instability may be associated with secondary ankle valgus and eventual degenerative change. Conversely, realignment of a deformed ankle can alter the foot position and adversely or positively affect function of other joints, particularly the subtalar joint. If compensatory foot deformities are identified on examination, their passive, manual correctability has to be assessed.

Tendons should be palpated to identify potential sources of pain. Finding the point of maximal tenderness during the examination may help in diagnosis. A vascular examination should be performed with palpation of pulses and assessment of the distal capillary refill, and a neurologic assessment looking for motor or sensory deficits rounds out the examination. It is important to identify patients with impaired balance.

Diagnostic Imaging

Radiographs should be done weight bearing if possible. The four radiographic views we use in our clinic to evaluate ankle pain include the anteroposterior, lateral, mortise, and hindfoot alignment views. Radiographs of the degenerative ankle can show joint space narrowing, osteophyte formation, subchondral sclerosis, and subchondral cysts. The hindfoot alignment view is important in the evaluation hindfoot varus or valgus and ankle deformity in the coronal plane.[18] It is taken with the patient standing on a platform facing a collector that angles away from the platform at 20 degrees. The x-ray tube is posterior to the ankle, with the beam perpendicular to the plane of the film at the level of the ankle. The source-to-collector distance is 40 inches. On average, the most inferior aspect of the calcaneus lies just medial to the longitudinal midaxis of the tibia (Fig. 17-4). Magnetic resonance imaging (MRI) has limited usefulness unless the examiner suspects an osteochondral lesion of the talus, osseous necrosis, or ligamentous abnormality that will alter patient care. In such cases, MR arthrography may be advantageous. Computed tomography (CT) is the better choice for three-dimensional bony imaging, and it allows visualization near hardware, unlike MRI. Noninvasive joint distraction plus air-contrast arthrography enhances visualization of the ankle's articular features.[19]

Selective fluoroscopically guided injections can be helpful in diagnosing patients who have clinical or radiographic findings that suggest more than one source of pain. It is reasonable to expect 75% pain relief in an area that is injected.[20] It is important to identify the patients' ankle pain as global (i.e., affecting most of the joint) or focal (i.e., affecting a specific region), because this distinction may guide the treatment options. It is essential to identify patients with coexisting subtalar pain, because that population needs to be counseled more intensely about the risks of residual pain and progression of adjacent joint arthritis.

TREATMENT

Nonoperative and operative treatments can help reduce symptoms and improve the function of painful ankle arthritis. There are no well-designed retrospective or prospective clinical trials reporting on nonoperative treatment of diffuse ankle arthritis. Our experience is that nonsteroidal anti-inflammatory drugs have variable efficacy in addressing the pain of ankle arthritis. The judicious use of corticosteroid injections may provide temporary relief and be beneficial in acute exacerbations in someone who has tolerable steady-state pain. Clinical trials suggest that hyaluronate-based injectables may diminish ankle pain and improve function in patients with ankle osteoarthritis, and additional trials exploring this treatment modality are being conducted.[21,22]

Nonoperative interventions primarily focus on mechanical unloading and immobilization. Devices that address this goal include the cane, ankle foot orthoses (AFOs), and the leather ankle lacer with an embedded polypropylene shell.[23] To fully unload the ankle joint requires a rigid linkage between the acceptance of force on the sole of the foot and the leg above the ankle. The prototypic device, a weight-bearing patellar brace (PTB), is poorly tolerated because load transfer irritates the soft tissues in front of the knee. Adding a rocker-bottom sole to a shoe or the use of a solid ankle-cushioned heel (SACH) may also provide relief by reducing ankle excursion with gait.

Operative intervention should be considered only after failure of nonoperative treatment methods. The surgeon should identify the cause of the patient's problem and to what extent ligamentous instability, malalignment, or other foot deformity contributes to the perceived pain from ankle arthritis. When planning surgical interventions, recreating normal foot alignment can encourage improved foot function, regardless of the chosen surgical technique. Surgical options for end-stage degenerative ankle arthritis include osteotomies about the ankle, débridement, distraction, ankle arthroplasty, and ankle arthrodesis. Ankle arthrodesis can be performed in a variety of ways, including open, mini-open, and arthroscopic techniques.

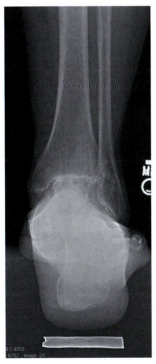

FIGURE 17-4 Hindfoot alignment view demonstrates no significant coronal malalignment.

If arthrodesis is the surgical treatment of choice, the next step is ensuring appropriate alignment at the fusion site, which takes into account the alignment of the entire limb. Malalignment or angulation of the tibia may require special consideration. Adjustment may need to be made in the position of the fusion to ensure a plantigrade foot if the foot has significant forefoot varus or valgus or other foot malalignment. For example, if a patient has significant fixed forefoot varus, the ankle joint needs to be positioned in a little more valgus so a plantigrade foot can be created. Concomitant knee and ankle arthritis and deformity should be fully assessed, and realignment at the knee is a priority before ankle arthrodesis.

General indications for ankle arthrodesis include degenerative arthritis with significant pain unresponsive to nonoperative interventions, end-stage arthritis due to other causes (e.g., rheumatoid arthritis, pseudogout, postinfectious arthritis, hemachromatosis), large osteochondral defects not amendable to other interventions, osseous necrosis of the talus, failed total ankle replacement, and malalignment or instability from a paralytic deformity. Absolute contraindications to ankle arthrodesis include active infection and active Charcot arthropathy. However, after appropriate treatment of an infection and resolution of the metabolic issues associated with Charcot arthropathy, arthrodesis is an acceptable treatment for these problems. Some surgeons may consider active smoking by the patient a relative contraindication.

In terms of arthroscopic ankle arthrodesis, the indications remain the same, with the exception of a failed total ankle replacement. Well-aligned ankles and those that are easily realigned are excellent candidates for arthroscopic fusion. Patients with soft tissue compromise (e.g., those with prior trauma, burn victims, patients with skin grafts) or vasculopathy are strongly considered for an arthroscopic approach. In the past, it was thought that ankle varus or valgus greater than 5 degrees was an absolute contraindication to arthroscopic arthrodesis. However, later reports suggested that substantial ankle varus or valgus is a relative contraindication rather than an absolute one.[24,25] The investigators consider any ankle that can be re-aligned properly after arthroscopic débridement appropriate but acknowledge that patients should be counseled that conversion to an open approach is prudent if an extensive capsulotomy is required to achieve correct alignment. Additional contraindications for the arthroscopic procedure are significant focal bone loss and deformity and extremely rigid ankles. In general, the desired position of the arthrodesis is neutral dorsiflexion, 5 degrees of ankle valgus, equal or slightly greater external rotation compared with the contralateral leg, and placement of the anterior aspect of the talar dome at the level of the anterior aspect of the tibia.

Arthroscopic ankle arthrodesis was first developed in the mid-1980s. Myerson and Quill reported the first comparative series, with 17 arthroscopic procedures compared with 16 open procedures done with a medial malleolar osteotomy.[7] They found an average fusion time of 8.7 weeks in the arthroscopic group and 14.5 weeks in the open group, with similar fusion rates for both groups. Their criteria for clinical union included an absence of tibiotalar motion, crepitus, or pain with ambulation or on examination. Radiographic union was defined as the appearance of osseous trabeculae across the tibiotalar arthrodesis site and incorporation of bone graft into the fusion mass when bone graft was used.

One of the first long-term series was published in 1996 by Glick and colleagues.[6] They reported 34 cases with an average follow-up of 8 years. Fusion rates were 97%, and good or excellent results were reported for 86% of patients. Three ankles in this series were rated poor because of subtalar pain and a nonunion, and a malunion accounted for the other poor results.

O'Brien and colleagues added support to arthroscopic arthrodesis by showing comparable fusion rates between 19 arthroscopically treated patients and 17 patients undergoing open arthrodesis using flat cuts.[8] The arthroscopic group had decreased operative times, decreased tourniquet times, less blood loss, and decreased hospital stays.

Since the publication of these three studies, the popularity of arthroscopic ankle arthrodesis has grown and the technique has evolved. Our current techniques are described subsequently in the context of individual cases.

Case 1

The patient is a 49-year-old woman with a history of rheumatoid arthritis and multiple left ankle sprains as a young adult. She has had increasing left ankle pain over the past few years. She underwent arthroscopic débridement of the ankle 3 years earlier, but the procedure did not improve her pain. An over-the-counter lace-up ankle brace did not ease the pain. She did get some relief with a corticosteroid injection in the left ankle, but the pain returned. Her pain was aggravated with walking and ascending and descending stairs.

On physical examination she had mild hindfoot varus and an ankle arc of motion of 15 degrees. She had a small ankle effusion, and palpation elicited tenderness along the medial, anterior, and lateral joint lines. The subtalar joint was not tender to palpation and had normal motion. The result of the anterior drawer test was negative. She was neurovascularly intact. A hindfoot alignment radiograph showed minimal varus (see Fig. 17-4). Anteroposterior, lateral, and mortise views showed loss of tibiotalar joint space and osteophyte formation (Fig. 17-5). The subtalar joint was preserved (Fig. 17-6).

Treatment options discussed with the patient included ankle arthrodesis and total ankle replacement. Given her young age and relatively poor motion, she was not considered to be a good candidate for ankle arthroplasty. Arthrodesis appeared to be the more reliable option, and the patient and surgeon decided to perform the procedure arthroscopically from an anterior approach.

Anterior Arthroscopic Ankle Arthrodesis
Room Setup

We recommend general anesthesia to relax the gastrocnemius-soleus complex, and it is augmented with a regional block to aid in postoperative pain control. At our center, a popliteal-level indwelling catheter and a single-shot saphenous block are placed with ultrasound guidance.

The bed is placed in a beach chair position and then in slight Trendelenburg so the operative leg is nearly parallel to the floor. The heel is positioned just off the edge of the table. The break in the bed should be positioned at the knee, so that when the end of the table is dropped, traction can be applied to the limb without moving the patient. This reflexed position provides sufficient

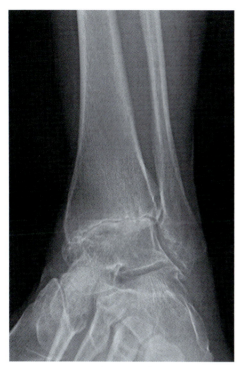

FIGURE 17-5 A mortise view shows significant narrowing of the tibiotalar joint space and involvement of the medial and lateral gutters.

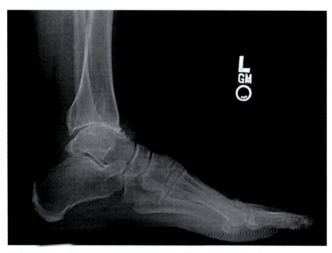

FIGURE 17-6 A lateral view shows significant tibiotalar degeneration but preservation of the subtalar joint.

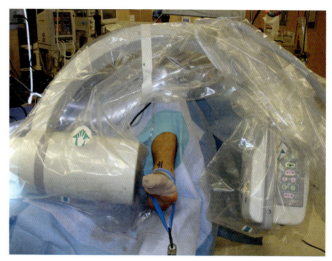

FIGURE 17-7 The position of the bed allows traction against the bed without using a well-leg holder. The fluoroscopic scanner can be positioned to enable easy visualization of the ankle joint.

visualization and navigation around the joint. If external strapping techniques are used to distract the joint, the force (usually less than 25 pounds) should be decreased during preparation of the anterior talar dome, because this takes tension off the anterior capsule, allowing easier access to the talar dome.

Joint Preparation

Use of thigh tourniquet is optional. Saltzman inflates a tourniquet only when needed for better visualization. An anteromedial approach is used to instill 15 to 20 mL of saline. A fluoroscope may be used to verify that the needle is correctly placed in the joint. With fluid injection, the ankle joint usually plantar flexes.

The medial portal is established just medial to the tibialis anterior tendon sheath and slightly distal to the ankle joint by incising the skin with a no. 15 blade and bluntly dissecting down to the capsule with a small, straight hemostat. The hemostat is then punched into joint, and the tips are used to spread the tissue to create a path for the arthroscope. The arthroscope is then introduced into the anterior ankle. The ankle is distended by turning on the fluid pump, and the entrance for the lateral portal is visualized with the camera. To avoid distending the soft tissues, the pump should always be run at the lowest possible flow rate and pressure to maintain adequate visualization. The lateral portal is made just lateral to the long extensor tendons and the peroneus tertius and just distal to the ankle joint. Placing portals too proximal, particularly if anterior osteophytes are present, should be avoided. The trajectory of the portal should be tested with an 18-gauge needle. We like to have a distance of 5 to 10 mm from the palpable branches of the superficial peroneal nerve when creating this portal. The joint is entered bluntly with the small hemostat, and a thin periosteal elevator is placed into the joint. If necessary, a shaver is used first and an anterior synovectomy is performed to improve visualization.

Any residual cartilage on the tibia and talus are removed with the shaver or curettes (Video 1). Having a set of thin-handled, angled curettes is helpful. If the lateral gutter does not show significant wear, the cartilage can be left in this location, and the fibula is excluded from the fusion. However, if there are degen-

resistance against the thigh to allow for distraction when traction is applied (Fig. 17-7). Preparing above the knee allows for assessment of rotational alignment. An alternative is to use a well-leg holder against the posterior thigh of the operative limb. We mark landmarks, including malleoli, branches of the superficial peroneal nerve, and the expected level of the tibiotalar joint space.

Instruments include a pump, a 4.5-mm arthroscope, a 4.5-mm aggressive shaver, and 4.0-mm burr and curettes. Distraction, noninvasive or invasive, may or may not be used. We find distraction helpful during the preparation of the articular surfaces because it allows easier movement of the instruments. We use a thin wire through the calcaneus attached to a custom distractor and apply 70 to 90 pounds of force to allow for better

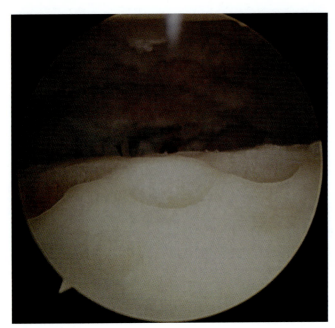

FIGURE 17-8 An intra-articular arthroscopic view reveals the pockmarked surface of the tibia and talus and shows that the overall congruency of the tibiotalar joint is preserved.

erative changes in this region, we remove all residual cartilage and incorporate the fibula into the fusion.

After all the cartilage is removed, a 3- to 4-mm burr is used to pockmark the subchondral surface so it looks like the surface of a golf ball (Fig. 17-8). It is crucial to do this across the entire undersurface of the tibia and the anterior two thirds of the talar dome. Distraction helps us to preserve the natural contours of the ankle joint. If the joint is unable to be débrided because it is too tight, the incision can be extended and a laminar spreader placed into the joint to facilitate cartilage removal to perform a mini-open procedure.[26] Adequacy of débridement is then determined by deflating the tourniquet, turning off the pump, and inspecting the joint for sufficient punctate bleeding.

Alignment

Aligning the foot correctly under the tibia is the critical step. Because most arthroscopic patients have a mild deformity, the goal is getting the foot plantigrade and neutral in the sagittal plane. This can sometimes be very challenging. We recommend placing the ankle in what is the best position clinically and temporarily fixing it with two large Kirschner wires or cannulated pins. Mechanically compressing the bones while the pins are placed can help to achieve proper compression.

During the next step, the assistant holds the leg without grabbing the foot and goes to the side of the patient to assess the sagittal position of the ankle with the foot gently dorsiflexed. The position must be perfect before moving onto fixation. The leg should be straightened to ensure proper coronal plane positioning and rotational alignment of the ankle.

Fixation

For the tibiotalar fusion, cannulated or solid screws can be used. We typically use two large, cannulated screws and check the

position and length of our guide pins with a fluoroscope before placing the screws.

The first pin is placed through a 2-cm incision placed on the anterior leg about 5 cm above the joint. This incision needs to be long enough to ensure that neither the superficial nor deep peroneal structures are injured by screw placement. The pin is placed on the anterolateral part of the tibia starting 3 cm above the joint, just superior and medial to Chaput's tubercle, and it is directed 10 to 20 degrees posterior from vertical into the posterior half of the talar dome. Lateral and anteroposterior views are needed to confirm pin placement before a large, cannulated, partially threaded compression screw (usually 6.5 mm) is used to pull the talus up into the mortise (Fig. 17-9).

A second screw is placed from a posteromedial position in the tibia to an anterocentral position in the talus (Fig. 17-10). The leg is placed in a figure-of-four position, and a 1-cm incision is made along the posteromedial edge of the tibia 3 cm above the joint line. Blunt dissection and retraction get the pin down to the bone. The pin should start at least 4 mm anterior to the sheath of the posterior tibial tendon and traverse the posteromedial corner of the ankle, coursing into the center of the neck of the talus (Fig. 17-11). Direct visualization of the posterior tibial tendon sheath is recommended to prevent injury to the tendon. After the guide pin is overdrilled, a partially threaded, large, cannulated screw is placed, which may slightly compress the construct back into the posteromedial corner.

If the lateral gutter (fibulotalar articulation) has no significant arthritis, it does not need to be débrided or fixed. However, if the

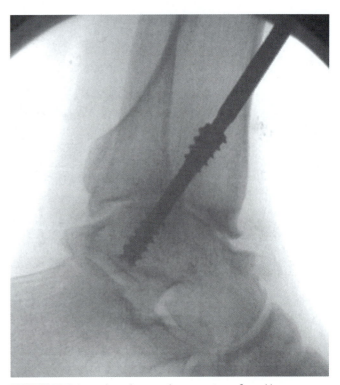

FIGURE 17-9 Anterolateral screw placement is confirmed by fluoroscopy. The screw is placed on the anterolateral part of the tibia starting 3 cm above the joint, just superior and medial to Chaput's tubercle, and it is directed 10 to 20 degrees posterior from vertical into the posterior half of the talar dome.

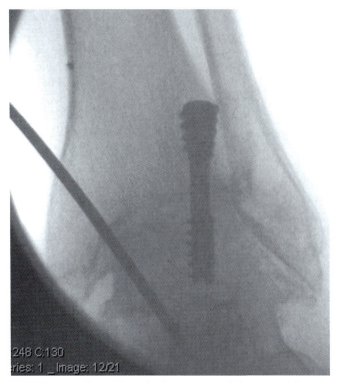

FIGURE 17-10 The guide pin for the posteromedial screw and the location of the anterolateral screw are seen on anteroposterior fluoroscopy.

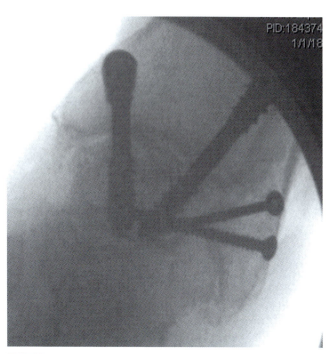

FIGURE 17-12 An anteroposterior view of the final construct demonstrates a downsized screw from the posterolateral fibula into the anterocentral neck of talus. An accessory screw was added from the fibula into the talar dome.

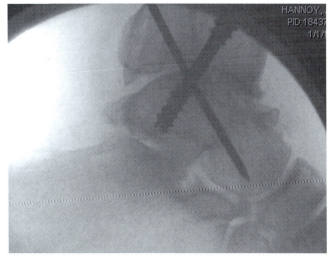

FIGURE 17-11 A lateral view shows the anteromedial pin starting 3 cm above joint line and coursing in the center of the neck of the talus. The pin should start at least 4 mm anterior to the sheath of the posterior tibial tendon.

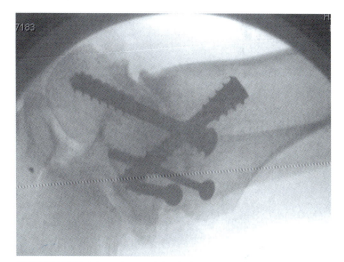

FIGURE 17-13 A lateral view of the final construct demonstrates incorporation of the lateral gutter into the fusion with a downsized posterolateral screw and accessory lateral screw.

fibulotalar joint is arthritic, a third screw is placed from a posterolateral position in the fibula to an inferocentral position in the talar neck and body. We often downsize the width of this screw to avoid cracking the fibula and add accessory screws directed from the fibula to the talar dome (Figs. 17-12 and 17-13). Another consideration is to perform a transverse osteotomy of the fibula a few centimeters proximal to the joint line to decouple forces from the proximal fibula to the distal fibular fragment.

This may enhance fusion of the syndesmotic region, and the distal fibular fragment can be secured with the same screw arrangement described earlier.

Small gaps usually exist between the bony surfaces after fixation. If the lateral malleolus is included in the fusion, there is often a small gap laterally because the medial screw may pull the talus medially. We inject about 5 to 10 cc of demineralized bone matrix into these small gaps through our portals. Alternatively, the demineralized bone matrix can be placed after the guide pins are placed, but it should be done before final screw placement.

Postoperative Care

The ankle is placed in a well-padded posterior splint. The splint and sutures are removed after 10 to 14 days, and a below-knee cast is placed. We allow patients 5 to 10 pounds of heel weight bearing so they can maintain their balance. Others allow full weight bearing at this point.[27] Our group has no experience with early weight bearing, and we remain concerned about increasing the rate of nonunion.

At 6 to 8 weeks, radiographs are taken. At this point, we hope to see early bridging, which has a ground-glass appearance in the joint space. If there is doubt about the adequacy of the fusion, CT can be used to better visualize the joint. If fusion is apparent and the patient has minimal pain in the joint, the leg is placed into a removable boot. It should be worn at all times except for sleeping, bathing, and sitting. The patient then begins progressive weight bearing as tolerated in the boot, as long as there is no significant pain.

At 10 weeks, a second set of radiographs is obtained. If the radiographs show increased bridging and the patient has no pain with standing, he or she is weaned from the boot. Formal physical therapy is not mandated, but a 4- to 8-week course of balance and gait training after removal of the boot seems to speed recovery, particularly in elderly patients.

PEARLS & PITFALLS

PEARLS
- Set up the arthroscopic procedure so fluoroscopy imaging is easy.
- Use mechanical distraction to open the joint space for débridement.
- Use a periosteal elevator *first* to remove cartilage.
- Spread the screws so each has mechanical independence.
- After preliminary fixation, observe alignment from a distance, and do not trust fluoroscopy imaging for clinical alignment.

PITFALLS
- Taking on irreducible deformities
- Injury to branches of the superficial peroneal nerve
- Placing the medial screw through the posterior tibial tendon sheath
- Ignoring the anterior talus during débridement
- Accepting suboptimal ankle alignment

Case 2

A 33-year-old man had an injury to the left ankle caused by automobile-pedestrian accident 2 years before presentation. The initial injury was suspected to be a large talar dome fracture, which was addressed by internal fixation. Two years after the injury, the patient underwent partial removal of hardware and subsequently became infected. He was treated with irrigation and débridement and with antibiotics. He was finishing antibiotic therapy at the time of presentation.

The patient had much ankle pain and hindfoot pain. Examination revealed that he had three healed incisions about the ankle. It was diffusely tender to palpation, and the ankle and subtalar range of motion was limited. Radiographs and CT scans demonstrated osseous necrosis of the medial half of the

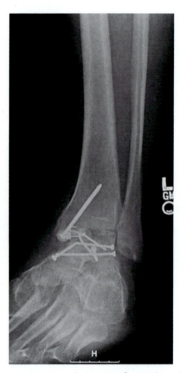

FIGURE 17-14 A mortise view shows significant tibiotalar degenerative disease and partial osseous necrosis of the talus.

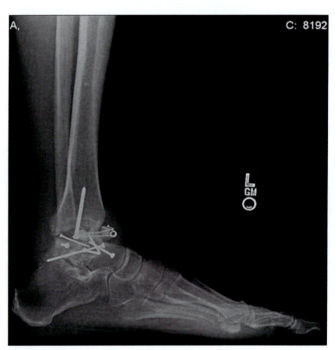

FIGURE 17-15 A lateral view shows additional degenerative disease of the subtalar joint.

talus, including the dome and the body, and arthrosis of the tibiotalar and subtalar joints (Figs. 17-14 and 17-15). The patient's overall alignment was well preserved (Fig. 17-16). Because the patient had numerous prior incisions, there was concern that his soft tissue envelope might be compromised. He was considered for a combined prone arthroscopic ankle and subtalar arthrodesis.

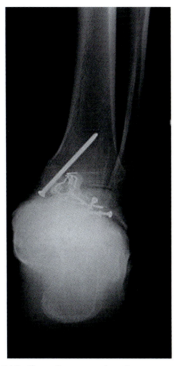

FIGURE 17-16 A hindfoot alignment view demonstrates preservation of the coronal alignment.

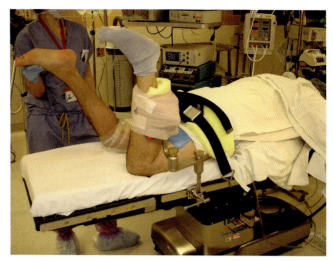

FIGURE 17-17 The setup for posterior ankle arthroscopy is shown. The nonoperative limb is flexed to 90 degrees at the knee.

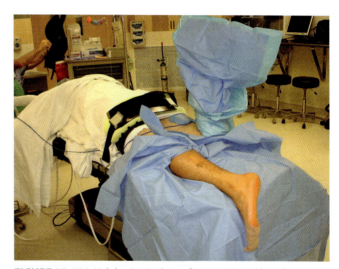

FIGURE 17-18 Initial draping is shown for posterior ankle arthroscopy. The Mayo stand cover is placed over the nonoperative limb.

Combined Posterior Arthroscopic and Subtalar Arthrodesis

Room Setup

The patient is positioned in the prone position, with the involved ankle placed approximately 10 cm distal to end of the table. We sling the safety strap posterior and inferior to the buttocks to resist the force of distraction. General anesthesia and a regional nerve block are used. Instruments include a custom distraction device; a 2.7-mm, 30-degree angled arthroscope; a larger, 4.0-mm arthroscope; thin periosteal elevators; long and thin-handled curettes; aggressive shavers; and a 4.0 mm burr. Before standard preparation and draping, the nonoperative limb is flexed to about 90 degrees at the knee and held in this position for the duration of the surgery (Figs. 17-17 and 17-18). This allows full access to the operative limb. On the operative side, the Achilles tendon, the medial and lateral malleoli, the sural nerve, the posteromedial neurovascular bundle, and the estimated levels of the tibiotalar and subtalar joints are marked with a surgical pen.

Joint Preparation

A transosseous, 1.6- to 1.8-mm wire is placed medial to lateral through the calcaneus and attached to a foot plate of a ring fixator or a modified traction bale to allow distraction with a hand-driven winch (Video 2). Posterolateral and posteromedial portal sites immediately adjacent to the Achilles tendon and equidistant between the ankle and subtalar joints are established.

The posterolateral portal is established first. An 18-gauge needle is used to inject 10 mL of normal saline into the subtalar joint and 10 mL into the tibiotalar joint under fluoroscopic guidance. The joints are observed to distract with fluid injection. A small,

longitudinal incision is then made through the skin (previously marked) just lateral to the Achilles. A short, straight hemostat is the used to dissect to the lateral aspect of the subtalar joint. The hemostat is used to penetrate the joint capsule, and then the 2.7-mm, 30-degree angled arthroscope is inserted. An arthroscopic pump controls the fluid flow and is held to a minimum flow rate to allow visualization. Next, an 18-gauge needle is inserted at the site marked for the posteromedial portal and directed toward the central aspect of the subtalar joint. The needle is visualized, making sure that it is lateral to the flexor hallucis longus. All work is performed lateral to the flexor hallucis longus to avoid injuring the posteromedial neurovascular structures. Visualization and clear delineation of the flexor hallucis longus is the first step in this procedure. The needle is then removed, and the posteromedial portal is established, directing all instruments centrally. At this point, the 4.0-mm arthroscope can be used to improve fluid flow and visualization during the procedure.

If necessary, a third portal is established approximately 1 cm proximal and 1 cm posterior to the tip of the lateral malleolus.

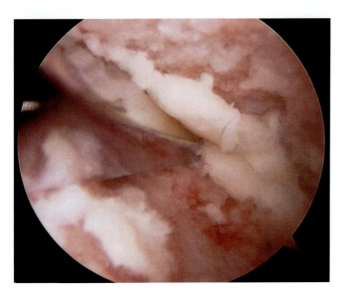

FIGURE 17-19 A periosteal elevator is used for débridement of residual cartilage from the subtalar joint.

The sural nerve is at risk, and caution is required when inserting instruments. This portal gives greater access to the posterior facet of the subtalar joint. Most of the procedure is done with the arthroscope in the posterolateral portal and the instruments in the posteromedial portal, although both portals are used in an alternating fashion for viewing and for instrumentation. Arthroscopic cannulas may be used.

Synovectomy is performed first with the shaver to improve visualization. The residual articular cartilage of the entire posterior facet is then removed with a thin, curved periosteal elevator, curettes, and an aggressive shaver (Fig. 17-19). Visualization of the interosseous ligament signifies the anterior extent of the débridement, and by staying posterior to this structure, the surgeon avoids the sinus tarsi vasculature. The bone surfaces are then pockmarked with the burr, as described for the ankle arthrodesis. It is best to preserve the overall congruency of the joint during the débridement and pockmarking to get good opposition of the joint during fixation.

Instruments are removed from the subtalar joint, and the tibiotalar joint is entered. A hemostat is used to bluntly enter the ankle from the lateral side, and all work is performed lateral to the flexor hallucis longus tendon. Using the same order of instruments described previously, the ankle is débrided of residual cartilage, and the bony surfaces are prepared. Depending on the angle of entry to the tibiotalar joint, an additional proximal portal that is in line with the other portals may be required for adequate instrument access. Demineralized bone matrix can be inserted by means of a small cannula through the posterolateral portal into the ankle and subtalar joints, and traction is released.

Fixation

Three choices are available for fixation: screws, intramedullary rod, and ring fixation. We typically use only screws when the bone is of good quality. Fixation of the subtalar joint can be achieved using two large, cannulated, 6.5- or 7.3-mm, partially threaded cancellous screws placed under fluoroscopic guidance. The initial guide

pin is started at the posterolateral calcaneus and is angled anterosuperior to the talus neck or body. It is placed proximal to the weight-bearing surface of the heel and distal to the initial attachment of the Achilles. A second guide pin is placed medially in a similar direction to the first. The pins are then overdrilled and the cannulated screws placed. Alternatively, the second screw can be directed from the inferolateral portion of the calcaneus into the head and neck region of the talus. We use a 4.5-mm screw for this purpose.

The tibiotalar joint is fixed first with a compression screw in a posterior to anterior direction. Having the patient prone makes placement of the first pin easier. The first pin is placed from a posterolateral position in the tibia to an anterocentral position in the talus. A 1-cm incision is made along the posterolateral edge of the Achilles 5 cm above the joint line. Blunt dissection and retraction are necessary to get the pin down to the bone and avoid injury to the sural nerve. The pin should traverse the posterior centrolateral distal tibia and end in the center of the neck of the talus. After the guide pin is overdrilled, a partially threaded, large, cannulated screw is placed, which usually compresses the construct back into the posterior malleolus. A second posteromedially based screw is placed from just anterior to the posterior tibial tendon, as described for the anterior ankle arthrodesis.

If the lateral gutter has no significant arthritis, it does not need to be débrided or stabilized. However, if the fibulotalar joint is arthritic, a third screw is placed across the tibiotalar joint from the fibula to inferocentral in the talar neck and body. Addition of a fully threaded screw from the plantar lateral calcaneus into the tibia allows enhanced stabilization.

Another option for fixation is a tibiotalocalcaneal fusion nail. After the joints are débrided and alignment verified, the nail can be placed with fluoroscopic guidance. We prefer a transverse incision in the heel, and care is taken to avoid the plantar nerves. Typically, the incision is placed mostly on the lateral half of the heel fat pad at the junction between the middle and distal thirds. Fluoroscopic confirmation is essential. The dissection down to the calcaneus is done bluntly, and retractors are used to prevent injury to the local neurovascular structures. The nail is inserted with reaming. The construct is compressed before final interlocking screws are placed (Figs. 17-20 and 17-21). Postoperative instructions are the same as for the ankle fusion described previously.

CLINICAL RESULTS

Many clinical series published since 1990 have reported the outcomes of arthroscopic ankle arthrodesis. All the studies are retrospective in nature, and only a few have compared the outcomes of arthrodesis with those of open treatment. Myerson and Quill published the first comparison of arthroscopic with open techniques.[7] Seventeen patients were treated with arthroscopic ankle arthrodesis, and 16 patients were treated with an open technique (i.e., medial malleolar osteotomy). The investigators found that the arthroscopic group had a shorter average time to fusion (8.7 vs. 14.5 weeks) and a much shorter hospital stay (1.5 vs. 4 days). The arthroscopic group had one pseudoarthrosis, for a fusion rate of 94.1% ,compared with 100% in the open group. However, this study was not controlled, and the two groups were dissimilar, with the open group having patients with greater deformity and bone loss.

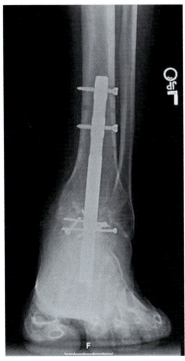

FIGURE 17-20 Postoperative, anteroposterior radiograph demonstrates fusion using a tibiotalocalcaneal fusion nail.

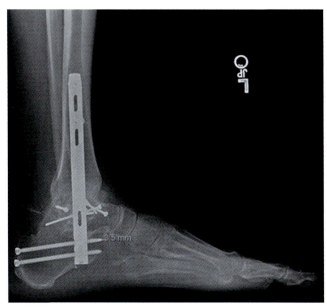

FIGURE 17-21 Postoperative, lateral radiograph demonstrates the neutral position of the ankle and fusion across the ankle and subtalar joints using a tibiotalocalcaneal fusion nail.

O'Brien and colleagues attempted to devise a better study by having two comparable groups in regard to the amount of deformity.[8] Nineteen patients were treated arthroscopically, and 17 were treated with open arthrodesis with flat cuts. The investigators reported an 84% fusion rate for the arthroscopic group and an 82% rate for the open group. They found the arthroscopic group had a shorter operative time by 12 minutes (166 vs. 184 minutes) and a significantly shorter hospital stay (1.6 vs. 3.4 days). The complication rate was similar for both groups.

The following results are compiled from an additional 13 clinical series (Table 17-1). Reported fusion rates range from 70% to 100%.[5,6,24,25,27-36] Five studies reported 100% fusion rates, and the other eight studies had rates ranging from 89% to 97%, with only one study reporting a fusion rate below 89%.[36] A common definition for fusion is an ankle that is clinically stable on examination and pain free on weight bearing, and it has radiographic signs of bridging trabeculae. Five studies reported mean fusion times of less than 10.5 weeks, with the fastest mean time to fusion reported at 8.9 weeks.[6,29,34-36] The other studies reported mean fusion times ranging from 11 to 16 weeks.

Five of the series reported the clinical outcomes of patients, with good or excellent results for 80% to 95% of patients and with follow-up ranging from 14 months to 18 years.[5,6,25,33,36] In the largest of the studies, Winson and colleagues reported good or excellent results for 83 (80%) of 104 patients at an average follow-up of 5.4 years.[25] Other studies have reported satisfaction rates of 95% to 100%.[34,35]

No studies have reported on arthroscopic tibiotalocalcaneal fusions. However, Amendola and colleagues described the technique and early results of posterior arthroscopic subtalar arthrodesis

(PASTA).[37] They reported 11 feet in 10 patients that underwent PASTA. Ten of the 11 joints fused by 10 weeks, with one patient going on to nonunion. Eight patients were very satisfied with the results, one was satisfied, and one patient was not satisfied with the results of subtalar fusion. The patients demonstrated a 50-point improvement in their modified American Orthopaedic Foot and Ankle Society (AOFAS) score (i.e., 36 to 86 points). Other than the one nonunion, there were no postoperative complications.

COMPLICATIONS

Complications with the arthroscopic procedure usually compare favorably with those reported with open techniques. Complications rates in the literature range from 0% to 55%. However, prominent or painful hardware is responsible for many of the reported complications that eventually result in additional procedures. In an early study that focused on complications in arthroscopic ankle fusion, Crosby and associates reported an overall complication rate of 55% in a series of 42 patients. There were three (7%) nonunions, two (5.1%) delayed unions, two stress fractures at the tibial pin sites used for distraction, five infections (i.e., four superficial infections at the sites pins were used and one deep infection), and six (14%) cases of painful hardware (four patients elected to have the screws removed), and four patients went on to have painful subtalar arthritis.[30] The amount of subsequent subtalar arthritis is similar to that reported in other studies.[24,25,28] Other reported complications include cutaneous nerve injury,[29,33] deep peroneal nerve palsy,[27] malunion, dorsalis pedis pseudoaneurysm,[6] and deep venous thrombosis with nonfatal pulmonary embolism.[25]

TABLE 17-1   Published Series of Arthroscopic Ankle Arthrodesis

Myerson and Quill,[7] 1991	17 (arthroscopic)	59%	94%	8.7 wk	11.7%
	16 (open)	75%	100%	14.5 wk	18.7%
O'Brien et al,[8] 1999	19 (arthroscopic)	63%	84%	Not reported	16%
	17 (open)	82%	82%		18%
Ogilvie-Harris et al,[33] 1993	19	74%	89%	12 weeks	26%
Dent et al,[32] 1993	8	60%	100%	Not reported	0%
De Vriese et al,[31] 1994	10		70%	4 mo	30%
Turan et al,[35] 1995	8 (10 ankles)	0% (all rheumatoid)	100%	10 wk	0%
Corso and Zimmer,[29] 1995	16	75%	100%	9.5 wk	12.5%
Glick and Morgan,[6] 1996	34		97%	9 wk	5.8%
Crosby et al,[30] 1996	42	90%	93%	5.5 mo	55%
Cameron and Ullrich,[28] 2000	15	33%	100%	11.5 wk	40%
Zvijac et al,[36] 2002	21	90%	95%	8.9 wk	4%
Cannon et al,[27] 2004	36	55%	100%	77% at 8 wk 100% at 16 wk	33%
Saragas,[34] 2004	26	92%	96%	10.5 wk	34%
Ferkel et al,[5] 2005	35	77%	97%	11.8 wk	23%
Winson et al,[25] 2005	116 (118 ankles)	57%	92%	12 wk	32%
Gougoulias et al,[24] 2007	74 (78 ankles)	49%	97%	12.5 wk	31%
Totals or averages	502 ankles	62%	88%	11.7 wk	22%

CONCLUSIONS

Reported series of arthroscopic ankle arthrodesis usually have comparable or improved rates of fusion, patient satisfaction, and adverse outcomes compared with the results of traditional open fusion techniques. It is an excellent option for patients with minimal deformity in the coronal plane and those with a compromised soft tissue envelope. Postoperative morbidity is less than with an open approach, patients spend less time in the hospital after treatment, and patient satisfaction is high. For surgeons with the proper skills, arthroscopic ankle arthrodesis is a good option for treating patients with end-stage ankle degenerative disease. Arthroscopic tibiotalocalcaneal fusion from a posterior approach is a promising procedure for patients with ankle and subtalar degenerative disease, but additional investigation is required before firm conclusions can be drawn regarding its efficacy.

REFERENCES

1. Huch K, Kuettner KE, Dieppe P. Osteoarthritis in ankle and knee joints. *Semin Arthritis Rheum.* 1997;26:667-674.
2. Muehleman C, Bareither D, Huch K, et al. Prevalence of degenerative morphological changes in the joints of the lower extremity. *Osteoarthritis Cartilage.* 1997;5:23-37.
3. van der Schoot DK, Den Outer AJ, Bode PJ, et al. Degenerative changes at the knee and ankle related to malunion of tibial fractures: 15-year follow-up of 88 patients. *J Bone Joint Surg Br.* 1996;78:722-725.
4. Cushnaghan J, Dieppe P. Study of 500 patients with limb joint osteoarthritis. I. Analysis by age, sex, and distribution of symptomatic joint sites. *Ann Rheum Dis.* 1991;50:8-13.
5. Ferkel RD, Hewitt M. Long-term results of arthroscopic ankle arthrodesis. *Foot Ankle Int.* 2005;26:275-280.
6. Glick JM, Morgan CD, Myerson MS, et al. Ankle arthrodesis using an arthroscopic method: long-term follow-up of 34 cases. *Arthroscopy.* 1996; 12:428-434.
7. Myerson MS, Quill G. Ankle arthrodesis. A comparison of an arthroscopic and an open method of treatment. *Clin Orthop Relat Res.* 1991;(268):84-95.
8. O'Brien TS, Hart TS, Shereff MJ, et al. Open versus arthroscopic ankle arthrodesis: a comparative study. *Foot Ankle Int.* 1999;20:368-374.
9. Kempson GE. Age-related changes in the tensile properties of human articular cartilage: a comparative study between the femoral head of the hip joint and the talus of the ankle joint. *Biochim Biophys Acta.* 1991; 1075:223-230.
10. Chubinskaya S, Huch K, Mikecz K, et al. Chondrocyte matrix metalloproteinase-8: up-regulation of neutrophil collagenase by interleukin-1 beta in human cartilage from knee and ankle joints. *Lab Invest.* 1996; 74:232-240.
11. Demetriades L, Strauss E, Gallina J. Osteoarthritis of the ankle. *Clin Orthop Relat Res.* 1998;(349):28-42.
12. Harrington KD. Degenerative arthritis of the ankle secondary to long-standing lateral ligament instability. *J Bone Joint Surg Am.* 1979; 61:354-361.
13. Saltzman CL, Salamon ML, Blanchard GM, et al. Epidemiology of ankle arthritis: report of a consecutive series of 639 patients from a tertiary orthopaedic center. *Iowa Orthop J.* 2005;25:44-46.
14. Schafer D, Hintermann B. Arthroscopic assessment of the chronic unstable ankle joint. *Knee Surg Sports Traumatol Arthrosc.* 1996;41:48-52.
15. Wyss C, Zollinger H. The causes of subsequent arthrodesis of the ankle joint. *Acta Orthop Belg.* 1991;57(suppl 1):22-27.
16. Ateshian GA, Soslowsky LJ, Mow VC. Quantitation of articular surface topography and cartilage thickness in knee joints using stereophotogrammetry. *J Biomech.* 1991;24:761-776.
17. Athanasiou KA, Niederauer GG, Schenck RC Jr. Biomechanical topography of human ankle cartilage. *Ann Biomed Eng.* 1995;23:697-704.
18. Saltzman CL, el-Khoury GY. The hindfoot alignment view. *Foot Ankle Int.* 1995;16:572-576.

19. El-Khoury GY, Alliman KJ, Lundberg HJ, et al. Cartilage thickness in cadaveric ankles: measurement with double-contrast multi-detector row CT arthrography versus MR imaging. *Radiology.* 2004;233:768-773.

20. Khoury NJ, el-Khoury GY, Saltzman CL, Brandser EA. Intraarticular foot and ankle injections to identify source of pain before arthrodesis. *AJR Am J Roentgenol.* 1996;167:669-673.

21. Carpenter B, Motley T. The role of viscosupplementation in the ankle using hylan G-F 20. *J Foot Ankle Surg.* 2008;47:377-384.

22. Luciani D, Cadossi M, Tesei F, et al. Viscosupplementation for grade II osteoarthritis of the ankle: a prospective study at 18 months' follow-up. *Chir Organi Mov.* 2008;92:155-160.

23. Saltzman CL, Shurr D, Kamp J, Cook TA. The leather ankle lacer. *Iowa Orthop J.* 1995;15:204-208.

24. Gougoulias NE, Agathangelidis FG, Parsons SW. Arthroscopic ankle arthrodesis. *Foot Ankle Int.* 2007;28:695-706.

25. Winson IG, Robinson DE, Allen PE. Arthroscopic ankle arthrodesis. *J Bone Joint Surg Br.* 2005;87:343-347.

26. Paremain GD, Miller SD, Myerson MS. Ankle arthrodesis: results after the miniarthrotomy technique. *Foot Ankle Int.* 1996;17:247-252.

27. Cannon L. Early weight bearing is safe following arthroscopic ankle arthrodesis. *Foot Ankle Surg.* 2004;10:135-139.

28. Cameron SE, Ullrich P. Arthroscopic arthrodesis of the ankle joint. *Arthroscopy.* 2000;16:21-26.

29. Corso SJ, Zimmer TJ. Technique and clinical evaluation of arthroscopic ankle arthrodesis. *Arthroscopy.* 1995;11:585-590.

30. Crosby LA, Yee TC, Formanek TS, Fitzgibbons TC. Complications following arthroscopic ankle arthrodesis. *Foot Ankle Int.* 1996;17:340-342.

31. De Vriese L, Dereymaeker G, Fabry G. Arthroscopic ankle arthrodesis. Preliminary report. *Acta Orthop Belg.* 1994;60:389-292.

32. Dent CM, Patil M, Fairclough JA. Arthroscopic ankle arthrodesis. *J Bone Joint Surg Br.* 1993;75:830-832.

33. Ogilvie-Harris DJ, Lieberman I, Fitsialos D. Arthroscopically assisted arthrodesis for osteoarthritic ankles. *J Bone Joint Surg Am.* 1993;75:1167-1174.

34. Saragas N. Results of arthroscopic arthrodesis of the ankle. *Foot Ankle Surg.* 2004;10:141-143.

35. Turan I, Wredmark T, Fellander-Tsai L. Arthroscopic ankle arthrodesis in rheumatoid arthritis. *Clin Orthop Relat Res.* 1995(320):110-114.

36. Zvijac JE, Lemak L, Schurhoff MR, et al. Analysis of arthroscopically assisted ankle arthrodesis. *Arthroscopy.* 2002;18:70-75.

37. Amendola A, Lee KB, Saltzman CL, Suh JS. Technique and early experience with posterior arthroscopic subtalar arthrodesis. *Foot Ankle Int.* 2007;28:298-302.

SUGGESTED READING

Sitler DF, Amendola A, Bailey CS, et al. Posterior ankle arthroscopy: an anatomic study. *J Bone Joint Surg Am.* 2002;84A:763-769.

Arthroscopic Fusion for Degenerative Arthritis of the Subtalar Joint

James P. Tasto ● John H. Brady

Arthrodesis of the subtalar joint is an accepted treatment option for many problems of the hindfoot, such as post-traumatic and primary arthritis, posterior tibial tendon dysfunction, symptomatic congenital deformities, and inflammatory arthritis.[1-3] Although sometimes viewed as a salvage procedure, results from subtalar fusions have been reported to be good or excellent in many patients.[4-6]

Historically, several other procedures for subtalar pathology have been described, including arthroscopy, arthroplasty, triple arthrodesis, and sinus tarsi exploration. Open reduction and internal fixation of calcaneal fractures has gained acceptance because the procedure aims to restore the normal anatomic alignment of the joint surfaces in an effort to avoid the sequelae of post-traumatic, degenerative subtalar arthritis. However, surgical and nonsurgical approaches to calcaneal fractures continue to be plagued with long-term changes in the subtalar joint, including post-traumatic degenerative arthritis and arthrofibrosis.

The many advantages of isolated subtalar arthrodesis compared with triple arthrodesis and other salvage procedures have been recognized. The major advantage of isolated fusion compared with triple arthrodesis or pantalar arthrodesis is that isolated subtalar fusion preserves motion in adjacent joints.[7] In a study of 48 isolated subtalar arthrodeses, Mann found that preserving motion of the transverse tarsal joints decreased the incidence of clinically significant symptoms of arthritis.[6]

ANATOMY

The subtalar joint is composed of three articulations: the posterior, middle, and anterior joints or facets (Figs. 18-1 and 18-2). Several extra-articular ligaments stabilize the subtalar joint. The major ligaments encountered during subtalar arthroscopy are the intra-articular components, which consist of the interosseous, lateral, and anterior talocalcaneal ligaments. These components coalesce to form the division between the posterior and the middle facets of the subtalar joint. The interosseous ligament is a broad, stout structure that

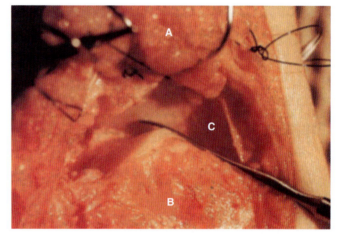

FIGURE 18-1 Gross dissection of the lateral posterior subtalar joint shows the talus (A), calcaneus (B), and subtalar joint (C).

is approximately 2.5 cm wide from its medial to lateral side. It marks the arthroscopic boundary for posterior subtalar arthroscopy.

Open subtalar arthrodesis has historically been the fusion method of choice, and results have generally been favorable. Studies reporting the results of open fusion techniques have all described similar results for fusion rate, time to union, and complications, such as nonunion or malunion, infection, and symptomatic hardware problems.[8-12] Open procedures entail removal of the interosseous ligaments and their vasculature and a lateral incision that can result in nerve dysfunction. Nonunion rates of 5% to 16% have been reported.[4,6] The successful results of arthroscopic ankle fusion have stimulated the development of an arthroscopic approach for subtalar joint arthrodesis, which has the advantages of reduced perioperative morbidity and preservation of the blood supply.[13-15]

Arthroscopic subtalar arthrodesis was designed to improve traditional methods by using a minimally invasive technique. Subtalar arthroscopy has been described by several investigators, but few

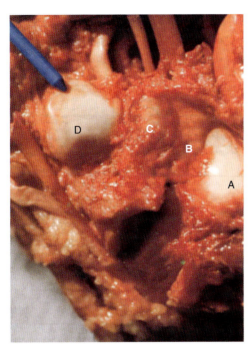

FIGURE 18-2 A view of the posterior subtalar joint shows the undersurface of the talus (A), the middle facet of the talus (B), the anterior facet of the talus (C), and the superior surface of calcaneus (D).

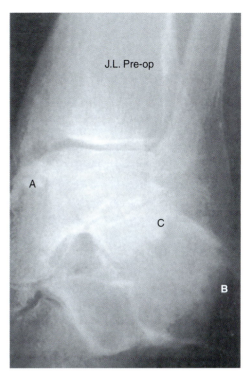

FIGURE 18-3 A Broden view of an arthritic posterior subtalar joint shows the talus (A), the calcaneus (B), and the subtalar joint (C).

reports of arthroscopic subtalar fusion have been published.[16] The development of an arthroscopic technique for subtalar arthrodesis was intended to lower morbidity using techniques and principles similar to those used for arthroscopic ankle fusion. It was hypothesized that perioperative morbidity could be reduced, blood supply preserved, and proprioceptive and neurosensory input enhanced. These theoretical advantages prompted us to initiate a prospective study to document the effectiveness of the procedure and to determine the time until complete fusion, the incidence of delayed unions and nonunions, and the incidence of complications.

PATIENT EVALUATION

History and Physical Examination

Subtalar pathology is often difficult to diagnose. The patient may have a history of lateral hindfoot pain that can easily be confused with ankle pathology. A clue that helps direct the clinician toward subtalar pathology is an increase in symptoms with weight bearing or ambulating on uneven terrain. A history of calcaneal fracture should immediately alert the physician to the possibility of subtalar pathology. Clinical findings consist of pain over the sinus tarsi and the posterolateral subtalar joint. Physical examination may reproduce these symptoms with inversion and eversion of the subtalar joint with the ankle locked in dorsiflexion. Differential injections continue to be a valuable diagnostic tool to confirm and distinguish ankle pain from subtalar pain.

Diagnostic Imaging

Evaluation for subtalar pathology should include plain radiographs of the ankle and subtalar joints. The Broden view pro-

vides the best visualization of the posterior subtalar joint and may be sufficient to confirm the diagnosis of subtalar pathology (Fig.18-3). Profound degenerative radiographic changes in the joint are not needed to confirm a diagnosis, because only small alterations in the biomechanics of this joint can produce significant symptoms. Computerized tomography (CT) is best able to define the bony anatomy, and with thin sections, scanning reconstructions in the axial, coronal, and sagittal planes can be performed. Magnetic resonance imaging (MRI) can be used to confirm associated bony changes such as subchondral bone edema and may be useful in evaluating the adjacent soft tissues to rule out other causes of hindfoot pain. Bone scanning and arthrography are usually not required, and these studies have largely been replaced by MRI.

TREATMENT

Indications and Contraindications

Arthroscopic subtalar arthrodesis is indicated for patients with intractable subtalar pain from a variety of conditions. Most of the earlier literature on subtalar surgery addressed the stabilization of paralytic deformities caused by poliomyelitis. However, most patients currently requiring this procedure have post-traumatic and primary arthritic conditions. A small number of patients who require subtalar arthrodesis have posterior tibial tendon dysfunction or a talocalcaneal coalition.

The contraindications to arthroscopic subtalar arthrodesis include prior failed subtalar fusions, gross malalignment requiring correction, infection, and significant bone loss. A patient with moderate malalignment may be a candidate for in situ stabilization. Although significant bone loss has not frequently been encountered, moderate bone loss has not presented a serious problem in a study of arthroscopic ankle arthrodesis.[15]

Conservative Management

Severe subtalar joint pain should initially be treated conservatively with nonsurgical treatments. Conservative treatments include orthotics, nonsteroidal anti-inflammatory drugs, activity modification, and corticosteroid injections into the subtalar joint. Patients who have not been successfully treated with nonsurgical management may be considered for arthroscopic subtalar fusion. These individuals should also be advised that an open procedure may still be indicated if the arthroscopic approach is found to be unsafe or not technically feasible.

Arthroscopic Technique

Our preferred method begins by placing the patient in the lateral decubitus position and lying on the unaffected side. We place two pillows between the legs while the affected ankle and subtalar joint hang over a blanket roll in a natural position of plantar flexion and neutral version. The patient is prepared and draped, after which the anatomic landmarks and portal sites are identified and marked with a surgical pen. A thigh tourniquet is then inflated.

Establishing the portal sites is one of the more challenging aspects of the procedure. It is critical to predetermine the angles of the subtalar joint, because its unique geometry and limited access requires precise determination to prevent error. Fluoroscopy should be used to confirm portal location if necessary.

The anterolateral and the posterolateral portals are conventionally used. An accessory portal usually needs to be established approximately 1 cm posterior to the anterolateral portal (Fig. 18-4).

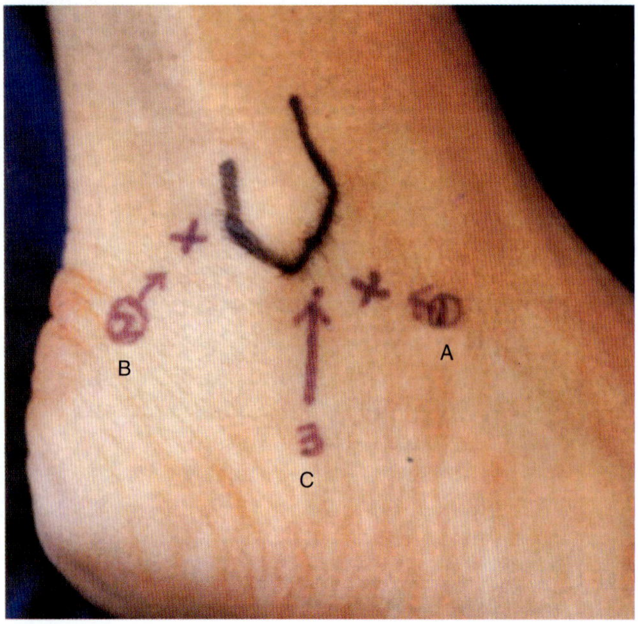

This portal can be used for debridement or for outflow enhancement and may occasionally be used for visualization. The anterolateral and posterolateral portals are used in an alternating manner for viewing and for instrumentation. If significant arthrofibrosis makes entry and visualization difficult, the accessory anterolateral portal is quite useful.

A 2.7-mm, wide-angle, small joint arthroscope should be used for this procedure. It should be equipped with a choice of sheaths to accommodate limited or increased flow. The blunt trocar and sheath are introduced through the anterolateral portal. The posterolateral portal can be established at this time, as can an accessory anterolateral portal. In patients who were initially treated with this procedure, a small laminar spreader was used in the anterolateral portal to increase access. This technique is no longer routinely used, but may be useful if subtalar joint distraction is a problem. Arthroscopic resection of the interosseous ligament also may provide additional distraction.

It is important to confirm that the arthroscope is in the subtalar joint and that the ankle joint or the fibular talar recess have not been inadvertently entered. All débridement and decortication is done posterior to the interosseous ligament because only the posterior facet is fused (Fig. 18-5). The middle and anterior facets are not seen under normal circumstances unless the interosseous ligament is absent. Most of the procedure is performed with the arthroscope in the anterolateral portal and the instruments in the posterolateral portal. The remaining débridement is accomplished by alternating the use of these portals.

At the beginning of the procedure, a primary synovectomy and debridement are necessary for visualization, usually through the accessory anterolateral portal (Fig. 18-6). The articular surface is debrided, making the joint more capacious and making the use of instrumentation easier. Complete removal of the articular surface down to subchondral bone is performed next (Figs. 18-7 and 18-8). The unique talocalcaneal geometry requires a variety of instruments, including straight and angled curettes and a complete set of shavers and burrs.

FIGURE 18-4 Standard portal placement for subtalar arthrodesis includes the anterolateral portal (A), posterolateral portal (B), and accessory lateral portal (C).

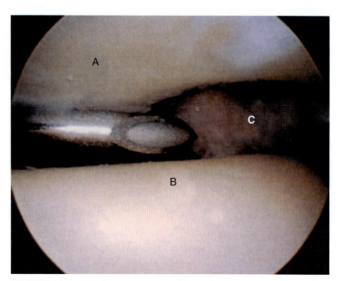

FIGURE 18-5 An arthroscopic view of the subtalar joint shows the talus (A), calcaneus (B), and posteromedial corner (C).

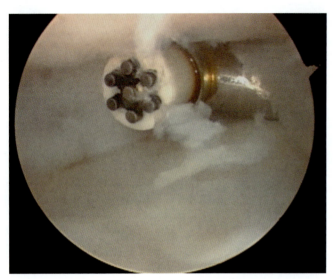

FIGURE 18-6 Electrocautery is used for soft tissue débridement of the subtalar joint. The scope is viewing from the anterolateral portal, and the electrocautery device is working through the posterolateral portal.

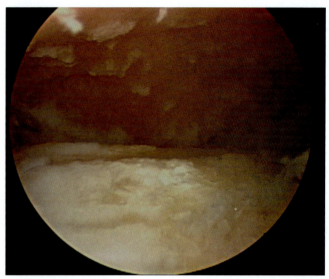

FIGURE 18-8 The subtalar joint is ready for arthrodesis after soft tissue and bony decortication.

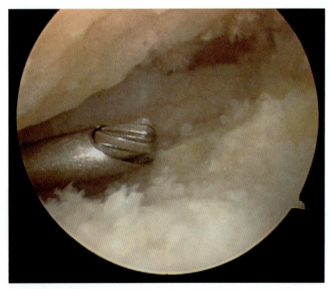

FIGURE 18-7 The remaining articular cartilage within the subtalar joint is removed with an arthroscopic burr. The scope is viewing from the posterolateral portal, and the burr is working through the anterolateral portal.

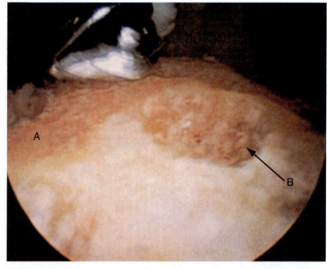

FIGURE 18-9 The superior surface of the calcaneus (A) is shown after decortication and "spot welding" (B).

After the articular cartilage has been resected, approximately 1 to 2 mm of subchondral bone is removed to expose the highly vascular cancellous bone. Care must be taken not to alter the articular surface geometry and not to remove excessive bone because this will lead to poor coaptation of the joint surfaces. After the subchondral plate is removed, small "spot-weld" holes approximately 2 mm deep are fashioned on the surfaces of the calcaneus and talus to create vascular channels (Fig. 18-9). Careful assessment of the posteromedial corner must be made, because residual bone and cartilage can interfere with talocalcaneal coaptation. The curette often safely breaks down this corner and can provide the surgeon with tactile feedback. The neurovascular bundle is located in the posteromedial corner, and it must be protected throughout the procedure.

After viewing from both portals to ensure complete débridement and decortication, the tourniquet is released, and the vascularity of the calcaneus and talus is carefully assessed. The joint is then thoroughly irrigated to remove bone fragments and debris. Autogenous bone graft or bone substitute are not needed for this procedure.

The fusion is fixed with a large, cannulated, 7.5-mm screw. The guide pin is started at the dorsal anteromedial talus and angled posterior and inferior to the posterolateral calcaneus; however, it does not violate the calcaneal cortical surface. Using fluoroscopy, the guidewire is placed with the ankle in maximum dorsiflexion to avoid screw head encroachment or impingement on the anterior lip of the tibia (Fig. 18-10). After the guidewire is placed, the ankle

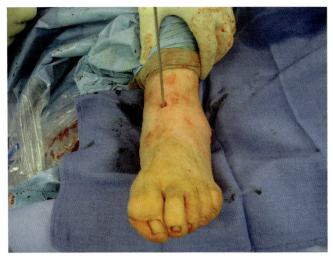

FIGURE 18-10 A guidewire is passed through the subtalar joint in an anterior to posterior direction in preparation for screw fixation.

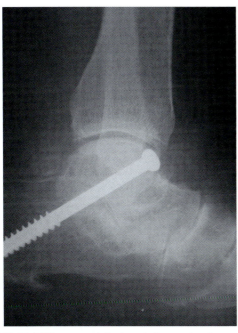

FIGURE 18-11 A 7.3-mm, partially threaded, cannulated screw is used to achieve fixation across the subtalar joint.

can be relaxed, the screw inserted under fluoroscopic control, and the fusion site compressed (Fig. 18-11). The screw runs along the natural axis of rotation of the subtalar joint using this technique. Starting the screw from the dorsal and medial aspect of the talus avoids painful screw head prominence over the calcaneus and reduces the need for a second procedure to remove the screw. There have been no fractures or complications with this particular fixation technique.[15] An alternate method of fixation uses a single screw placed from the calcaneus into the talus in the appropriate direction.

PEARLS & PITFALLS

PEARLS

- Extensive synovectomy may be necessary to establish visualization. Triangulate the arthroscope in the anterolateral portal and a shaver in the accessory portal. Touch the shaver to the shaft of the scope and walk the shaver to the tip of the scope. Shave the synovium to establish the space.
- Have a selection of straight and angled curettes in an assortment of sizes to approach all portions of the articular surface.
- Do not get bogged down in one area. Move the scope and instruments to access all areas of the joint.
- Débride only the subchondral bone to the level of viable bleeding bone, which is documented by deflating the tourniquet and visualizing punctate bleeding. Maintain the normal contours of the joint surfaces to maximize the surface area of joint coaptation.

PITFALLS

- Be certain that the degenerative problem is limited to the subtalar joint by thoroughly reviewing plain radiographs and correlating with a CT or MRI. The presence of significant talonavicular or calcaneocuboid arthritis requires triple arthrodesis rather than isolated subtalar arthrodesis.
- Use differential diagnostic injections into the ankle joint and subtalar joint to ensure that the problem is limited to the subtalar joint.
- Assess for a fixed hindfoot deformity, which may require an osteotomy to realign the hindfoot. Persistent hindfoot deformity results in failure to relieve clinical symptoms and may result in transfer of stress to other parts of the foot and ankle.

Postoperative Rehabilitation Protocol

Sterile adhesive wound closure strips are used instead of sutures to allow adequate drainage. A bulky dressing and a short-leg bivalved cast are applied. The patient is discharged from the surgical center and may return home after appropriate circulatory checks are completed in the recovery room.

The first clinical evaluation takes place in the physician's office within 48 hours. At approximately 1 week postoperatively, the cast is removed, and the patient is fitted with an ankle-foot orthosis (AFO) if swelling is minimal. Full weight bearing is permitted and encouraged immediately after surgery. In general, patients can tolerate full weight bearing without crutch support within 7 to 14 days after surgery. Patients should wear the AFO 24 hours per day, except for bathing and exercising the ankle and foot through a range of motion without the brace. The brace is removed when full union has been achieved. For follow-up assessment, the standard three views of the ankle plus a Broden view are the radiographs of choice.

RESULTS OF TREATMENT AND COMPLICATIONS

Since September 1992, we have followed 25 consecutive patients undergoing arthroscopic subtalar fusion, and there has been sufficient follow-up time to determine the effectiveness of the procedure. Fusion rate, time until complete union, surgical technique,

and the complication rate were analyzed. One standard surgical procedure was used, and the method of internal fixation was consistent throughout this study. The posterior subtalar joint was the only joint fused during this procedure. Three of the 25 patients had a combined arthroscopic ankle and subtalar fusion. In this study, 8 patients had osteoarthritis, 10 had post-traumatic arthritis, 4 had posterior tibial tendon dysfunction, 2 had rheumatoid arthritis, and 1 patient had a talocalcaneal coalition. Every patient had a radiographic evaluation at 2-week intervals to determine the rate and quality of fusion. Clinical and radiographic forms of evidence were required to categorize an arthrodesis as completely fused. The parameters required for a successful arthrodesis are evidence of bone consolidation across the subtalar joint, no motion at the screw, the absence of pain with weight bearing, and pain-free forced inversion and eversion. The mean follow-up time was 22 months (range, 6 to 92 months). The subtalar joint of all 25 patients had united clinically and radiographically; the average time until complete fusion was 8.9 weeks (range, 6 to 16 weeks).[15]

There have been no additional operations, with the exception of two screw removals. Two patients had some residual anterolateral pain with some radiographic and clinical evidence of minor degenerative joint disease in the ankle. These findings were documented on preoperative films. One patient had complete pain relief after a diagnostic and therapeutic steroid and lidocaine injection into the ankle joint. One patient eventually underwent arthroscopic ankle arthrodesis because of preexisting osteoarthritis of the ankle. Valgus tilting of the ankle joint after subtalar arthrodesis has been reported, but it is unclear whether this results from the fusion or is merely a natural progression of the disease (TC Fitzgibbons, MD, Dublin, Ireland, personal communication, 1995).

Two patients are not included in this study because the procedure could not be completed arthroscopically because of significant malformation of the calcaneus and arthrofibrosis of the subtalar joint. These patients underwent a modified mini-open posterior subtalar arthrodesis. Identical screw fixation and postoperative protocol was used in these two patients. Skin complications about the hindfoot can be catastrophic and are minimized using the arthroscopic technique. No patients in this study had superficial or deep infections. All arthroscopic procedures have been associated with reduced rates of infection. Those who favor arthroscopic subtalar arthrodesis believe that the same trends seen in other arthroscopic procedures will be demonstrated for the subtalar joint.

COMPARISON OF PROCEDURES

Arthroscopic subtalar fusion has many advantages compared with open procedures. It is a minimally invasive technique that theoretically preserves the blood supply of the calcaneus and talus, which is especially important because many of these patients have had previous open procedures. Conventional open procedures by definition interrupt the blood supply and compromise vascular ingrowth and eventual fusion. Avoidance of incisions coupled with early range of motion and weight bearing helps to avoid stress depravation and enhances proprioception, reducing the devastating effects of complex regional pain syndrome.

Glanzmann conducted a prospective analysis of 41 consecutive arthroscopic subtalar arthrodeses. The average modified American Orthopaedic Foot and Ankle Society (AOFAS) ankle-hindfoot score improved from 53 points (range, 22 to 69) preoperatively to 84 points (range, 41 to 94) at the final follow-up assessment (average, 55 months). Union was achieved in all cases.[17] These data echo the results demonstrated by Tasto and colleagues,[22] showing reproducible excellent results with arthroscopic subtalar fusion.

In a comparison of open and arthroscopic isolated subtalar arthrodesis, Scranton reported a union rate of 100% in the five arthroscopic procedures and one nonunion in the 17 open procedures.[12] This was a small study with limited statistical power, and a larger, prospective, randomized trial is needed before a direct comparison of open versus arthroscopic subtalar arthrodesis can be made. However, some studies show a trend toward higher fusion rates with the use of arthroscopic procedures. Easley and coworkers[4] reported a union rate of 84% for 148 patients who had isolated open subtalar arthrodesis, compared with the 100% rate of union in the two arthroscopic studies performed by Tasto and Glanzmann.[22] Smoking, the presence of more than 2 mm of avascular bone at the arthrodesis site, and the failure of a previous operative procedure were identified as factors contributing to a less favorable union rate.[4] Perhaps the observed higher fusion rate in the arthroscopic cohort reflects the preservation of the blood supply and the ability to initiate early weight bearing. One disadvantage of arthroscopic subtalar arthrodesis is that it requires a high level of experience in ankle and subtalar arthroscopy.

In the original technique for arthroscopic subtalar arthrodesis reported by Tasto,[22] the arthroscope enters the subtalar joint from the lateral position. This approach has been demonstrated to be safe and reliable.[15] Amendola has added to the literature by describing a posterior arthroscopic subtalar arthrodesis.[18,19]

There are advantages to prone positioning. Parisien and Vagsness[14] found that posterior lesions and loose bodies were seen and treated more effectively through two posterior portals when the limb was situated prone. There is concern, however, that the tibial nerve, the posterior tibial artery, and the medial calcaneal nerve are at risk when the posteromedial portal is used.[20-23] Voto and colleagues[23] found that the posteromedial portal is "potentially hazardous" even if placed adjacent to the Achilles tendon. Ferkel[21] reported a series of 612 ankle arthroscopies with a neurologic complication rate of 4.4%. He recommended against use of anterocentral, trans-Achilles, and posteromedial portals.

Acevedo and coworkers[24] demonstrated that coaxial posteromedial and posterolateral portals were safe, effective, and reproducible. Sitler and colleagues,[25] in a cadaver study with the limb prone, demonstrated an average distance between the posteromedial portal and the tibial nerve, posterior tibial artery, and medial calcaneal nerve of 6.4 mm, 9.6 mm, and 17.1 mm, respectively. Based on these results, some consider the posteromedial portal to be safe, provided it is kept directly adjacent to the Achilles tendon and the patient is in the prone position.

CONCLUSIONS

Although open subtalar arthrodesis has historically proved to be safe and effective, the arthroscopic approach offers several advantages, including lower morbidity, preservation of the interosseous ligaments and vascularity, shorter hospital stay, early weight bearing, faster rehabilitation, and a better fusion rate. However, arthroscopic subtalar arthrodesis is a technically demanding procedure that requires advanced arthroscopic skills. Subtalar joint access is more difficult than other joints because of the complex, curved articular surfaces held by tight ligaments, and it requires the use of small joint instrumentation. Because deformities cannot be corrected using this arthroscopic technique, the procedure must be considered only for fusion in situ. There are relatively few patients who qualify for this procedure, and the learning curve for improving surgical skills is steep. Cadaveric surgical skills workshops are the most efficacious method of mastering this technique.

The results of arthroscopic subtalar arthrodesis appear to be excellent in terms of patient satisfaction, fusion rate, time until union, and postoperative morbidity. Continued research is needed to compare open and arthroscopic techniques, determine the safest and most reliable arthroscopic approach, and promote continuing education to help surgeons master these important skills.

REFERENCES

1. Goldner JL, Poletti SC, Gates HS, Richardson W. Severe open subtalar dislocations. *J Bone Joint Surg Am.* 1995;77A:1075-1079.
2. Huang PJ, Fu YC, Cheng YM, Lin SY. Subtalar arthrodesis for late sequelae of calcaneal fractures: fusion in situ versus fusion with sliding corrective osteotomy. *Foot Ankle Int.* 1999;20:166-170.
3. Rammelt S, Zwipp H. Calcaneus fractures: facts, controversies and recent developments. *Injury.* 2004;35:443-461.
4. Easley ME, Trnka HJ, Schon LC, Myerson MS. Isolated subtalar arthrodesis. *J Bone Joint Surg Am.* 2000;82A:613-624.
5. Lundeen RO. Arthroscopic fusion of the ankle and subtalar joint. *Clin Podiatr Med Surg.* 1994;11:395-306.
6. Mann RA, Beaman DN, Horton GA. Isolated subtalar arthrodesis. *Foot Ankle Int.* 1998;19:511-519.
7. Stroud CC. Arthroscopic arthrodesis of the ankle, subtalar, and first metatarsophalangeal joint. *Foot Ankle Clin.* 2002;7:135-146.
8. Amendola A, Lammens P. Subtalar arthrodesis using interposition iliac crest bone graft after calcaneal fracture. *Foot Ankle Int.* 1996;17:608-614.
9. Buch BD, Myerson MS, Miller SD. Primary arthrodesis for the treatment of comminuted calcaneal fractures. *Foot Ankle Int.* 1996;17:61-70.
10. Crosby LA, Yee TC, Formanek TS, Fitzgibbons TC. Complications following arthroscopic ankle arthrodesis. *Foot Ankle Int.* 1996;17:340-342.
11. Dahm DL, Kitaoka HB. Subtalar arthrodesis with internal compression for post-traumatic arthritis. *J Bone Joint Surg Br.* 1998;80B:134-138.
12. Scranton PE. Comparison of open isolated subtalar arthrodesis with autogenous bone graft versus outpatient arthroscopic subtalar arthrodesis using injectable bone morphogenic protein-enhanced graft. *Foot Ankle Int.* 1999;20:162-165.
13. Godberger MI, Conti SF. Clinical outcome after subtalar arthroscopy. *Foot Ankle Int.* 1998;19:462-465.
14. Parisien JS, Vangsness T. Arthroscopy of the subtalar joint: an experimental approach. *Arthroscopy.* 1985;1:53-57.
15. Tasto JP, Frey C, Laimans P, et al. Arthroscopic ankle arthrodesis. *Instr Course Lect.* 2000;49:259-280.
16. Ferkel RA. *Arthroscopic Surgery: The Foot and Ankle.* Philadelphia, PA: Lippincott-Raven; 1996.
17. Glanzmann MC, Sanhueza-Hernandez R. Arthroscopic subtalar arthrodesis for symptomatic osteoarthritis of the hindfoot. *Foot Ankle Int.* 2007;28:2-7.
18. Amendola A, Lee KB, Saltzman CL, Sub JS. Technique and early experience with posterior arthroscopic subtalar arthrodesis. *Foot Ankle Int.* 2007;28:298-302.
19. Lee KB, Saltzman CL, Suh JS, et al. A posterior 3 portal arthroscopic approach for isolated subtalar arthrodesis. *Arthroscopy.* 2008;24:1306-1310.
20. Feiwell LA, Frey C. Anatomic study of arthroscopic portal sites of the ankle. *Foot Ankle.* 1993;14:142-147.
21. Ferkel RD. Complications in ankle and foot arthroscopy. In: Ferkel RD, Whipple TL, eds. *Arthroscopic Surgery: The Foot and Ankle.* Philadelphia, PA; Lippincott-Raven; 1996:291-304.
22. Tasto JP. Subtalar arthroscopy. In: McGinty JB, Burkhart SS, Jackson RW, et al, eds. *Operative Arthroscopy.* 3rd ed. New York: Lippincott Williams & Wilkins; 2002:944-952.
23. Voto SJ, Ewing JW, Fleissner PR. Ankle arthroscopy: neurovascular and arthroscopic anatomy of standard and trans-Achilles tendon portal placement. *Arthroscopy.* 1989;5:41-46.
24. Acevedo JI, Busch MT, Ganey TM, et al. Coaxial portals for posterior ankle arthroscopy: an anatomic study with clinical correlation on 29 patients. *Arthroscopy.* 2000;16:836-842.
25. Sitler DF, Amendola A, Bailey CS, et al. Posterior ankle arthroscopy: an anatomic study. *J Bone Joint Surg Am.* 2002;84A:763-769.

SUGGESTED READINGS

Ferkel RD. Subtalar arthroscopy. In: Whipple TL ed. *Arthroscopic Surgery: The Foot and Ankle.* Philadelphia, PA: Lippincott-Raven; 1996:231-254.
Frey C, Gasser S, Feder K. Arthroscopy of the subtalar joint. *Foot Ankle Int.* 1994;15:424-428.

Complex Ankle, Subtalar, and Triple Fusions

Alastair S.E. Younger

Arthroscopy allows surgeons to perform foot and ankle procedures that would otherwise be contraindicated because of the risks of an open approach. Although early in their development and more time-consuming than their open counterparts, combined arthroscopic subtalar and ankle fusion and arthroscopic triple arthrodesis have increasing roles to play in treating complex conditions in patients who are not candidates for an open procedure.

Arthroscopic ankle arthrodesis can be extended to include cases with some bone deformity or extensive osteophyte formation if the surgeon is patient and experienced with simpler cases.[1] These cases should be performed after the surgeon has achieved proficiency with arthroscopic ankle and subtalar fusion. When the soft tissue envelope is compromised, the additional time required for the more complex operation may be justified by the prevention of soft tissue complications.

NORMAL AND PATHOLOGIC ANATOMY

Anatomic considerations are addressed in Chapter 17. Talonavicular arthritis with deformity or subtalar arthritis is a clear indication for triple arthrodesis. Isolated talonavicular arthritis may be amenable to isolated talonavicular fusion. However, an isolated talonavicular fusion is more likely to progress to a nonunion because there may be motion across the joint despite two screws being used for fixation. Because no significant gain in motion is achieved with an isolated talonavicular fusion compared with a full triple arthrodesis, a triple arthrodesis may be preferable because a larger fusion mass is obtained and better stabilization performed.

Usually, these procedures are performed open. However, for patients with bleeding problems (e.g., hemophilia), poor wound healing, or preexisting scar, a less invasive procedure may be preferable. For patients with anticipated wound-healing problems who are not candidates for an open procedure, an arthroscopic fusion is an ideal alternative.

PATIENT EVALUATION
History and Physical Examination
Location of Pain

To allow the patient to correctly identify the area of discomfort, both feet and ankles should be exposed during the physical examination. Patients with isolated ankle arthritis present with pain localized anteriorly in the ankle between the malleoli. Swelling may occur in the same area, and the pain is localized above and between the tips of the malleoli.

Talonavicular joint pain is localized anterior to the ankle and malleoli and down toward the tuberosity of the navicular. Swelling occurs anterior to the ankle and onto the dorsum of the foot. Because the superior joint margin of the talonavicular joint is only 1 to 2 cm in front of the anterior margin of the ankle joint, talonavicular arthritis can be confused with ankle arthritis.

Subtalar joint pain is localized in the sinus tarsi inferior to the lateral malleolus. Medially, pain is localized directly inferior to the medial malleolus.

Degree of Disability

Patients should be assessed for their degree of disability. Their walking tolerance and standing tolerance are good indicators of disability. They might have had to stop work because of the hindfoot pain. Sports might have been permanently discontinued or restricted due to pain or instability. Before treatment, the degree of disability should be outlined to determine success of intervention.

Comorbidities

Patients with hemophilia should be followed closely by the hematologist if surgery is contemplated. Their ability to be anticoagulated before and after surgery should be assessed.

Patients with rheumatoid arthritis should be optimized with regard to medical treatment. Other joint involvement should be assessed and the degree of associated disability known. Only in exceptional circumstances should the foot or ankle undergo fusion if another joint is more symptomatic.

Extra-articular manifestations of rheumatoid arthritis include iritis, cardiomyopathy, conduction delays, respiratory disease, and skin breakdown. A systemic evaluation is required.

Physical Examination

Both extremities should be exposed to the knee. While standing, alignment of the hindfoot and forefoot is assessed from behind and in front of the patient.

Gait is observed, concentrating on stance and swing phases. Pain is associated with a reduced stance phase on the painful side and failure to toe-off. On inspection, the location and size of scars, calluses, and ulcers are recorded.

Palpation is used to determine the area of maximum tenderness. In ankle arthritis, this is localized on the anterior and posterior joint margins between the malleoli. For the subtalar joint, the pain is under the fibula, toward the sinus tarsi, behind and inferior to the ankle, and under the medial malleolus. For the talonavicular joint, tenderness is localized medially behind and above the navicular tubercle and just anterior to the ankle joint.

Assessing range-of-motion deficits may assist in determining the painful joints. To isolate the ankle, the examiner should move the talus on the tibia and palpate the joint margin at the same time. For the subtalar joint, the calcaneus is moved on the talus, and for the talonavicular joint, the navicular is moved on the talus. Absolute motion is difficult to measure, but pain and loss of motion (i.e., normal, mild, moderate, or severe restriction) is more instructive than the actual degree of motion.

Special tests include a single-leg heel raise to determine the integrity of the tibialis posterior tendon and the foot's ability to act as a lever arm. Pulses and sensation should be assessed and recorded.

Diagnostic Imaging

Standing anteroposterior and lateral views of the ankle and foot should be obtained if the patient has hindfoot arthritis. For ankle arthritis, the status of the talonavicular joint should be determined on an anteroposterior view of the foot. An ankle fusion may increase the load on a compromised joint and lead to symptoms. Similarly, the condition of the ankle joint should be determined if a triple arthrodesis is considered.

If the plain radiographs do not clearly identify the status of these joints, helical computed tomography (CT) is the appropriate imaging technique to better define the anatomy of the hindfoot. Occasionally, magnetic resonance imaging (MRI) can be performed, but it tends to be oversensitive for this assessment. Single photon emission computed tomography (SPECT) can assist in defining the precise location of bone turnover in patients with undiagnosed pain.

Differential local anesthetic blocks are beneficial. However, care should be taken in their interpretation, because there may be flow between joints that confuses the result.

TREATMENT

Indications and Contraindications

Combined arthroscopic ankle and subtalar fusion is indicated for the patient with combined symptomatic ankle and subtalar arthritis with a risk of soft tissue complications. These patients may have post-traumatic arthritis with extensive soft tissue damage, hemophiliac arthropathy of the ankle and subtalar joints, or rheumatoid arthritis with a history of poor wound healing. Patients with scleroderma are also at risk for wound healing problems, and they may benefit from an arthroscopic approach. Patients with psoriatic arthritis with plaques around the ankle are at risk for wound complications and can benefit from an arthroscopic procedure.

Patients with arthritis of the talonavicular joint in isolation or with other hindfoot involvement may benefit from an arthroscopic talonavicular or arthroscopic triple arthrodesis. The indications for patients at risk for wound healing complications are the same as outlined previously.

Many patients have contraindications for these procedures. Major bone defects require grafting or osteotomies, and an arthroscopic procedure is not possible. Patients with avascular necrosis require bone resection of an amount that cannot be performed through the arthroscope. Patients with Charcot arthropathy have a combination of bone defect and avascular necrosis that requires resection beyond the capabilities of arthroscopy.

Conservative Management

Nonoperative treatment of ankle and hindfoot arthritis involves activity modification, bracing and orthotics, analgesia, or a combination of these methods. Activity modification may include the use of a cane and avoiding activities that cause discomfort.

Braces beneficial in hindfoot arthritis should reduce the range of motion of the affected joint. Some may be designed to also off load the limb. An off-the-shelf ankle-stabilizing brace is a cost-effective start. If this fails, a custom brace, ankle-foot orthotic, or Richie Brace may assist in reducing motion and correcting any associated deformity. Orthotics can correct the foot shape and reduce impingement or eccentric loading. The orthotic can be combined with a brace (e.g., Richie Brace).

Complex Arthroscopic Ankle Fusion

Bone Deformity

When there is erosion of the medial or lateral side of the joint, a standard arthroscopic fusion can be performed and augmented by correction of the deformity by sculpting of the prominent side of the joint with a burr to allow correction of the varus or valgus plane deformity. Removal of some of the tip of the medial or lateral malleolus may be required to allow joint compression. The edge of the bone deformity often is located within the joint and can indicate where to start applying the burr to reduce the deformity. The degree of bone removal can be estimated using intraoperative fluoroscopy.

After correction is achieved in the varus and valgus plane, the talus can be corrected using a Kirschner wire or drill from the lateral or medial malleolus. Any defect left gapping on one side can be filled with bone graft or bone graft substitute. A screw is first placed through the malleolus to the talus to hold the correction, and the opposite side of the ankle is compressed with two or three compression screws.

Extensive Osteophyte Formation

In cases with extensive osteophyte formation, the joint may be difficult to instrument with an arthroscope. This situation usually requires an open procedure, but in cases in which the soft tissue complications may merit arthroscopic fusion, it can be performed. However access to the joint may take some time and patience.

Osteophytes can be identified for removal by fluoroscopy before arthroscopy (Fig. 19-1). The osteophytes can be removed through the standard anteromedial and anterolateral arthroscopic portals using a small metatarsal osteotome. The bone fragments must be removed with care so as not to damage the deep branch of the peroneal nerve or its superficial branches. Alternatively, a 3.5- to 4.0-mm, round burr may be used from the medial and lateral approaches to remove the bone spurs under direct visualization. It may be useful to decrease the joint distraction and to dorsiflex the ankle, which allows the anterior joint capsule to relax during removal of anterior tibial and talar neck osteophytes.

The Tight Joint

In some cases, the tight ankle cannot be easily accessed for an arthroscopic fusion. After release of the osteophytes as described

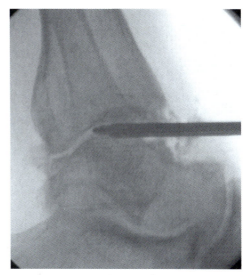

FIGURE 19-2 The C-arm is used to identify the joint line during arthroscopy in a tight joint (same patient as in Fig. 19-1).

earlier, the joint may have to be instrumented with the assistance of fluoroscopy. The joint line can be hard to find, and gradual opening of the joint is required until the arthroscope can be inserted (Fig. 19-2).

Combined Arthroscopic Ankle and Subtalar Fusion

Arthritic ankle and subtalar joints can be fused simultaneously. Fixation can be achieved by using a combination of lag screws or a retrograde intramedullary nail. Use of the arthroscope reduces considerably the size of wounds and therefore the potential for postoperative bleeding complications.

Instrumentation

A 2.7-mm-diameter arthroscope works well for the ankle joint but may be a tight fit for the subtalar fusion, and a 1.9-mm-diameter arthroscope should be available. It is useful to have arthroscopes with 30- and 70-degree viewing angles available for small joint arthroscopy. Otherwise, the surgeon should have a 3.5-mm shaver and a selection of small, straight and angled curettes available. These instruments usually fit the ankle and subtalar joints. Intraoperative fluoroscopy is essential for the procedure.

Technique

The patient is positioned on the operating table with the hip on the surgical side elevated to allow access to the lateral ankle and subtalar joint (Fig. 19-3).[3] Distraction can be performed using an external distraction device to improve access to the joint. Alternatively, distraction can be performed for the ankle fusion using an Ace Wrap around the surgeon's waist.

The ankle joint is approached first. The anteromedial and anterolateral portals are used to débride the anterior ankle joint. Posterior débridement requires a posterior portal. I use a portal just behind the medial malleolus. Anatomic dissections have documented that this portal passes posterior to the tibialis posterior tendon and usually passes anterior to the flexor digitorum longus. Alternatively, a

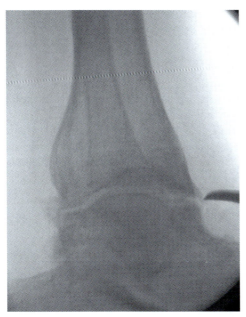

FIGURE 19-1 C-arm view shows osteophyte removal before arthroscopy in a tight joint.

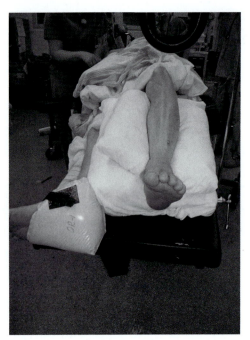

FIGURE 19-3 Positioning is shown for arthroscopic ankle and subtalar fusion. Notice the position of the foot, with the toes pointing toward the ceiling.

standard posterior lateral portal can be used. This approach requires working around the fibula. However, care should be taken not to damage the tibial nerve during the use of both posterior portals. The posterior joint is difficult to débride without using a posterior portal in all but the most lax ankle joints.

After the ankle joint has been completely débrided, the subtalar joint is approached from the lateral portals. Anterolateral, direct lateral, and posterolateral portals are used. The foot is inverted to allow access while the surgeon sits on the lateral side of the table while working the portals of the subtalar joint. Sequential débridement is performed of the posterior facet of the subtalar joint using standard techniques.

After both joints have been débrided, the instruments are withdrawn, and the joints are held in a neutral position. A retrograde rod is the preferred method of fixation in these cases, because its insertion requires minimal exposure while providing a strong mechanical construct.

Retrograde Rod Technique

An incision is made on the plantar aspect of the foot directly in line with the long axis of the tibia with the foot in the corrected position. The starting point can be confirmed on anteroposterior and lateral image views before the incision is made. The starting point usually is 1 to 2 cm behind the calcaneocuboid joint and on the medial slope of the calcaneus (Fig. 19-4). Care should be taken when exposing this part of the calcaneus from the plantar side to ensure that the tibial nerve is not damaged. The nerve lies on the medial side of the approach. Deep dissection should be performed bluntly and the medial soft tissues retracted.

A Kirschner wire is inserted through the calcaneus and into the central aspect of the tibia. A wire inserted off center will result in malreduction of the joint during insertion of the nail. For

example, if the wire hits the anterior cortex and bends, reaming the calcaneus and talus in this position will result in a greater degree of flexion than was anticipated. Similarly, extension will occur if the wire hits the posterior cortex.

Some nails have a bend on the distal end that allows more lateral placement of the starting point in the calcaneus, potentially improving calcaneal fixation. Nail designs vary by the fixation achieved (i.e., lateral versus lateral and posterior screw fixation on the distal end), length (i.e., 150 to 300 mm), and compression techniques.

The tibia should be sequentially reamed until appropriate cortical chatter is obtained. The nail is sized for 1 mm less than the last reamer diameter. The reamer should be passed beyond the planned length of the nail to ensure that the nail does not bind in the tibia before being fully seated.

The surgeon should ensure that there is no stress riser at the tip of the nail. Occasionally, the drill for the proximal locking screw passes posterior to the nail and creates a stress riser. In this case, a longer nail should be used to bypass the stress riser.

The retrograde nail should be correctly seated to ensure that the distal locking screws are correctly located within the talus and calcaneus. Compression may be achieved through the fusion site by dynamic proximal fixation. Distal fixation can be performed first, the nail impacted, and then proximal fixation performed. Alternatively, proximal fixation can be achieved first and then distal compression performed on the nail or using an external compression device. Regardless of the sequence, the surgeon should perform some form of compression and should understand the nail system being used. Compression should be performed across the ankle first, followed by the subtalar joint. Failure to compress the joint may result in nonunion. Additional fixation using compression screws around the nail can be performed if the surgeon thinks that additional fixation is required.

Fluoroscopic views are obtained at the end of the procedure. The wounds are closed, and the patient is immobilized during the postoperative period.

Arthroscopic Triple Arthrodesis

Arthroscopic triple arthrodesis is performed for indications similar to those outlined for arthroscopic combined ankle and subtalar fusion. I have found that the primary indication for the arthroscopic procedure is joint degeneration in patients with rheumatoid or psoriatic arthritis who have a good potential for poor wound healing.

Contraindications to the arthroscopic procedure include significant bone loss. Patients with significant deformity requiring correction, such as a cavus foot or planovalgus foot, may not be correctable through an arthroscopic approach. A subtle planovalgus foot is easier to correct than a subtle cavus foot, because a flexible foot is required to allow appropriate instrumentation of the joints.

A patient with a stiff talonavicular joint may be difficult to instrument at the talonavicular and subtalar joints. The procedure should therefore be attempted only after the surgeon has gained expertise by performing arthroscopy on joints with easier access.

Instrumentation

The 1.9-mm-diameter arthroscope is best for the triple fusion because the joint capsules are tight. However, the fluid flow is

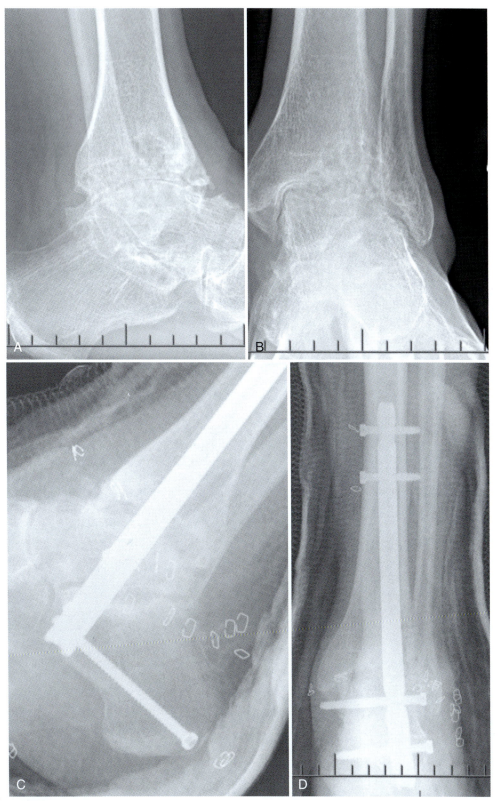

FIGURE 19-4 A and **B,** A hemophiliac patient has end-stage arthritic changes of the ankle and subtalar joints. **C** and **D,** Postoperative views.

inadequate for using the smaller arthroscope and canula for the débridement for this type of fusion, and a separate portal for inflow may be required.

The 3.5-mm or smaller shavers can be used. May colleagues and I used a small joint distractor in some of the earlier cases but have preferred no distraction for the more recent cases, because this allows easier motion around the joints, as recommended by Lui.[2]

Technique

The patient is positioned with the operative hip internally rotated on a beanbag or elevated on a bump. The leg is prepared and draped free.[2]

Subtalar Fusion. Three lateral portals are used for the subtalar fusion, as described earlier for the combined procedure.

Talonavicular Fusion. The talonavicular joint is best approached from a dorsal medial, plantar medial, and dorsal lateral portal. A trans-calcaneocuboid joint portal can assist in visualization of the plantar lateral aspect of the joint (Figs. 19-5 and 19-6).

Care should be taken not to damage the deep branch of the peroneal nerve that is closely apposed to the dorsal capsule of the joint. Palpation of the dorsalis pedis artery before inflation of the tourni-

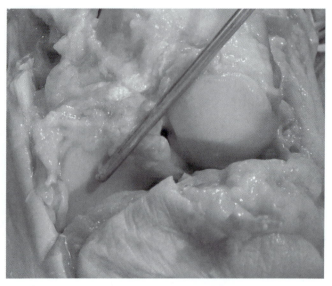

FIGURE 19-6 A trans-talonavicular portal can be used for the calcaneocuboid joint. Similarly, the talonavicular joint can be scoped from the calcaneocuboid joint.

quet should assist the surgeon in its correct localization. Confirmation of the position of the cannula by intraoperative fluoroscopy is required, particularly in patients with softer bone (Fig. 19-7).

The arthritic and mobile rheumatoid joint is quite easily instrumented and often requires minimal débridement. When the joint is hard to distract, cautious release of the capsule with a meniscectomy knife may be required. If the joint is stiff, it may be hard to identify. Fluoroscopic confirmation of correct positioning of the cannula is wise, because inadvertent insertion of the cannula into an osteopenic navicular in an arthritic patient can occur. If required, the portal can be expanded to 1 cm, and

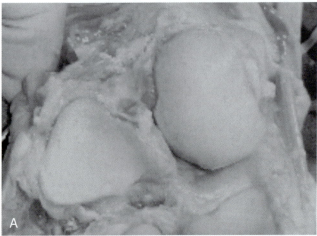

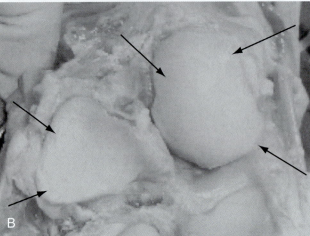

FIGURE 19-5 A cadaver view of the calcaneocuboid and talonavicular joints shows the position of the portals (arrows).

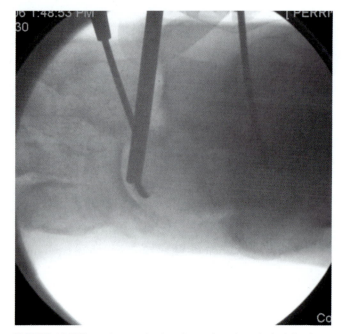

FIGURE 19-7 The arthroscopic view shows the talonavicular joint. In this case, a small external fixator was used to assist in distraction.

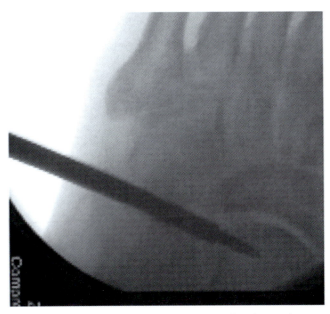

FIGURE 19-8 A cannulated drill is used to expose the talonavicular joint.

skin hooks can be used to retract while the joint capsule is released under direct visualization. Alternatively, after the joint is initially visualized, the joint capsule can be released using a meniscectomy blade or small osteotome under direct visualization.

An alternative technique uses a cannulated drill placed across the arthritic joint. The 5-mm drill from the cannulated hip screw set has a diameter to fit the 2.9-mm scope and canula. After the guidewire is placed under fluoroscopic control, the drill is placed across the joint under direct fluoroscopy (Fig. 19-8). Oblique drill placement is used. One drill hole can then be used for the scope and the other for the instruments. However, working outside these drill holes can be problematic for completing cartilage removal. Similarly, tight subtalar and calcaneocuboid joints can be drilled with a cannulated drill to facilitate exposure (Fig. 19-9).

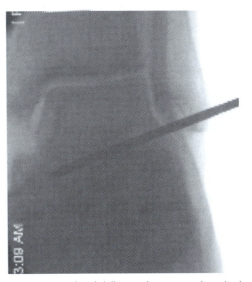

FIGURE 19-9 A cannulated drill is used to expose the subtalar joint.

Calcaneocuboid Joint Fusion. The calcaneocuboid joint is the tightest joint of the three joints to enter. The capsule, however, can be released to allow better access in a manner similar to that for the talonavicular joint.

Three portals offer the best access to the calcaneocuboid joint. A dorsal lateral portal, a plantar lateral portal, and a transtalonavicular portal allow access to the dorsomedial side of the joint.

Fluoroscopic views may be required to confirm correct positioning of the cannula before insertion of the arthroscope. The calcaneocuboid joint is hard to access because of its sinusoidal shape, making it hard to triangulate within the joint. Release of the capsule can be performed by using skin hooks in one lateral portal and dissecting the joint lining off the bone or by inserting an osteotome within the joint and, by feel or visualization through the scope, teasing the joint capsule off the bone on the proximal or distal side of the joint.

Double Fusions. A double fusion may suffice in some cases. A combined subtalar and calcaneocuboid fusion may be performed for patients with minimal loss of calcaneal height after calcaneal fracture if both joints are stiff and painful and if the talonavicular joint is relatively well preserved. I have experience with one patient who had a poor soft tissue envelope that prevented lateral exposure of both joints; a double fusion was successful.

A double fusion of the talonavicular and subtalar joint may be appropriate in some cases of talonavicular arthritis. Although a double fusion can be performed for a planovalgus foot deformity, my colleagues and I have not performed an arthroscopic triple arthrodesis for this indication, because often other corrective fusions or osteotomies often are required at the same time.

Although an isolated talonavicular fusion can be performed, I have not done so because there is a risk of nonunion of the isolated talonavicular fusion. Addition of the subtalar fusion adds rigidity and support to the fusion mass and decreases this risk without significant loss of hindfoot motion. Appropriate percutaneous fixation may also be hard to achieve. Isolated calcaneocuboid fusions can be performed arthroscopically.

Fixation

Fixation of the arthroscopic triple arthrodesis follows the same screw placement as for the open procedure. Cannulated or solid screws can be used, depending on surgeon's preference (Fig. 19-10).

The subtalar fusion can be transfixed using two screws from the calcaneus into the talus. Care should be taken to ensure that the screws are within the body of the talus and not laterally placed. The starting point in the calcaneal tuberosity needs to be at the midpoint of the tuberosity or lateral to it to avoid medial penetration of the calcaneus and potential damage to the tibial nerve. Radiographs should include anteroposterior and lateral views of the foot, an anteroposterior view of the ankle, and an axial view of the calcaneus.

Fixation of the talonavicular joint can be performed percutaneously. Small fragment screws are used in all but the largest patients. A cannulated equivalent can also be used. The screws

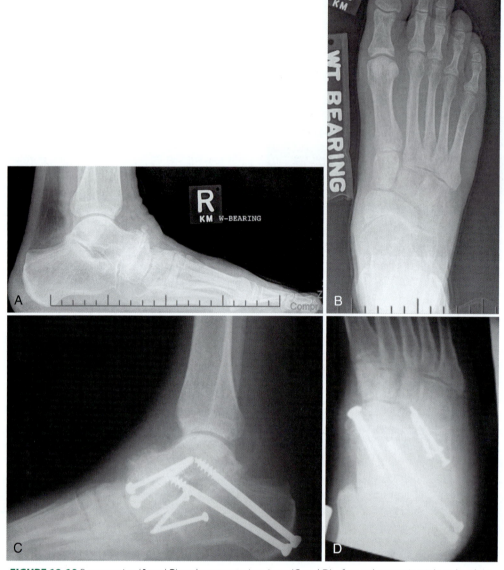

FIGURE 19-10 Preoperative (**A** and **B**) and postoperative views (**C** and **D**) of an arthroscopic triple arthrodesis.

can be inserted from the tuberosity of the navicular, which is easy to palpate. The screws also can be inserted from the dorsomedial and dorsolateral side. Care should be taken to avoid the direct dorsal approach because the deep branch of the peroneal nerve may be injured. The screws must be placed parallel to the plantar surface of the foot to ensure that they engage the talus. Two or three screws should be used on the talonavicular joint.

Fixation of the calcaneocuboid joint can be obtained by a small incision in the sinus tarsi, just behind the anterior process of the calcaneus. The fixation proceeds from just behind the anterior process into the body of the calcaneus. Care should be taken to ensure that the screws are pointing laterally and dorsally enough to engage the cuboid. Two screws are used, with an additional third screw inserted percutaneously from the cuboid into the calcaneus.

PEARLS & PITFALLS

- The use of some form of dynamic distraction allows the foot to be changed in position so that the joint can be accessed.
- The medial portal (just behind the medial malleolus) allows access to the posterior aspect of the ankle without the patient being placed prone.
- A 2.9-mm arthroscope works well in the ankle and has a high-flow canula that can assist in joint débridement.
- Aggressive shavers are required, and several may be required for the case. They are helpful for cartilage removal. They often block, break, or dull and should be changed often.
- Pituitary rongeurs applied through the portals are useful way of removing debris.
- Osteophytes may block access to the joint, and they should be removed at the beginning of the case under C-arm control, if necessary.

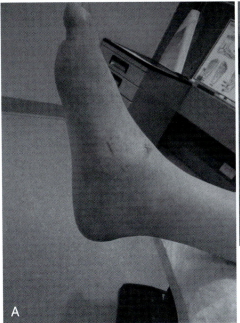

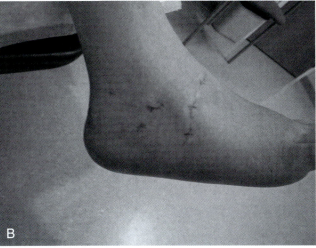

FIGURE 19-11 A and **B,** Clinical pictures were obtained 6 weeks after an arthroscopic triple arthrodesis.

- Curved curettes and osteotomes are invaluable for removing cartilage over the dome of the talus.
- The subtalar, talonavicular, and calcaneocuboid joints are hard to access because of the tight joint capsule. An internal capsulotomy helps to expose the joints and get the instruments in. A 1.9-mm arthroscope should be used.
- Screw fixation should include two screws crossing each joint to obtain stable fixation.
- For triple arthrodesis, the subtalar joint should be transfixed first, followed by the talonavicular joint then the calcaneocuboid joint.

Postoperative Care

Patients are immobilized in a plaster slab or walker boot at the time of surgery. At the 2-week review, the sutures are removed and range of motion initiated. For ankle or ankle and subtalar fusions combined, the patient is placed in a fiberglass cast for 6 weeks and not allowed to bear weight for 8 weeks. The arthroscopic technique reduces postoperative wound complications and swelling, assisting in recovery (Fig. 19-11). For an arthroscopic triple arthrodesis, the patient not permitted to bear weight for 6 weeks after surgery and can begin range-of-motion exercises at 2 weeks.

Patients are evaluated at the initiation of weight bearing, and radiographs are taken at that time. Remobilization is supervised by a physiotherapist, and final review is performed 3 months after surgery.

OUTCOMES

There are no outcome studies for arthroscopic combined fusions or arthroscopic triple arthrodesis. Outcomes for arthroscopic ankle arthrodesis and subtalar arthrodesis are covered in the relevant chapters.

REFERENCES

1. Gougoulias NE, Agathangelidis FG, Parsons SW. Arthroscopic ankle arthrodesis. *Foot Ankle Int.* 2007;28:695-706.
2. Lui TH. New technique of arthroscopic triple arthrodesis. *Arthroscopy.* 2006;22:464:e461-e465.
3. Sekiya H, Horii T, Kariya Y, Hoshino Y. Arthroscopic-assisted tibiotalocalcaneal arthrodesis using an intramedullary nail with fins: a case report. *J Foot Ankle Surg.* 2006;45:266-270.

SUGGESTED READINGS

Failace JJ, Leopold SS, Brage ME. Extended hindfoot fusions and pantalar fusions. History, biomechanics, and clinical results. *Foot Ankle Clin.* 2000; 5:777-798.
Lui TH. Arthroscopic triple arthrodesis in patients with Muller-Weiss disease. *Foot Ankle Surg.* 2009;15:119-122.
Thordarson DB. Fusion in posttraumatic foot and ankle reconstruction. *J Am Acad Orthop Surg.* 2004;12:322-333.

Great Toe Arthroscopy

Phinit Phisitkul • Tun Hing Lui

Arthroscopy of the first metatarsophalangeal joint (MTP-1) was originally described by Watanabe in 1972.[1] Because of the small size of the joint, the applicability of arthroscopy has been limited by the small number of clinical results reported in the literature. Advances in technology for visualization and instrumentation and the recent clinical experience of the surgeons have propelled small joint arthroscopy into a new era. Although arthroscopy in the MTP-1 has not been as widely used as arthroscopy in the knee or the shoulder, its value has been demonstrated, and its use continues to grow for the treatment of traumatic and degenerative conditions and for reconstructive procedures. With proper patient selection and familiarity with the technique, MTP-1 arthroscopy can be a useful addition to the surgeon's armamentarium.

NORMAL AND PATHOLOGIC ANATOMY

The MTP-1 is composed of the first metatarsal head and neck, proximal phalangeal base, and medial and lateral sesamoids. The first metatarsal articular surface is composed of two fields in continuity, the superior phalangeal and inferior sesamoidal fields. The former is smaller and convex, whereas the latter is larger and separated into two sloped surfaces by a small bony ridge or crista (Fig. 20-1). The proximal phalanx articular surface is oval, concave, and smaller than the corresponding articular surface of the metatarsal head. The base of the proximal phalanx serves as insertions of the extensor hallucis brevis and longus dorsally and the intrinsic muscles of the big toe and plantar plate plantarly.

The two sesamoids embedded in the thick plantar plate have two surfaces: the inferior, convex, nonarticular, insertional surface and the superior articular surface. The medial sesamoid is usually larger, ovoid, and elongated, whereas the lateral sesamoid is smaller and more circular. The articular surface of each sesamoid is convex in the coronal plane and concave in the sagittal plane and fits well with the corresponding trochlear surface.

The dorsomedial aspect of the joint contains a sizable synovial fold, with the average width of 7 mm and covering 29% of the joint.[2] It has abundant blood supply, but the nerve supply is found only in the periphery.

The stability of the joint is provided mainly by the capsuloligamentous complex. The medial and lateral collateral ligaments have two components, the metatarsophalangeal and the metatarsosesamoid suspensory ligaments. The latter components insert directly on the medial and lateral borders of the plantar plate. Balance of the joint is also affected by the function of the musculotendinous structures, including short and long flexors and extensors, abductor hallucis, and adductor hallucis.

At the level of the MTP-1, the distribution of the cutaneous nerve varies, but the dorsomedial and dorsolateral cutaneous branches usually originate from the medial dorsal cutaneous branch of the superficial peroneal nerve and the deep peroneal nerve, respectively (Fig. 20-2). The plantar medial and plantar lateral branches originate from the medial plantar nerve. The dorsomedial cutaneous nerve lies close to the dorsomedial portal and is on average 13.1 mm medial to the extensor hallucis longus tendon,[3] but it has been reported to be 2 to 5 mm from it.[4] The plantar medial hallucal nerve is on average 10.6 mm plantar to the midline, which is the location for the medial portal. Because of the variations of the nerves in the foot, all the arthroscopic portals should be handled as if a nerve was located directly underneath. The pathologic anatomy of various conditions of the MTP-1 that can be addressed arthroscopically or endoscopically are listed in Table 20-1.

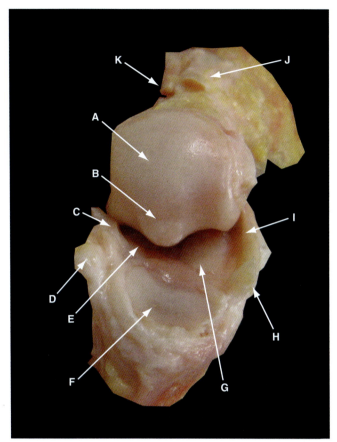

FIGURE 20-1 The anatomy of the first metatarsophalangeal joint is illustrated with the dorsal capsule and extensor tendons removed and the joint hyperflexed: superior phalangeal part of the first metatarsal articular surface (A); inferior sesamoidal part of the first metatarsal articular surface and the crista (B); metatarsophalangeal part of the lateral collateral ligament (C); lateral sesamoid (D); medial sesamoid (E); metatarsophalangeal part of the medial collateral ligament (F).

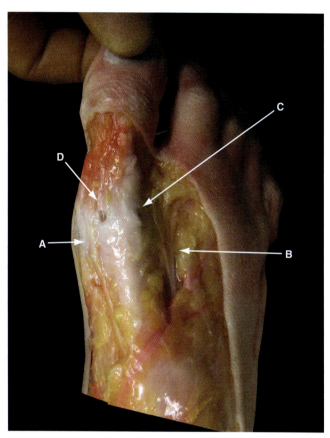

FIGURE 20-2 In the dissected specimen, the dorsomedial and dorsolateral portals are on the medial and lateral aspects of the extensor hallucis longus tendon. The dorsomedial and dorsolateral hallucal nerves are adjacent to the portals.

TABLE 20-1   Pathologic Conditions of the First Metatarsophalangeal Joint

Conditions	Pathologic Anatomy	Physical Findings	Arthroscopic Procedure
Hallux rigidus osteophytes	Synovitis, osteophytes, loose bodies, thickened joint capsule	Joint effusion, limited range of motion with pain, tenderness over osteophytes, possible associated flexor hallucis longus contracture	Synovectomy, cheilectomy, loose body removal, capsular release, arthroscopy-assisted first metatarsophalangeal joint fusion (advanced case)
Loose bodies	Cartilaginous or osteochondral loose bodies	Mild joint effusion, occasional crepitus	Loose body removal
Chondral and osteochondral lesions	Partial- or full-thickness cartilage damage, osteochondral fragments	Mild joint effusion, occasional crepitus	Débridement of unstable parts, microfracture for full-thickness or osteochondral defects
Arthrofibrosis	Contracted and thickened joint capsule, intra-articular adhesion	Global loss of motion, thickened joint capsule	Débridement of fibrotic tissue in the dorsal, medial, and lateral gutters and in the metatarsosesamoid compartment
Synovitis, pigmented villonodular synovitis	Synovial hyperplasia, hemosiderin-laden synovium in pigmented villonodular synovitis	Moderate joint swelling, pain on impingement test and thumb pressure on the dorsal joint line with dorsiflexion	Synovectomy

Continued

TABLE 20-1   Pathologic Conditions of the First Metatarsophalangeal Joint—cont'd

Conditions	Pathologic Anatomy	Physical Findings	Arthroscopic Procedure
Sesamoiditis, bipartite sesamoid	Sesamoid fragmentation, cartilage injury	Localized tenderness over the sesamoid	Sesamoidectomy
Hallux valgus	Contracted lateral capsule and adductor tendon, attenuated medial capsule, prominent medial eminence, synovitis	Reducibility of the first metatarsal adduction deformity, joint line tenderness, medial metatarsal tenderness	Lateral release, bunionectomy, medial capsule advancement, percutaneous positioning screw fixation of the first metatarsal base, arthroscopic débridement in patients with joint line pain
Gouty tophi	Tophi formation integrated into the joint capsule and intra-articular lesions	Subcutaneous tophi, skin breakdown, displacement of neurovascular structures, joint swelling and crepitus	Débridement

PATIENT EVALUATION

History and Physical Examination

Patients with MTP-1 problems usually present with forefoot pain. Obtaining a problem-focused history should include the characteristics of pain, swelling, deformities, associated injuries, preexisting diseases, shoewear, prior treatments, and a family history. Athletic activities and expectation are also important factors. Systemic diseases can be associated with increased uric acid and urate crystal arthropathy, which is a common cause of MTP-1 pain.[5]

Physical examination is the cornerstone of all clinical judgments. We always perform a systematic and thorough examination of all patients with foot and ankle problems, starting with gait, skin, motor, motion, palpation, and special tests. Patients with considerable pain in the MTP-1 may walk on the lateral border of the foot. The forefoot should be observed for deformities, swelling, and discoloration. Active and passive motion of the MTP-1 should be evaluated and compared with the contralateral side. The average passive motion of the MTP-1 in men older than 45 years is 87 degrees, with 67 degrees of dorsiflexion and 20 degrees of plantar flexion.[6] Patients with decreased range of motion of the MTP-1 should be differentiated by the characteristics of stiffness. Arthrofibrosis or osteoarthrosis may result in global loss of motion, whereas an early hallux rigidus may produce primarily limited dorsiflexion. Pseudo-hallux rigidus can mimic or be associated with a hallux rigidus, but the tightness from the flexor hallucis longus tendon contracture can usually be decreased by ankle plantar flexion.[7] Occasionally, crepitus can be differentiated from arthritis, osteochondral injury, or loose bodies. Pain can be provoked with forced dorsiflexion in patients with hallux rigidus or soft tissue impingement. Bony landmarks, such as the head of the first metatarsal and the base of the proximal phalanx, are superficial and easily palpable. Pain in daily activities often can be reproduced by direct palpation over the osteophytes or the sesamoids.

Soft tissue landmarks should be palpated, including the dorsomedial hallucal nerve at the dorsomedial edge of the medial eminence and the plantar medial hallucal nerve just medial and dorsal to the medial sesamoid. The sensory branches of the deep peroneal nerve supplying the first web space are small and usually not palpable.

In hallux valgus, the first metatarsal adduction can be evaluated if it can be manually corrected, which is a requirement for an endoscopic correction of hallux valgus deformity.[8] Sometimes, complete correction may not be achieved because of obstruction by the dislocated fibular sesamoid bone in the web space. This is not a contraindication for the procedure, because the sesamoid bone can be reduced after lateral release, and the intermetatarsal space can then be closed. Specific physical examinations for various pathologies of the MTP-1 that are amendable to arthroscopic treatment are listed in Table 20-1.

Diagnostic Imaging

We use standard weight-bearing anteroposterior, lateral, and axial sesamoid views for initial evaluation of all patients with forefoot problems (Fig. 20-3). Osteophytes, joint space narrowing, and loose bodies usually can be demonstrated.

Elevation of the first metatarsal in relation to the lesser metatarsals can be associated with hallux rigidus.[9] Inflammatory arthropathy can develop juxta-articular osteopenia or joint destruction in the late stages, whereas gouty tophi often have juxta-articular punch-out lesions and soft tissue thickening. Hallux valgus requires measurements of the hallux valgus angle, intermetatarsal angle, distal metatarsal articular angle, and proximal phalanx articular angle. Oblique views may be helpful in visualizing dorsal MTP-1 osteophytes, the joint space, and the profile of an individual sesamoid.

Computed tomography (CT) is rarely indicated, but it can better visualize the osteochondral lesions or loose bodies with an osseous component. Magnetic resonance imaging (MRI) can demonstrate a bone bruise, cartilage defects, and synovial hyperplasia, especially with pigmented villonodular synovitis (PVNS), which has low signal intensity on T1-weighted and T2-weighted images.[10] MR images of a symptomatic, bipartite medial sesamoid are shown in Figure 20-4. Ultrasound imaging is advantageous in the forefoot because of its magnification power and real-time visualization.[11] It can identify loose bodies and small bone spurs. The probe can also be used to reproduce pain with direct pressure over the suspected location.

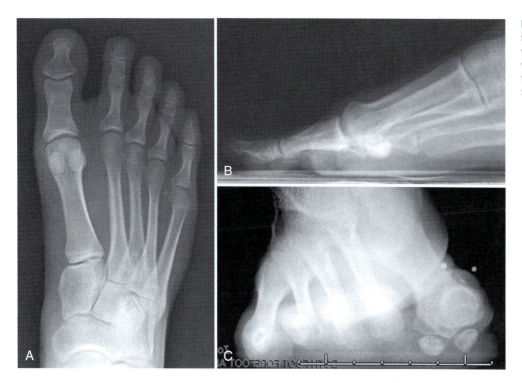

FIGURE 20-3 The standard forefoot radiographs include a weight-bearing anteroposterior view (**A**), a weight-bearing lateral view (**B**), and a weight-bearing sesamoid view (**C**).

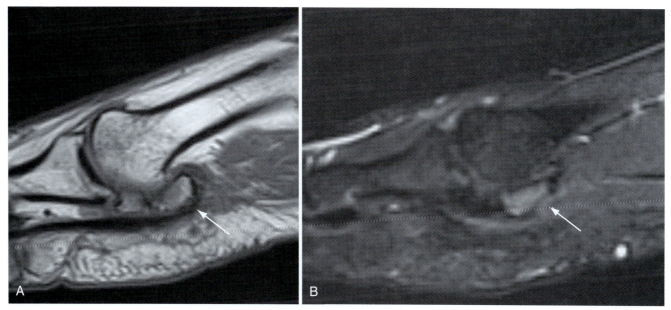

FIGURE 20-4 A bipartite sesamoid is shown in T1-weighted (**A**) and T2-weighted magnetic resonance images. The proximal part of the medial sesamoid has increased signal intensity on the T2-weighted image, indicating bone edema that is consistent with the location of maximum pain.

TREATMENT

Indications and Contraindications

Arthroscopic treatment of MTP-1 generally has the same indications as open operations, including failure of nonoperative treatment for 3 to 6 months. Indications are as follows:

1. Dorsal impingement from early hallux rigidus or osteoarthritis (arthroscopic decompression)[4,12]
2. Chondral and osteochondral lesions[4,13,14]
3. Loose bodies[4]
4. Synovitis and PVNS[4,15,16]
5. Advanced hallux rigidus or osteoarthritis (arthroscopy-assisted arthrodesis)[17,18]
6. Arthrofibrosis[4,16,19]
7. Hallux valgus[8,20,21]
8. Gouty tophi[5,16,22,23]
9. Sesamoidectomy[24,25]

Contraindications to arthroscopic treatment are as follows:

1. Severe joint ankylosis[4]
2. Hallux valgus with an abnormal distal metatarsal articular angle or interphalangeus deformity or irreducible intermetatarsal widening[8]
3. Overlying soft tissue infection[4]
4. Poor vascular status

Nonoperative Management

Immobilization is beneficial for most MTP-1 pathologies, including degenerative, traumatic, and inflammatory processes. In the acute setting, a walking cast or boot can be helpful. Taping can be applied before athletic activities. A cortisone injection may provide at least a temporary relief for the patient with pain from an inflammatory component, such as synovitis and osteoarthritis.

Shoes should have a low heel and a stable sole to decrease MTP joint motion and loading. A carbon-reinforced insert can be used to increase the rigidity of the sole. Unloading is the mainstay treatment for the sesamoid problems. A silicone gel pad can be placed to support the painful sesamoid and to produce medial posting to shift the load laterally. Shoes with a wide toe box are necessary for patients with MTP-1 osteoarthritis or tophi and hallux valgus.

Arthroscopic Technique

Positioning

We prefer to do the arthroscopy of the MTP-1 with the patient in a supine position and with both hips in abduction (Fig. 20-5). The surgeon has 360-degree access to the forefoot, but most of the procedures can be done with the surgeon at the end of the bed. Plantar portals, if needed, can be approached with the surgeon sitting between the patient's legs.

Traction

Manual traction is usually sufficient for visualization of the metatarsal head and the base of the proximal phalanx. We do not routinely use Chinese finger trap traction. Joint distraction, although opening up the distance between articular facets, obliterates the intra-articular

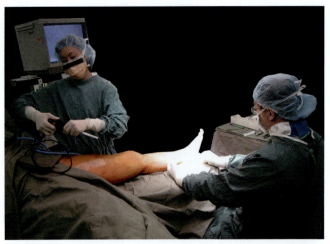

FIGURE 20-5 The preferred positioning for first metatarsophalangeal joint arthroscopy is shown. The ends of the bed are separated to allow both hips to be in abduction. The monitor and the arthroscopic tower are on the ipsilateral side.

gutters and decreases the maneuverability of the arthroscope and instruments. However, it can be useful for access to some osteochondral lesions and in arthroscopy-assisted arthrodesis, which requires passing instruments between the joint facets. The Chinese finger trap traction can be attached to 3- to 5-kg weights, or the limb can be suspended from a pole so that it is just off the operating table.

Instruments

A 1.9- or 2.7-mm, 30-degree, small joint arthroscope is used for most arthroscopic visualization of the MTP-1. The 1.9-mm arthroscope is used in tight joints, especially when no traction is applied, but it should be handled with care because of its fragility. A 4-mm, 30-degree arthroscope, which provides a wider field of view and easier orientation, is helpful in periarticular endoscopy, such as in a first web space release and gouty tophi excision. The gravity-driven inflow usually is adequate, and the arthroscopic pump is rarely required. An alternative is to use a 50-mL syringe with continuous irrigation controlled by an assistant. Small bone-cutting shavers allow soft tissue and bone débridement, which can minimize instrument switching. Equipment is listed Box 20-1 and Figure 20-6.

Box 20-1 Recommended Equipment for First Metatarsophalangeal Joint Arthroscopy

- Thigh tourniquet
- Sterile Chinese finger trap and shoulder traction apparatus with a 3- to 5-kg weight (optional)
- 21-gauge needle and 10-mL syringe (optional)
- 1.9- or 2.7-mm and 4.0-mm, 30-degree arthroscopes
- 3.0-mm full-radius shaver and abrader
- 2.0-mm full-radius shaver and abrader
- 2.0-mm probe
- 2.0-mm curette
- 2.0-mm baskets
- Small joint microfracture probe
- Small, curved and straight hemostats
- Retrograde knife

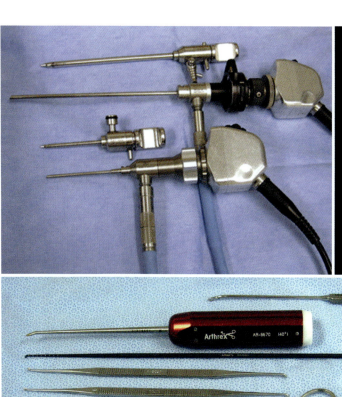

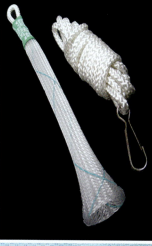

FIGURE 20-6 The required equipment is shown for first metatarsophalangeal joint arthroscopy.

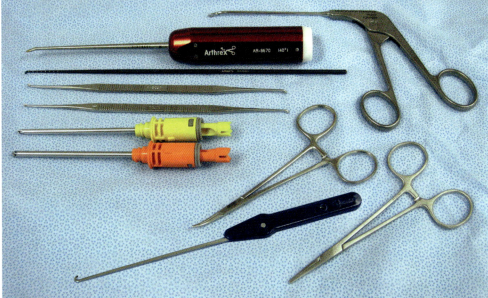

Portals

Dorsomedial and dorsolateral portals are commonly used as the main arthroscopic portals for most MTP-1 pathology (Fig. 20-7). The dorsomedial portal is at the level of joint line and just medial to the extensor hallucis longus tendon joint. The dorsolateral portal is at the same level, but it is just lateral to the extensor hallucis longus tendon. The dorsomedial and dorsolateral hallucal nerves can be directly beneath or can send off a branch close to the dorsal portals.[3] The medial portal is at the level of the joint line at the equator of the joint and is positioned away from neurovascular structures (Fig. 20-8). The portal is established through a thick medial capsule by making a longitudinal capsulotomy with a no. 15 blade.

The combination of dorsolateral and medial portals has been more commonly used as the main access route in our experience. It allows a wider distance between portals, reducing crowding of the instruments. The medial portal is particularly helpful in the visualization of the sesamoids, dorsal and plantar gutters, and parts of the metatarsal head.[4] The proxi-

mal medial portal is in line with the medial portal but is just proximal to the medial eminence. This portal is used for the medial exostectomy.[8] The plantar medial portal described for the instrumentation in the metatarsosesamoid compartment is located 4 cm proximal to the joint line and between the abductor hallucis tendon and the medial head of the flexor hallucis brevis.[13,19]

The toe web portal and the plantar portal are required for endoscopic lateral release of the hallux valgus correction and for lateral sesamoidectomy.[8,13] The toe web portal is just dorsal to the first web space. The plantar portal is approximately 4 to 5 cm proximal to the web space created inside-out by a Wissinger rod from the toe web portal passing underneath the intermetatarsal ligament. The key to establishing the plantar portal is to make the portal wound just proximal to the point where the rod penetrated the plantar aponeurosis, minimizing the length of the subcutaneous tunnel of the portal tract, which is not the working length of the tract. The toe web portal is relatively safe from the neurovascular structures, but the plantar

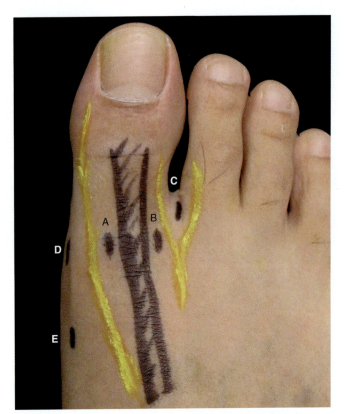

FIGURE 20-7 The diagram of the dorsal view of the foot shows the dorsomedial portal (A), the dorsolateral portal (B), the toe web portal (C), the medial portal (D), and the proximal medial portal (E) in relation to the dorsal cutaneous nerves.

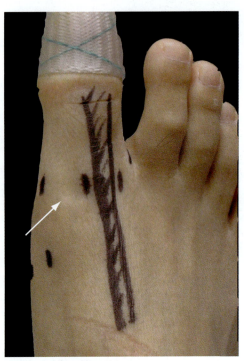

FIGURE 20-9 The skin overlying the joint line is puckered with traction of the great toe in a finger trap.

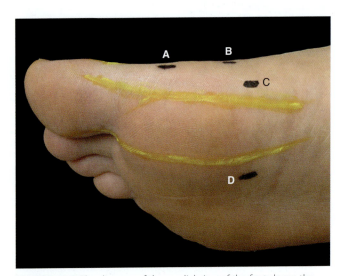

FIGURE 20-8 The diagram of the medial view of the foot shows the medial portal (A), the proximal medial portal (B), the plantar medial portal (C), and the plantar portal (D) in relation to the plantar cutaneous nerves.

portal is in the vicinity of the branches from the medial plantar nerve.

Arthroscopic Examination

The joint line is localized by puckering of the skin with straight traction of the great toe and by direct palpation (Fig. 20-9). The

dorsomedial portal is established at the previously described location by making a longitudinal, 3-mm incision followed by blunt dissection with a curved hemostat. The dorsolateral portal and the medial portal placement can be assisted by arthroscopic localization with a 21-gauge needle. Alternatively, the dorsolateral portal can be created first, followed by a medial portal made under direct visualization.

An easy way to introduce instruments without traction is shown in Figure 20-10. The 13-point examination of the joint has been described by Ferkel to systematically visualize intra-articular structures.[4] The areas visualized from the dorsomedial, dorsolateral, and medial portals are shown in Figures 20-11 through 20-13. A 2.0-mm probe is used to palpate the cartilage surface for the detection of softening, crevices, delamination, and osteochondral lesions. Loose bodies are removed with small, straight hemostats, which are preferable over the graspers because of the suction effect that pulls the loose body to the jaws when opened. Sometimes, a tight joint may require manual manipulation to enhance visualization, such as plantar flexion to open the metatarsosesamoid compartment or a combination of traction, plantar flexion, and varus stress for the lateral plantar recess.[16]

Treatment of Specific Conditions

Synovitis and Pigmented Villonodular Synovitis

Treatment of synovitis and soft tissue impingement had good results in a case series.[16] Successful treatment of a patient with

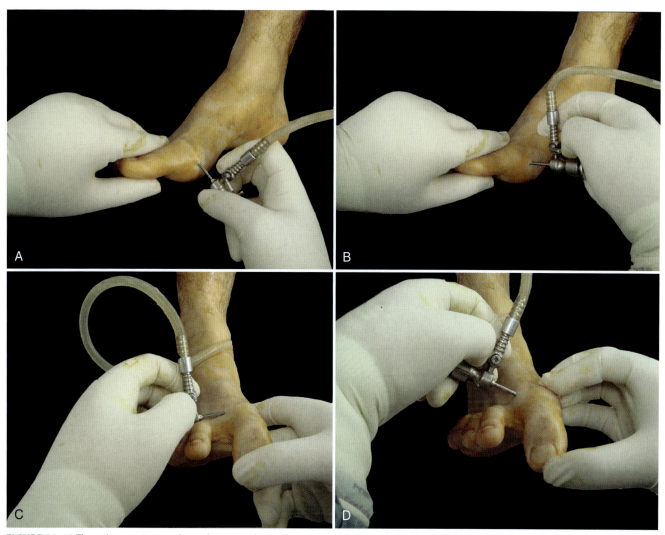

FIGURE 20-10 The arthroscopic cannula can be inserted into the metatarsophalangeal compartment by first introducing the instrument into the adjacent capsular gutter and then gently sliding its tip into the metatarsophalangeal compartment. The technique is demonstrated for the medial portal (**A** and **B**) and the dorsolateral portal (**C** and **D**).

PVNS of the MTP-1 with arthroscopic synovectomy has been reported.[15] Visualization of the (occasionally enlarged) dorsomedial synovial fold is more easily performed through the dorsolateral portal (Fig. 20-14).[2] Thorough débridement of the inflamed synovial tissue, which is usually a major pain generator, can be performed with a 3.0-mm, full-radius shaver. Traction is typically not required for a synovectomy. Suction is kept at minimum due to the limited inflow from the small arthroscopic cannula.

Hallux Rigidus and Osteophytes

Van Dijk and colleagues reported good or excellent results in 8 of 12 patients with dorsal impingement and in 2 of 5 patients with hallux rigidus at the 2-year follow-up assessment.[13] Iqbal and coworkers reported satisfactory results in all 15 patients with mild to moderate hallux rigidus.[12]

Small osteophytes can be easily removed with a bone-cutting shaver, with the round-tip abrader reserved for large ones or those with unusually hard bone. For an arthroscopic cheilec-tomy, the dorsal metatarsal head, including a small amount of articular cartilage, is decompressed until 50 to 70 degrees of dorsiflexion is achieved. If there is any question regarding the amount of the decompression, fluoroscopy can be used. A prominent osteophyte on the proximal phalangeal base should be evaluated and adequately decompressed (Fig. 20-15).

Osteoarthritis

Mild to moderate osteoarthritis of the MTP-1 with pain, which usually is caused by synovitis, is an appropriate indication for an arthroscopic treatment, especially when arthrodesis or arthroplasty is not indicated (Fig. 20-16). However, patients with advanced osteoarthritis with midrange pain have not had lasting benefit from arthroscopic débridement.[16,26] Cases with large osteophytes (>5 mm) may have obliteration of the dorsal joint space. This can be handled arthroscopically by first stripping the dorsal capsule with a small periosteal elevator through the dorsal portals to increase the working space (Fig. 20-17).

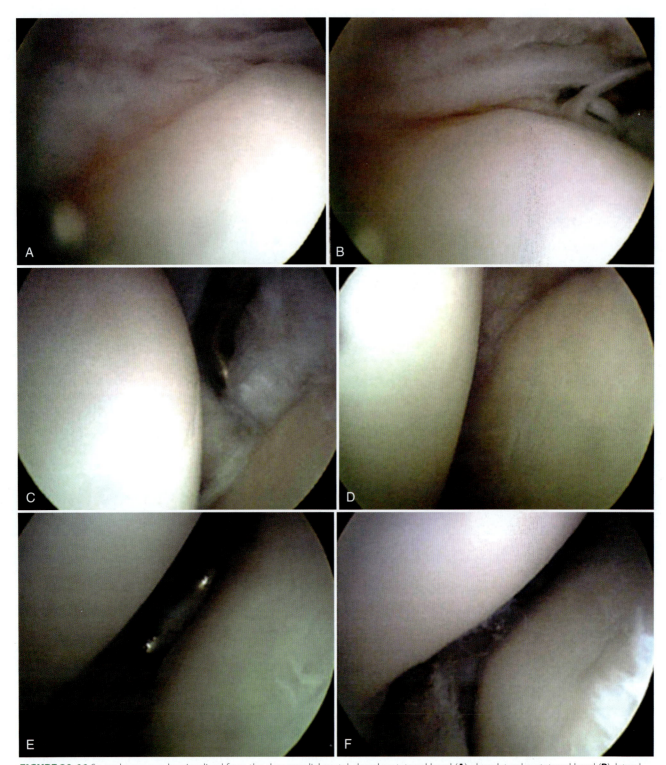

FIGURE 20-11 Several areas can be visualized from the dorsomedial portal: dorsal metatarsal head (**A**), dorsolateral metatarsal head (**B**), lateral gutter (**C**), lateral metatarsophalangeal compartment (**D**), central metatarsophalangeal compartment (**E**), and medial metatarsophalangeal compartment (**F**).

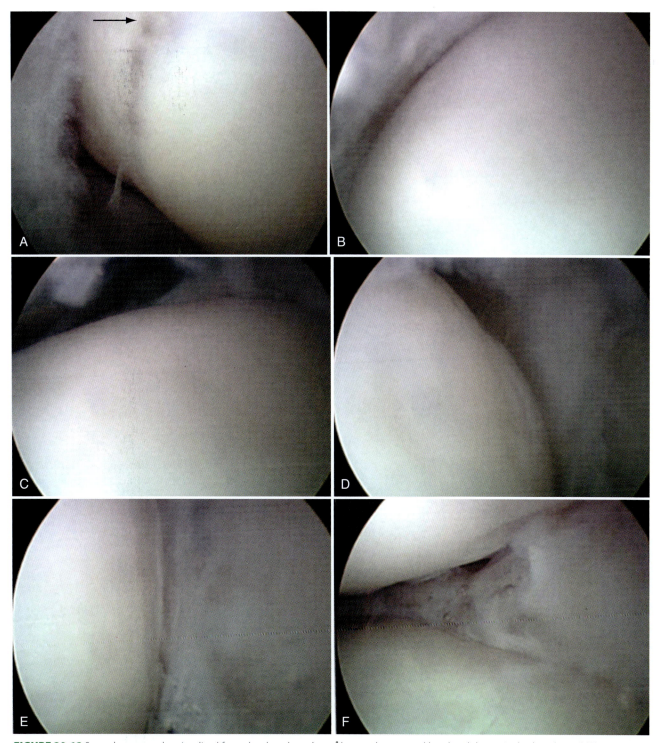

FIGURE 20-12 Several areas can be visualized from the dorsolateral portal: central metatarsal head and the sagittal sulcus *(arrow)* (**A**), dorsomedial metatarsal head and medial gutter (**B**), dorsocentral metatarsal head (**C**), dorsolateral metatarsal head (**D**), lateral gutter (**E**), and lateral metatarsophalangeal compartment (**F**).

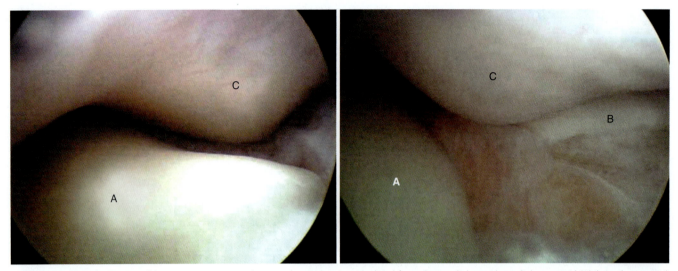

FIGURE 20-13 Several areas of the metatarsosesamoid compartment can be visualized from the medial portal: medial sesamoid (A), lateral sesamoid (B), and crista of the metatarsal head (C).

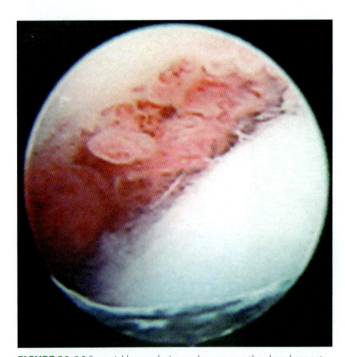

FIGURE 20-14 Synovial hyperplasia can be seen on the dorsal aspect of the first metatarsophalangeal joint.

The dorsomedial and dorsolateral portals can be established farther away from the extensor tendons at the dorsomedial and the dorsolateral corners of the joint (see Fig. 20-17B). This allows better access for débridement of the osteophytes in the dorsal, medial, and lateral gutters while avoiding crowding of the instruments. For example, the medial osteophytes can be débrided with the dorsolateral portal used as the visualization portal and the dorsomedial portals used as the instrumentation portals. In the event of a large, overhang osteophyte at the metatarsal head, an accessory proximal dorsal portal can be established at the proximal end of the osteophyte. If adequate débridement is not possible arthroscopically, the decision should be made to perform an open débridement.

Arthroscopy-assisted arthrodesis has been described for end-stage disease without gross deformity or bone loss.[17,18] Dorsomedial, dorsolateral, and medial portals are used together with finger trap traction. Residual cartilage is débrided using curettes, shavers, or abraders. The preserved subchondral bone is microfractured using a small chondral pick (Fig. 20-18). The position of the fusion is 15 degrees of valgus and 20 degrees of dorsiflexion. The provisional fixation is made with a Kirschner wire, and the position is confirmed with fluoroscopy. When the foot is placed flat on a metal tray, the interphalangeal joint should be slightly elevated from the surface. Crossed cannulated screws are inserted under fluoroscopic guidance.

Chondral and Osteochondral Lesions

Chondral and osteochondral lesions have been successfully treated arthroscopically, and the benefits included less pain, less stiffness, and reduced rehabilitation time (Fig. 20-19).[13,14,16] In cases with cartilage lesions, the aims are to remove the source of pain, stimulate fibrocartilaginous regeneration, and eliminate mechanical symptoms.

Partial-thickness cartilage injury can be treated with a radiofrequency probe to provide smooth edges. We recommend a microfracture technique using a small joint microfracture probe or a Kirschner wire for a full-thickness cartilage loss or an osteochondral defect. For the in situ osteochondral lesion, the overlying cartilage may look deceptively normal, but with careful palpation with a probe, the lesion can be identified. A curette can be used to remove the osteochondral fragments, although we have found the 2.0-mm probe causes less trauma to the surrounding tissue. Softened cartilage can be easily penetrated and cut with the tip of the probe. The probe can then be used as a hook to pull the fragment loose. The fragment can be débrided with a shaver or removed with hemostats. The defect is further débrided until fresh cancellous surface is uncovered. Microfracture is then performed. The joint is mobilized through range of motion, and any potential location that can provide mechanical catching is smoothed with a radiofrequency probe. A corresponding lesion

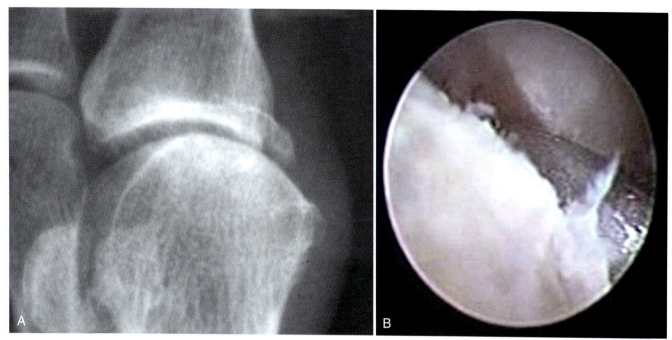

FIGURE 20-15 A, The radiograph shows osteophytes on the dorsal aspect of the metatarsal head and the base of the proximal phalanx. **B,** The arthroscopic view shows an instrument interposed between the osteophytes.

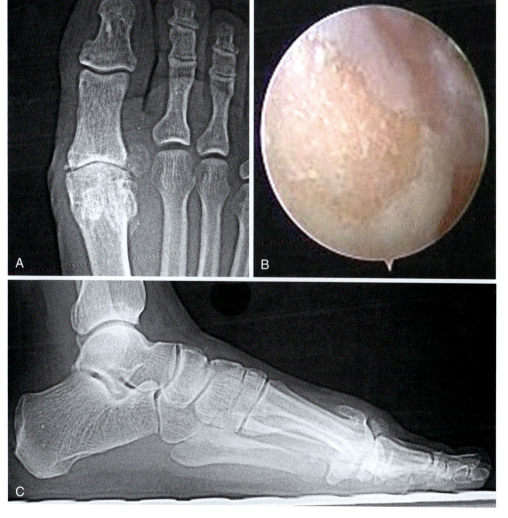

FIGURE 20-16 Anteroposterior (**A**) and lateral (**C**) radiographs of a foot with moderate osteoarthritis show dorsal osteophytes and loose bodies at the first metatarsophalangeal joint. Eburnation of the cartilage is seen on the dorsal aspect of the metatarsal head (**B**).

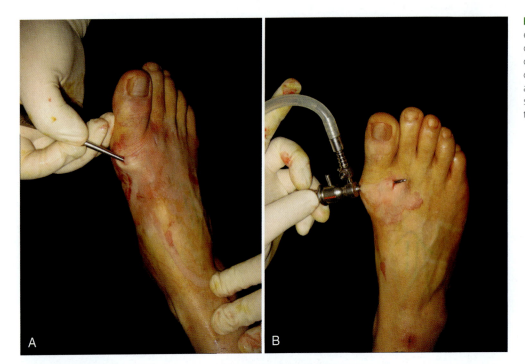

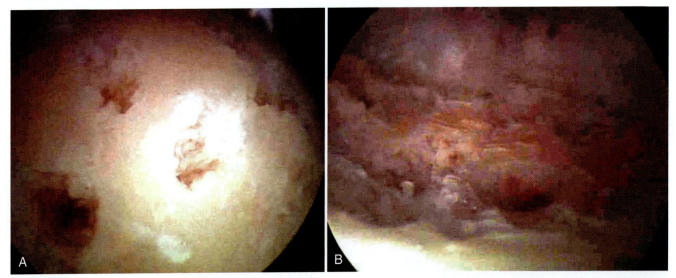

FIGURE 20-18 The metatarsal (**A**) and proximal (**B**) phalangeal facets have been prepared by cartilage débridement and microfracture of subchondral bone.

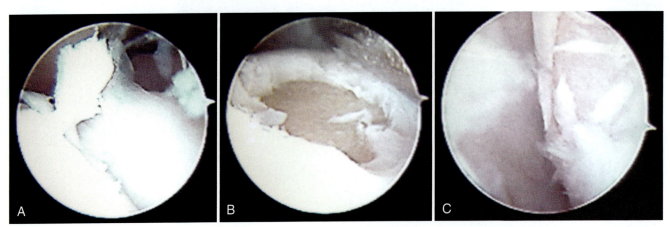

FIGURE 20-19 A full-thickness cartilage lesion on the dorsum of the metatarsal head is visualized before (**A**) and after (**B**) débridement. A kissing lesion (**C**) can be seen in the metatarsosesamoid compartment.

that may manifest on the proximal phalangeal base should be observed and treated.[27]

Arthrofibrosis

Arthroscopic lysis of the MTP-1 arthrofibrosis has been reported.[19,26] It has the potential advantage of early postoperative rehabilitation, because there is less pain associated with the procedure. Arthroscopic visualization in the joint can be limited by advanced arthrofibrosis.

The routine dorsomedial and dorsolateral portals are employed for the débridement of the dorsal, medial, and lateral gutters. At the initial portal placement, the trocar should be used to free the dorsal fibrotic tissue by sweeping in a back-and-forth fashion. Soft tissue release can involve stripping the medial capsule from the metatarsal head if overplication has occurred from a hallux valgus reconstruction. The sesamoid apparatus can be examined from the medial portal, and a plantar medial working portal is created under direct visualization for the débrider (Fig. 20-20). Plantar flexion of the joint opens the metatarsosesamoid compartment for easier instrumentation. Manual manipulation to achieve maximum range of motion is usually performed after the release.

Sesamoidectomy

The medial and lateral sesamoids can be accessed from the combination of dorsomedial, dorsolateral, medial, and plantar medial portals.[24] The evidence is limited, with only case reports presented in the literature. The lateral sesamoid has been removed using the medial portal or the toe web portal for visualization and the plantar medial portal for instrumentation.[25] The medial sesamoid has been removed using the dorsolateral portal for visualization and the medial portal for instrumentation.[24] The sesamoid can be excised in piecemeal with a pituitary rongeur or a 2.0-mm, round abrader. The ligamentous attachments are preserved. Van Dijk and colleagues found the medial sesamoid excision to be less successful, and an open excision was used in all three cases in their series.[13] Excision of both sesamoids is not recommended because of the risk of a cock-up deformity.

Gouty Tophi

Percutaneous soft tissue shaving of gouty tophi has produced good aesthetic results in 17 patients, with 2 patients having partial skin necrosis and no reported nerve injuries.[23] An endoscopy-assisted technique has been described to minimize wound breakdown and persistent drainage.[22] A study by Wang and colleagues[5] showed superior reduction in the number of acute attacks (5.4 vs. 1.9) and an increase in the American Orthopaedic Foot and Ankle Society (AOFAS) score (20.9 vs. 4.0) after endoscopic débridement (n = 15) compared with medication alone (n = 13) at a minimum of 2 years' follow-up.

Two portals are localized at the proximal and distal ends of the tophi (Fig. 20-21). A trocar is used to make a tunnel

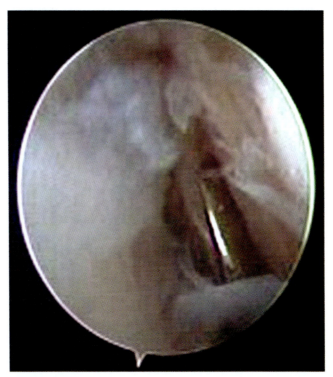

FIGURE 20-20 The arthroscopic view demonstrates complete release of the metatarsosesamoid compartment.

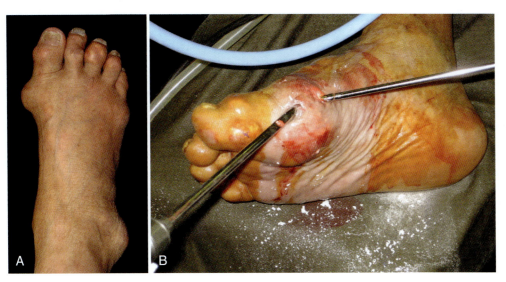

FIGURE 20-21 A, The patient has difficulty with shoewear because of large tophi overlying the first metatarsophalangeal joint. **B,** Débridement is performed using two medial portals.

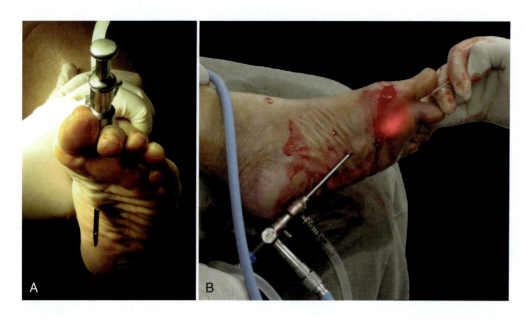

FIGURE 20-22 A, The plantar portal is established inside-out from the toe web portal. **B,** The arthroscope is positioned through the plantar portal while the intermetatarsal ligament is being released with a retrograde knife from the toe web portal.

through the tophi that joins both portals. The portals can be used interchangeably for visualization or instrumentation. The tophaceous material is removed with a shaver, progressing from the tunnel toward the pseudocapsule at the periphery. Part of the medial capsule may need to be removed. Great care is used to avoid injury to the dorsomedial hallucal nerve superficial to the pseudocapsule. The dorsolateral portal can be added for intra-articular débridement. The use of warm irrigation fluid is recommended to increase the solubility of the urate and prevent the system from clogging.[23] Postsurgical gout attack can be prevented by presurgical control of serum uric acid and prophylactic perioperative administration of colchicine.[28,29]

Hallux Valgus

Patients with hallux valgus can develop pain at the joint line without bunion pain or difficulties due to the deformity. In a case series of 30 feet, arthroscopic synovectomy through the standard dorsomedial and dorsolateral portals achieved complete pain relief in 22, significant pain relief in 5, and persistent pain in 3 at 5 years' follow-up.[20] Five patients developed bunion pain and required further arthroscopy-assisted correction. For patients with a painful joint line and a hallux valgus requiring correction, synovectomy performed through the described portals can be used in conjunction with deformity correction.

The arthroscopy-assisted correction of hallux valgus deformity has been reported by Lui and associates in a series of 94 patients with reducible 1-2 intermetatarsal angle and normal distal metatarsal articular angle.[8] The average hallux valgus angle improved from 33 ± 7 degrees to 14 ± 5 degrees, and the intermetatarsal angle improved from 14 ± 3 degrees to 9 ± 2 degrees°. The postoperative AOFAS score was 93, and the satisfaction rate was 95.7%. Complications included hallux varus, skin impingement, screw breakage, and MTP-1 stiffness.

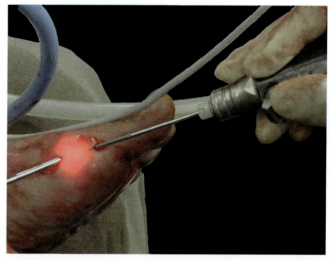

FIGURE 20-23 The exostectomy is performed through the medial and proximal medial portals.

The lateral release is performed through the toe web and the plantar portals. Under arthroscopic visualization through the plantar portal, the intermetatarsal ligament, adductor hallucis tendon, and lateral capsule are released with a retrograde knife (Fig. 20-22). Manipulation is performed to bring the toe to at least neutral alignment. The sesamoid reduction can be evaluated from the toe web portal or the medial portal. The medial portal and the proximal medial portal are used interchangeably for the arthroscope and the round abrader for the medial exostectomy (Fig. 20-23). The sagittal sulcus is a landmark that can be visualized from the dorsolateral portal. Through the medial and proximal medial portals, the medial capsule is percutaneously plicated with a no. 1 PDS suture to pull the distal plantar part toward the proximal dorsal part. The intermetatarsal angle is manually closed, and fixation with a 4.0 cannulated screw is performed under fluoroscopic guidance (Fig. 20-24).[30] The PDS suture is tied afterward (Fig. 20-25).

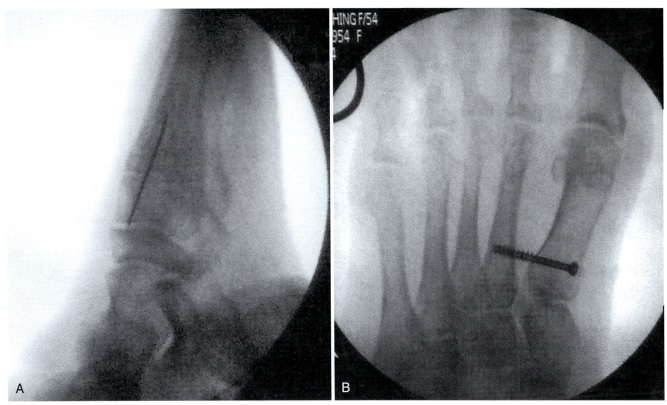

FIGURE 20-24 A cannulated screw is placed to stabilize the first and second metatarsals. **A,** The guide pin is placed into the center of the second metatarsal from the lateral aspect. **B,** Satisfactory reduction of the intermetatarsal angle is demonstrated.

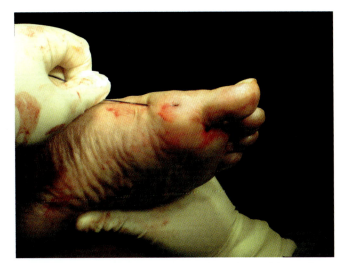

FIGURE 20-25 The PDS suture is used to plicate the medial capsule. The suture is tied from the proximal medial portal under proper tension to achieve further correction of the valgus and pronation deformity.

PEARLS *&* PITFALLS

PEARLS
- All portals are made carefully with a sharp incision through only the skin. Small, curved hemostats should be used to spread the soft tissue, puncture the joint capsule, feel the joint and the cartilage, dilate the portals, and occasionally strip the fibrotic joint capsule.

- Joint distraction may be used as needed for work that must be done between the articular facets, such as fusion of an osteochondral lesion.
- When the arthroscope is superficial, it is held such that one of the surgeon's fingers sits on the cannula at the skin level of the portal to prevent pistoning or dislodgment of the arthroscope.
- Percutaneous suture technique is performed by passing the curved eyed-needle through a portal into a structure and out through the intact skin for both ends of the suture. The suture ends are then retrieved from the plane just superficial to that structure with small, curved hemostats. Both suture ends are used to anchor to another structure in the same way before tying.

PITFALLS
- The MTP-1 joint can sometimes be so stiff and fibrotic that arthroscopic maneuvers can do harm by damaging the articular cartilage or the instruments. Consent must be obtained from patients, who must be informed that an open procedure may be required as a backup plan.
- Small joint arthroscopy has steep learning curve. Arthroscopic laboratory training can be helpful.
- Superficial nerves, especially the dorsomedial hallucal nerve, can be injured from portal placement, instrument passing, or suture placement. The surgeon should be aware of the location of the nerve and possible anatomic variations.
- For the lateral release in treating hallux valgus, the retrograde knife should be introduced through the toe web portal only, without passing through the plantar portal. The retrograde knife and the shaver should be kept away from the fat tissue plantar to the intermetatarsal ligament.

Postoperative Rehabilitation Protocol

Bulky dressing and a postoperative shoe are routinely used for 5 to 7 days. Bearing weight on the heel is allowed. The patient gradually increases weight bearing and range of motion as tolerated. For a hallux valgus correction, a toe web spacer is used, and the screw is removed at week 8 under local anesthesia. For an arthrodesis, full weight bearing in a stiff-sole shoe is allowed after crossing of the trabeculae at 6 to 8 weeks. Swelling can persist for a few months but usually to a lesser degree than with open procedures. For a medial sesamoid excision, the hallux is strapped into slight varus for 3 weeks to prevent hallux valgus deformity.

CONCLUSIONS

Arthroscopy can be helpful in selected cases of MTP-1 pathologies. Because of the steep learning curve for the technique, basic small joint arthroscopic skills and some laboratory training are recommended. Considered as an alterative to open procedures, MTP-1 arthroscopy allows magnified visualization, minimally invasive treatment, and diminution of postoperative pain and scarring. Familiarity with the topographic anatomy of the forefoot and awareness of nerve variations can minimize complications. Because of the limited amount of information about MTP-1 arthroscopy, evidence-based recommendations and guidelines must be developed.

REFERENCES

1. Watanabe M. *Selfox-Arthroscope (Wantantabe No. 24 Arthroscope)*. Tokyo, Japan: Teishin Hospital, 1972.
2. Lidtke RH, George J. Anatomy, biomechanics, and surgical approach to synovial folds within the joints of the foot. *J Am Podiatr Med Assoc.* 2004;94:519-527.
3. Solan MC, Lemon M, Bendall SP. The surgical anatomy of the dorsomedial cutaneous nerve of the hallux. *J Bone Joint Surg Br.* 2001;83:250-252.
4. Ferkel R. Great-toe arthroscopy. In: Whipple T, ed. *Arthroscopic Surgery: The Foot & Ankle*. Philadelphia, PA: Lippincott-Raven; 1996:255-272.
5. Wang CC, Lien SB, Huang GS, et al. Arthroscopic elimination of monosodium urate deposition of the first metatarsophalangeal joint reduces the recurrence of gout. *Arthroscopy.* 2009;25:153-158.
6. Browne K, Lee J. The appreciation of passive movement of the metatarsophalangeal joint of the great toe in man. *J Physiol.* 1954;123:10-1P.
7. Michelson J, Dunn L. Tenosynovitis of the flexor hallucis longus: a clinical study of the spectrum of presentation and treatment. *Foot Ankle Int.* 2005;26:291-303.
8. Lui TH, Chan KB, Chow HT, et al. Arthroscopy-assisted correction of hallux valgus deformity. *Arthroscopy.* 2008;24:875-880.
9. Roukis TS. Metatarsus primus elevatus in hallux rigidus: fact or fiction? *J Am Podiatr Med Assoc.* 2005;95:221-228.
10. Masih S, Antebi A. Imaging of pigmented villonodular synovitis. *Semin Musculoskelet Radiol.* 2003;7:205-216.
11. Fessell DP, van Holsbeeck M. Ultrasound of the foot and ankle. *Semin Musculoskelet Radiol.* 1998;2:271-282.
12. Iqbal MJ, Chana GS. Arthroscopic cheilectomy for hallux rigidus. *Arthroscopy.* 1998;14:307-310.
13. van Dijk CN, Veenstra KM, Nuesch BC. Arthroscopic surgery of the metatarsophalangeal first joint. *Arthroscopy.* 1998;14:851-855.
14. Bartlett DH. Arthroscopic management of osteochondritis dissecans of the first metatarsal head. *Arthroscopy.* 1988;4:51-54.
15. Borton DC, Peereboom J, Saxby TS. Pigmented villonodular synovitis in the first metatarsophalangeal joint: arthroscopic treatment of an unusual condition. *Foot Ankle Int.* 1997;18:504-505.
16. Debnath UK, Hemmady MV, Hariharan K. Indications for and technique of first metatarsophalangeal joint arthroscopy. *Foot Ankle Int.* 2006;27:1049-1054.
17. Carro LP, Vallina BB. Arthroscopic-assisted first metatarsophalangeal joint arthrodesis. *Arthroscopy.* 1999;15:215-217.
18. Stroud CC. Arthroscopic arthrodesis of the ankle, subtalar, and first metatarsophalangeal joint. *Foot Ankle Clin.* 2002;7:135-146.
19. Lui TH. Arthroscopic release of first metatarsophalangeal arthrofibrosis. *Arthroscopy.* 2006;22:906.e1-4.
20. Lui TH. First metatarsophalangeal joint arthroscopy in patients with hallux valgus. *Arthroscopy.* 2008;24:1122-1129.
21. Lui TH, Ng S, Chan KB. Endoscopic distal soft tissue procedure in hallux valgus surgery. *Arthroscopy.* 2005;21:1403.
22. Lui TH. Endoscopic resection of the gouty tophi of the first metatarsophalangeal joint. *Arch Orthop Trauma Surg.* 2008;128:521-523.
23. Lee SS, Lin SD, Lai CS, et al. The soft-tissue shaving procedure for deformity management of chronic tophaceous gout. *Ann Plast Surg.* 2003; 51:372-375.
24. Perez Carro L, Echevarria Llata JI, Martinez Agueros JA. Arthroscopic medial bipartite sesamoidectomy of the great toe. *Arthroscopy.* 1999; 15:321-323.
25. Chan PK, Lui TH. Arthroscopic fibular sesamoidectomy in the management of the sesamoid osteomyelitis. *Knee Surg Sports Traumatol Arthrosc.* 2006;14:664-667.
26. Ferkel R, Buecken KV. Great toe arthroscopy: indications, technique and results. Presented at the Arthroscopy Association of North America, April, 1991; San Diego, CA.
27. Shonka TE. Metatarsal phalangeal joint arthroscopy. *J Foot Surg.* 1991; 30:26-28.
28. Kang EH, Lee EY, Lee YJ, et al. Clinical features and risk factors of postsurgical gout. *Ann Rheum Dis.* 2008;67:1271-1275.
29. Linton RR, Talbott JH. The surgical treatment of tophaceous gout. *Ann Surg.* 1943;117:161-182.
30. Friscia DA. Distal soft tissue correction for hallux valgus with proximal screw fixation of the first metatarsal. *Foot Ankle Clin.* 2000;5:581-589.

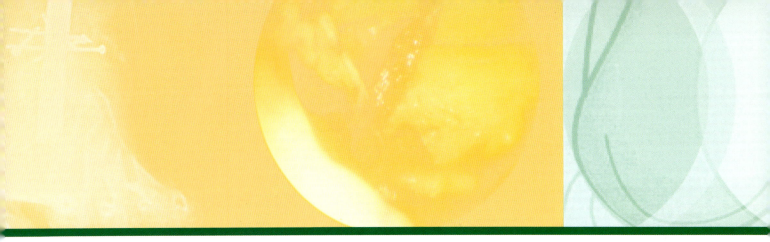

Index

Note: Page numbers followed by f refer to figures; page numbers followed by b refer to boxes.

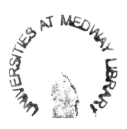